Multicultural Health

THIRD EDITION

Lois Ritter
University of Nevada, Reno

Donald H. Graham
Attorney and Consultant, Health Care

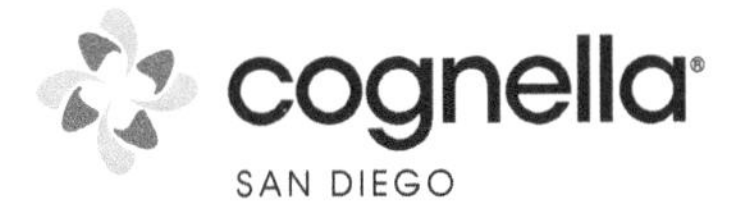

Bassim Hamadeh, CEO and Publisher
Amanda Martin, Publisher
Amy Smith, Senior Project Editor
Shannon Egan, Production Editor
Emely Villavicencio, Senior Graphic Designer
Kylie Bartolome, Licensing Coordinator
Kim Scott, Interior Designer
Stephanie Adams, Senior Marketing Program Manager
Natalie Piccotti, Director of Marketing
Kassie Graves, Senior Vice President, Editorial
Jamie Giganti, Director of Academic Publishing

Printed in the United States of America.

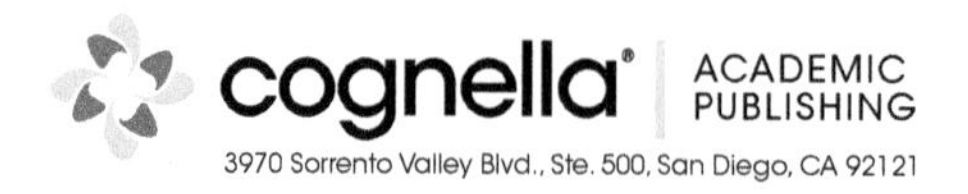

To Randy, Emma, and Samantha, for the love and laughter

—LR

To Sarah

—DG

Brief Contents

Detailed Contents

UNIT II Specific Cultural Groups 133

Preface

Your mind is like a parachute ... it functions only when open.
—AUTHOR UNKNOWN

Health care professionals work in a diverse society that presents both opportunities and challenges, so being culturally competent is essential to their role. Although knowing about every culture is not possible, having an understanding of various cultures can improve effectiveness. *Multicultural Health* provides an introduction and overview to some of the major cultural variations related to health.

Throughout this text, those engaged in health care can acquire the knowledge necessary to improve their effectiveness when working with diverse groups, regardless of the predominant culture of the community in which they live or work. The content of this book is useful when working in the field on both individual and community levels. It serves as a guide to the concepts and theories related to cultural issues in health and as a primer on health issues and practices specific to certain cultures groups.

New to This Edition

A second case study has been added to all chapters. Statistics, legal, and health information, such as COVID-19, has been updated and/or added throughout the book.

- Chapter 1: Incorporated new laws related to same-sex marriage and the gender binary law.
- Chapter 2: Added the sunrise model.
- Chapter 3: This chapter is a combination of the worldview and religion chapters in the previous editions.
- Chapter 4: Expanded to include cannabis information.
- Chapter 5: Communication information related to social media added, as well as a new section on health literacy.
- Chapters 6–10: Updated to include information on COVID-19 and health disparities information.
- Chapter 11: Expanded to included rural-urban and generational cultures.
- Chapter 12: New chapter expanding on the cultures of commerce and address the cultures of class and capitalism in relation to health.
- Chapter 13: Updated Healthy People content to 2030.

About This Book

Multicultural Health is divided into three units.

Unit I, The Foundations, includes Chapters 1 through 5 and focuses on the context of culture, cultural beliefs regarding health and illness, health disparities, models for cross-cultural health and communication, and approaches to culturally appropriate health promotion programs and evaluation.

- Chapter 1, Introduction to Multicultural Health, discusses the reasons for becoming knowledgeable about the cultural impact of health practices. It defines terminology and key concepts that set the foundation for the remainder of the text. The chapter addresses diversity in the United States and the racial makeup of the country, health disparities and their causes, laws designed to protect minorities, and ethics.
- Chapter 2, Theories and Models Related to Multicultural Health, addresses theories regarding the occurrence of illness and its treatment. Terms and theoretical models related to cultural competence are provided. Individual and organizational cultural competence assessments are included.
- Chapter 3, Worldview and Health, explores the worldview on illness and treatment and cultural influences that affect health. Differences in worldview and how that affects perceptions about health, health behaviors, and interactions with health care providers are described. Verbal and nonverbal communication considerations are explained as well as how worldview influences specific areas of health, such as the use of birth control. The chapter then turns to focus on religion and rituals and how they impact health.
- Chapter 4, Complementary and Alternative Medicine, provides an introduction to complementary and alternative medicine and health practices. It explores the major non-Western medicine modalities of care, including Ayurvedic medicine, traditional Chinese medicine, herbal medicine, and holistic and naturopathic medicine. The history, theories, and beliefs regarding the source of illness and treatment modalities are described.
- Chapter 5, Public Health, includes information about culturally sensitive communication strategies used in public health. Considerations to making health care campaigns using various communication channels, such as social media, appropriate for diverse audiences are explained. Information about health literacy and public health models are included.

Unit II, Specific Cultural Groups, includes Chapters 6 through 12. Chapters 1 through 11 address the history of specific U.S. cultural groups' beliefs regarding the causes of health and illness, healing traditions and practices, common health problems, and health promotion and program planning for the various cultural groups.

Chapter 12 describes the overarching commercial and economic culture that affects everyone in the country.

- Chapter 6: Hispanic and Latino American Populations
- Chapter 7: American Indian and Alaskan Native Populations
- Chapter 8: African American Populations
- Chapter 9: Asian American Populations
- Chapter 10: European and Mediterranean American Populations
- Chapter 11: Nonethnic Cultures
- Chapter 12: The Macro Cultures Related to Health and the Health Care System

Unit III, Looking Ahead, outlines priority areas in health disparities and strategies to eliminate them.

- Chapter 13, Closing the Gap: Strategies for Eliminating Health Disparities, explores the implications of diversity growth in the United States in relation to future disease prevention and treatment. It further addresses diversity in the health care workforce and its impact on care, as well as the need for ongoing education in cultural competence for health care practitioners.

Features and Benefits

Each chapter includes a "Did You Know?" and "What Do You Think?" section to stimulate critical thinking and classroom discussions. Also included are chapter review questions, related activities, and two case studies. Key concepts are listed, and their definitions are provided in the glossary.

We hope the information contained in *Multicultural Health* will introduce you to the rich and fascinating cultural landscape in the United States and the diverse health practices and beliefs of various cultural groups. This book is not intended to be an end point; rather, it is a starting point in the journey to becoming culturally competent in health care.

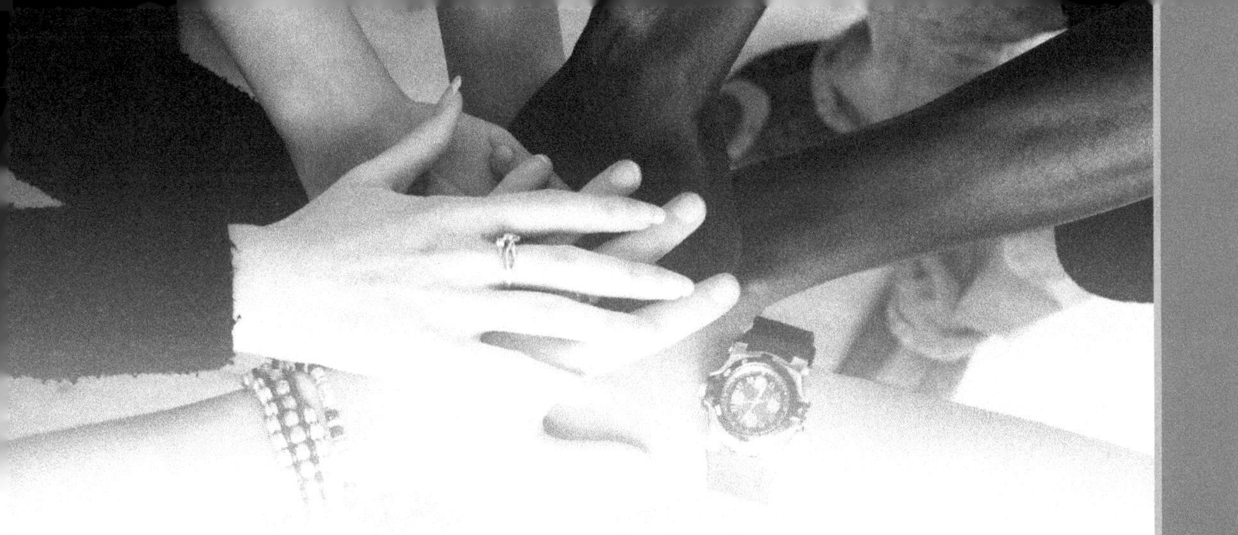

UNIT I

The Foundations

CHAPTER 1

Introduction to Multicultural Health

We have become not a melting pot but a beautiful mosaic.

—JIMMY CARTER

One day our descendants will think it incredible that we paid so much attention to things like the amount of melanin in our skin or the shape of our eyes or our gender instead of the unique identities of each of us as complex human beings.

—AUTHOR UNKNOWN

KEY CONCEPTS

Acculturation
Assimilation
Autonomy
Beneficence
Cultural adaptation
Cultural competence
Cultural ethnocentricity
Cultural relativism
Culture
Discrimination
Dominant culture
Ethics
Ethnicity
Fidelity
Health disparity
Healthy People 2030
Heritage consistency
Hill–Burton Act
Justice
Minority
Multicultural health
Morality
Nonmaleficence
Race
Racism
Respect
Stereotype
Veracity

LEARNING OBJECTIVES

After reading this chapter, you should be able to do the following:

1. Explain why cultural considerations are important in health care.
2. Describe the processes of acculturation and assimilation.
3. Define race, culture, ethnicity, ethnocentricity, cultural relativism, stereotype, and discrimination.
4. Explain what cultural adaptation is and why it is important in health care.
5. Explain what health disparities are and their related causes.
6. List the five elements of the determinants of health and describe how they relate to health disparities.
7. Explain key legislation related to health and minority rights.

Why do we need to study multicultural health? Why is culture important if we all have the same basic biological makeup? Isn't health all about science? Shouldn't people from different cultural backgrounds just adapt to the health care system and perspectives in the United States?

For decades, the role that culture plays in health was virtually ignored, but the links have now become more apparent. As a result, the focus on the need to educate health care professionals about the important role that culture plays in health has escalated. Health is influenced by factors such as genetics, the environment, and socioeconomic status, as well as by other cultural and social forces. Culture affects people's perception of health and illness, how they pursue and adhere to treatment, their health behaviors, beliefs about why people become ill, how symptoms and concerns about the problem are expressed, what is considered a health problem, and ways to maintain and restore health. Recognizing cultural similarities and differences is an essential component for delivering effective health care services. To provide quality care, health care professionals need to provide services within a cultural context, which is the focus of multicultural health.

Multicultural health is the phrase used to reflect the need to provide health care services in a sensitive, knowledgeable, and nonjudgmental manner with respect for people's health beliefs and practices when they are different from our own. It entails challenging our own assumptions, asking the right questions, and working with the patient and the community in a manner that respects the patient's lifestyle and approach to maintaining health and treating illness. Multicultural health integrates different approaches to care and incorporates the culture and belief system of the health care recipient while providing care within the legal, ethical, and medically sound practices of the practitioner's medical system.

Knowing the health practices and cultures of all groups is not possible, but becoming familiar with various groups' general health beliefs and preferences can be very beneficial and improve the effectiveness of health care services. In this text, generalizations about cultural groups are provided, but it is important to realize that many subcultures exist within those cultures, and people vary in the degree to which they identify with the beliefs and practices of their culture of origin. Awareness of general differences can help health care professionals provide services within a cultural context, but it is important to distinguish between stereotyping (the mistaken assumption that everyone in a given culture is alike) and generalizations (Juckett, 2005). Generalizations can serve as a starting point but do not preclude factoring in individual characteristics such as education, nationality, faith, and level of cultural adaptation. Stereotypes and assumptions can be problematic and can lead to errors and ineffective care. Remember, every person is unique, but understanding the generalizations can be beneficial because it moves people in the direction of becoming culturally competent.

Cultural competence refers to an individual's or an agency's ability to work effectively with people from diverse backgrounds. *Culture* refers to a group's integrated patterns of behavior, and *competency* is the capacity to function effectively. Cultural competence occurs on a continuum, and this text is geared toward helping you progress along the cultural competence continuum.

Specific terms related to multicultural health, such as *race* and *acculturation*, need to be clarified, and this chapter begins by defining some of these terms. Following that is a discussion of the demographic landscape of the U.S. population and how it is changing, types and degrees of cultural adaptation, and health disparities and their causes. The chapter concludes with information about legislation related to health care that is designed to protect minorities.

Key Concepts and Terms

Some of the terminology related to multicultural health can be confusing because the differences can be subtle. This section clarifies the meaning of terms such as *culture, discrimination, race, ethnicity, ethnocentricity,* and *cultural relativism.*

Culture

There are countless definitions of culture. The short explanation is that culture is everything that makes us who we are. E. B. Tylor (1871/1924), who is considered the founder of cultural anthropology, provided the classical definition of culture: "Culture, or civilization, taken in its broad, ethnographic sense, is that complex whole which includes knowledge, belief, art, morals, law, custom, and any other capabilities and habits acquired by man as a member of society" (p. 1). Tylor's definition is still widely cited today. A modern definition of culture is "group membership, such as racial, ethnic, linguistic or geographical groups, or as a collection of beliefs, values, customs, ways of thinking, communicating, and behaving specific to a group" (Centers for Disease Control and Prevention [CDC], 2021).

Culture is learned, changes over time, and is passed on from generation to generation. It is a very complex system, and many subcultures exist within each culture. For example, universities, businesses, neighborhoods, age groups, the gay and lesbian community, athletic teams, and musicians are subcultures of the dominant American culture. Dominant culture refers to the primary or predominant culture of a region and does not indicate superiority. People simultaneously belong to numerous subcultures, because we can be students, fathers or mothers, and bowling enthusiasts at the same time.

Race and Ethnicity

Race refers to a person's physical characteristics, but race is not a scientific construct. Race is a social construct that was developed to categorize people, and it was based on the notion that some "races" are superior to others. Many professionals in the fields of biology, sociology, and anthropology have determined that race is a social construct and not a biological one because not one characteristic, trait, or gene distinguishes all the members of one so-called race from all the members of another so-called race. "There is more genetic variation within races than between them, and racial categories do not capture biological distinctiveness" (Williams et al., 1994).

Why is race important? Because society makes it important. Race shapes social, cultural, political, ideological, and legal functions in society. Race is an institutionalized concept that has had devastating consequences. Race has been the basis for deaths from wars and murders and suffering caused by discrimination, violence, torture, and hate crimes. The ideology of race has been the root of suffering and death for centuries, even though it has little scientific merit.

The 2020 U.S. Census questions related to ethnicity and race can be found in **Figures 1.1** and **1.2**. **Box 1.1** explains how these race terms were defined in the 2020 census. The U.S. government declared that Hispanics and Latinos are an ethnicity and not a race.

Is this person of Hispanic, Latino, or Spanish origin?

- **No**, not of Hispanic, Latino, or Spanish origin
- Yes, Mexican, Mexican Am., Chicano
- Yes, Puerto Rican
- Yes, Cuban
- Yes, another Hispanic, Latino, or Spanish origin – *Print, for example, Salvadoran, Dominican, Colombian, Guatemalan, Spaniard, Ecuadorian, etc.*

Figure 1.1 U.S. Census origin question, 2020.

It is important to note that there is great variation within each of the racial and ethnic categories. For example, American Indians are grouped together even though there are variations between the tribes. It is essential to be aware of the differences that occur

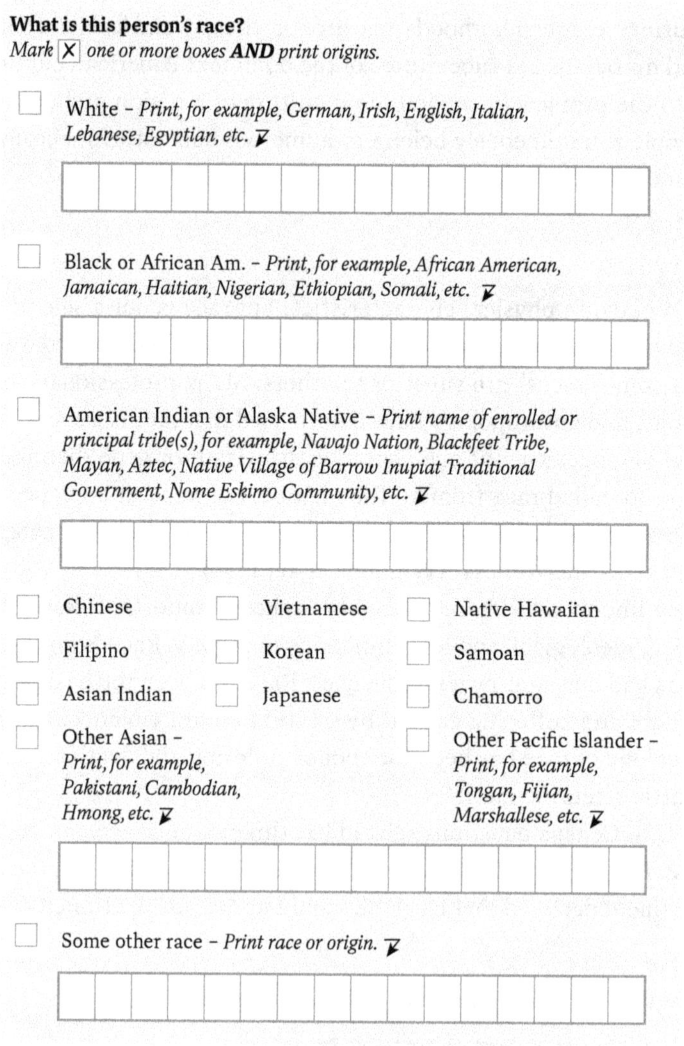

What is this person's race?
Mark ☒ *one or more boxes* ***AND*** *print origins.*

☐ White – *Print, for example, German, Irish, English, Italian, Lebanese, Egyptian, etc.*

☐ Black or African Am. – *Print, for example, African American, Jamaican, Haitian, Nigerian, Ethiopian, Somali, etc.*

☐ American Indian or Alaska Native – *Print name of enrolled or principal tribe(s), for example, Navajo Nation, Blackfeet Tribe, Mayan, Aztec, Native Village of Barrow Inupiat Traditional Government, Nome Eskimo Community, etc.*

☐ Chinese ☐ Vietnamese ☐ Native Hawaiian

☐ Filipino ☐ Korean ☐ Samoan

☐ Asian Indian ☐ Japanese ☐ Chamorro

☐ Other Asian – *Print, for example, Pakistani, Cambodian, Hmong, etc.*

☐ Other Pacific Islander – *Print, for example, Tongan, Fijian, Marshallese, etc.*

☐ Some other race – *Print race or origin.*

Figure 1.2 U.S. Census race question, 2020.

within these groups and not to stereotype people. Stereotyping people by their race and ethnicity is a form of racism. **Racism** is the belief that some races are superior to others by nature. Discrimination occurs when people act on that belief and treat people differently as a result. Discrimination can occur because of beliefs related to factors such as race, sexual orientation, dialect, religion, or gender.

Ethnicity is the socially defined characteristic of a group of people who share common cultural factors such as race, history, national origin, religious belief, or language. So how is ethnicity different from race? Race is primarily based on physical characteristics, whereas ethnicity is based on social and cultural identities. For example, consider these terms in relation to a person born in Korea to Korean parents but adopted by a French family in France as an infant. Ethnically, the person may feel French: the person eats French food, speaks French, celebrates French holidays, and learns French history and culture. This

BOX 1.1 Definition of Race Categories Used in the U.S. Census (2020)

White

The category "White" includes all individuals who identify with one or more nationalities or ethnic groups originating in Europe, the Middle East, or North Africa. Examples of these groups include, but are not limited to, German, Irish, English, Italian, Lebanese, Egyptian, Polish, French, Iranian, Slavic, Cajun, and Chaldean.

Black or African American

The category "Black or African American" includes all individuals who identify with one or more nationalities or ethnic groups originating in any of the Black racial groups of Africa. Examples of these groups include, but are not limited to, African American, Jamaican, Haitian, Nigerian, Ethiopian, and Somali. The category also includes groups such as Ghanaian, South African, Barbadian, Kenyan, Liberian, and Bahamian.

American Indian or Alaska Native

The category "American Indian or Alaska Native" includes all individuals who identify with any of the original peoples of North and South America (including Central America) and who maintain tribal affiliation or community attachment. It includes people who identify as "American Indian" or "Alaska Native" and includes groups such as Navajo Nation, Blackfeet Tribe, Mayan, Aztec, Native Village of Barrow Inupiat Traditional Government, and Nome Eskimo Community.

Asian

The category "Asian" includes all individuals who identify with one or more nationalities or ethnic groups originating in the Far East, Southeast Asia, or the Indian subcontinent. Examples of these groups include, but are not limited to, Chinese, Filipino, Asian Indian, Vietnamese, Korean, and Japanese. The category also includes groups such as Pakistani, Cambodian, Hmong, Thai, Bengali, Mien, and so on.

There are individual Asian checkboxes for people who identify as one or more of the following:

- Chinese
- Filipino
- Asian Indian
- Vietnamese
- Korean
- Japanese
- Other Asian (e.g., Pakistani, Cambodian, and Hmong)

Native Hawaiian and Pacific Islander

The category "Native Hawaiian or Other Pacific Islander" includes all individuals who identify with one or more nationalities or ethnic groups originating in Hawaii, Guam, Samoa, or other Pacific Islands. Examples of these groups include, but are not limited

(continued)

BOX 1.1 Definition of Race Categories Used in the U.S. Census (2020) (*Continued*)

to, Native Hawaiian, Samoan, Chamorro, Tongan, Fijian, and Marshallese. The category also includes groups such as Palauan, Tahitian, Chuukese, Pohnpeian, Saipanese, Yapese, and so on.

There are individual Pacific Islander checkboxes for people who identify as one or more of the following:

- Native Hawaiian
- Samoan
- Chamorro
- Other Pacific Islander (e.g., Tongan, Fijian, and Mashallese)

Some other race: Defined by Census respondent

person knows nothing about Korean history and culture, but in the United States that person would likely be treated racially as Asian. Let's consider another example. The physical characteristics of Caucasians (a race) are typically light skin and eyes, narrow noses, thin lips, and straight or wavy hair. A person whose appearance matches these characteristics is said to be a Caucasian. However, there are many ethnicities within the Caucasian race such as Dutch, Irish, Greek, German, French, and so on. What differentiates these Caucasian ethnic groups from one another is their country of origin, language, cultural heritage and traditions, beliefs, and rituals.

How is ethnicity different from culture? One can belong to a culture without having ancestral roots to that culture. For example, people can belong to the hip-hop culture, but they were not born into the culture. With ethnicity, the culture is a part of the ethnic background, so culture is embedded within the ethnic group. Ethnic groups have shared beliefs, values, norms, and practices that are learned and shared. These patterned behaviors are passed down from one generation to another and are thus preserved.

Cultural Ethnocentricity and Cultural Relativism

Cultural ethnocentricity refers to people's belief that their culture is superior to another one. This can cause problems in the health care field. If professionals believe that their way is the better way to prevent or treat a health problem, health care workers may disrespect or ignore the patient's cultural beliefs and values. The health care professional may not take into consideration that the listener may have different views than the provider. This can lead to ineffective communication and treatment and leave listeners feeling unimportant, frustrated, disrespected, or confused about how to prevent or treat the health issue, and they might view the professional as uneducated, uncooperative, unapproachable, or closed-minded.

To be effective, one needs to see and appreciate the value of different cultures; this is referred to as cultural relativism. The phrase developed in the field of anthropology to refute the idea of cultural ethnocentricity. It posits that all cultures are of equal value and need to be studied from a neutral point of view. It rejects value judgments on cultures and holds the belief that no culture is superior to any other. Cultural relativism takes an objective view of cultures and incorporates the idea that a society's moral code defines whether something is right (or wrong) for members of that society.

WHAT DO YOU THINK?

Cultural imposition occurs when one cultural group, usually the majority group, forces their culture view on another culture or subculture. Can you provide examples of cultural imposition? Do you think it is ethical? Why or why not?

Diversity Within the United States

A great strength of the United States is the diversity of the people. Historically, waves of immigrants have come to the United States to live in the land of opportunity and pursue a better quality of life. Immigrants brought their traditions, languages, and cultures with them, creating a country that developed a very diverse landscape. Of course, some peoples, such as Native Americans, were already on the land, and others, such as African Americans, were forced to come to the United States. An unfortunate outcome was that despite its great advantages, this diversity contributed to racial and cultural clashes as well as imbalances in equality and opportunities that continue today. These positive and adverse consequences of diversity must be considered in our health care approaches, particularly because the demographics continue to change and the inequalities persist. The delivery of health care to individuals, families, and communities must meet the needs of the wide variety of people who reside in and visit the United States.

The percentage of the U.S. population characterized as White is decreasing (see **Table 1.1**). This is an important consideration for health care providers because ethnic minorities often experience poorer health status, which is usually due to economic disparities.

Cultural Adaptation

With this changing landscape in the United States, professionals are encouraged to consider the degree of cultural adaptation that the person has experienced. **Cultural adaptation** refers to the degree to which a person or community has adapted to the dominant culture or retained their traditional practices. Generally, first-generation people will identify more with their culture of origin than those from the third-generation. Therefore, when working with the first-generation person, health care professionals need to be more sensitive to issues such as language barriers, distrust, lack of understanding of the American medical system, and ties to traditional beliefs.

Acculturation relates to the degree of adaptation that has taken place, a process in which members of one cultural group adopt the beliefs and behaviors of another group.

TABLE 1.1 Population Data Related to Origin and Race

	2000 (n = 281,421,906)	2010 (n = 308,745,538)	2019 estimates* (n = 328,239,523)
	Percentage of total population	Percentage of total population	Percent of total population
Hispanic Origin and Race			
Hispanic or Latino	12.5	16.3	18.5
White non-Hispanic	75.1	72.4	60.1
Black or African American	12.3	12.6	13.4
American Indian and Alaska Native	0.9	0.9	1.3
Asian	3.6	4.8	5.9
Native Hawaiian and Other Pacific Islander	0.1	0.2	0.2
Two or more races[1]	2.4	2.9	2.8

[1]In the 2000 U.S. Census, an error in data processing resulted in an overstatement of the two or more races population by about 1 million people (about 15%) nationally, which almost entirely affected race combinations involving some other race. Therefore, data users should assess observed changes in the two or more races population and race combinations involving some other race between the 2000 Census and the 2010 Census with caution.

* U.S. Census Bureau. (n.d.).

Source: U.S. Census Bureau (2011).

Essentially, members of the minority cultural group take up many of the dominant culture's traits. Because of the great variety of peoples who have immigrated to the United States, the country is often said to be a melting pot. However, given the tendencies of cultural groups to locate together and maintain some familiar practices in a foreign land, the country also has been described as a salad bowl. Both these analogies reflect the process of cultural interaction.

Except for the Indigenous population, everyone in the United States is or is descended from immigrants and refugees. For instance, the Pilgrims of Plymouth Rock were refugees from religious persecution. Each group of people who traveled to America built on the strengths of their own culture while adapting to a new social and economic environment through acculturation. Acculturation can include adopting customs from one culture to another or direct change of customs as one culture dominates the other. Each of the cultures discussed in the text has adapted as new populations arrive, territory is acquired or conquered, or popular or useful practices and beliefs are invented and spread throughout the overall population. Some interactions between cultures generate discriminatory responses, individual stress, and family conflict, whereas others create an appreciation for variation as customs or practices are welcomed into other cultures. Whether melting or mixing, the interrelationship of cultures in the United States in constantly changing. The process continues as new people arrive in the country.

People can experience different levels of acculturation as illustrated in Berry's (1997) acculturation framework (see **Figure 1.3**). The acculturation framework identifies four levels of integration:

1. An **assimilated** individual demonstrates high-dominant and low-ethnic society immersion. This entails moving away from one's ethnic society and immersing fully in the dominant society (Stephenson, 2000). As a result, the minority group disappears through the loss of particular identifying physical or sociocultural characteristics. This usually occurs when people immigrate to a new geographic region and in their desire to be part of the mainstream give up most of their culture traits of origin and take on a new cultural identity defined by the dominant culture. Many people do not fully assimilate, however, and tend to keep some of their original cultural beliefs.

2. An integrated person has high-dominant and high-ethnic immersion. Integration entails immersion in both ethnic and dominant societies (Stephenson, 2000). An example of an integrated person is a Russian American who socializes with the dominant group but chooses to speak Russian at home and marries a person who is Russian.

3. Separated individuals have low-dominant and high-ethnic immersion. A separated individual withdraws from the dominant society and completely submerges into the ethnic society (Stephenson, 2000). An example is a person who lives in an ethnic community such as Little Italy or Chinatown.

4. A marginalized individual has low-dominant and low-ethnic immersion and does not identify with any particular culture or belief system.

Dominant immersion		
Assimilated	Integrated	**Ethnic immersion**
Marginal	Separated	

Figure 1.3 Acculturation framework.

Marginalized people tend to have the most psychological problems and the highest stress levels. These individuals often lack social support systems and are not accepted by the dominant society or their culture of origin. People in the separated mode are accepted in their ethnic society but may not be accepted by the dominant culture, leaving the person feeling alienated. The integrated and assimilated modes are considered the most psychologically healthy adaptation styles, although some individuals benefit more from one than from the other. Western Europeans and individuals whose families have been in the United States for a number of generations (and are not discriminated against) are most likely to adopt an assimilated mode, because they have many beliefs and attributes of the dominant society. Individuals who retain value structures from their country of origin and encounter discrimination benefit more from an integrated (bicultural) mode. To be bicultural one must be knowledgeable about both cultures and see the positive attributes of both.

The degree to which people identify with their culture of origin is sometimes referred to as **heritage consistency**. Some indicators that can help professionals assess the level of cultural adaptation are inquiring about how long the person has been in the country, how often the person returns to his or her culture of origin, what holidays the person celebrates, what language the person speaks at home, and how much knowledge the person has of his or her culture of origin.

Are people who have higher levels of cultural adaptation healthier? Despite increasing research on the relationships between acculturation and health, the answer to that question is not clear. Research on the influence of acculturation on health indicates contradictory results because the variables are complex. The answer is also dependent on which health habits are incorporated into one's lifestyle and which are lost. For example, acculturation can have detrimental effects on one's dietary patterns if a person is from a culture where eating fruits and vegetables is common and the person incorporates the habit of eating at fast-food restaurants, which is common in the United States. On the other hand, if someone moves from a culture where smoking is common to a culture where it is frowned upon, the person may stop smoking and reduce his or her chances of serious illness.

Acculturation from traditional, nonindustrialized cultures to a modern Westernized culture generally has been associated with higher rates of disease. An example of this is the rate of cardiovascular disease among Japanese males in the United States. Increasing levels of acculturation also have been associated with higher rates of specific mental disorders and with substance abuse, suggesting that these disorders result from acculturation. Increasing levels of acculturation are correlated with advancing socioeconomic status, and higher socioeconomic status is correlated with lower rates of disease and disorders. However, in some instances higher acculturation is correlated with higher rates of disease and disorders. What constitutes healthy acculturation, as contrasted with unhealthy acculturation, for which health outcomes, for whom, and under what conditions? Scientific answers to these questions may help empower diverse communities by promoting health and wellness in the presence of acculturation (González Castro, 2007).

Health Disparities

Health disparities "are differences in health outcomes and their determinants between segments of the population, as defined by social, demographic, environmental, and geographic attributes" (CDC, Division of Community Health, 2013, p. 4). Health disparities occur among groups who have persistently experienced historic trauma, social disadvantage, or discrimination. Research suggests that discrimination impacts health primarily through three major pathways: psychosocial stress, access to health and social resources, and violence and bodily harm. These pathways are related. For example, denied access to jobs and housing is a cause of psychosocial stress. Discrimination acts as both a stressor and a cause of other stressors and can directly and indirectly lead to harm for those who experience it (Davis, 2020).

Health disparities are widespread in the United States, as demonstrated by the fact that many minority groups in the United States have a higher incidence of chronic diseases, higher mortality, and poorer health outcomes when compared to Whites. Numerous other disparities exist such as the health of rural residents being poorer than urban residents and people with disabilities reporting poorer health compared to those without disabilities.

Eliminating health disparities is an important goal for our nation and is one of the five overarching goals of ***Healthy People 2030***:

1. Attain healthy, thriving lives and well-being, free of preventable disease, disability, injury and premature death.
2. Eliminate health disparities, achieve health equity, and attain health literacy to improve the health and well-being of all.
3. Create social, physical, and economic environments that promote attaining full potential for health and well-being for all.
4. Promote healthy development, healthy behaviors and well-being across all life stages.
5. Engage leadership, key constituents, and the public across multiple sectors to take action and design policies that improve the health and well-being of all (Office of Disease Prevention and Health Promotion, 2020).

Some examples of health disparities follow, but numerous statistics illuminate these differences as well:

- Unintentional injury deaths are approximately 50% higher in rural areas than in urban areas, partly due to greater risk of death from motor vehicle crashes and opioid overdoses (CDC, 2017).
- In 2017, non-Hispanic Whites had the lowest uninsured rate among race and Hispanic-origin groups (6.3%). The uninsured rates for Blacks and Asians were 10.6% and 7.3%, respectively. Hispanics had the highest uninsured rate (16.1%) (Berchick et al., 2018).

- African Americans have 2.3 times the infant mortality rate as non-Hispanic Whites (U.S. Department of Health and Human Services, Office of Minority Health, 2019).
- Hispanic women are 40% more likely to have cervical cancer and 20% more likely to die from cervical cancer than non-Hispanic White women (U.S. Department of Health and Human Services, Office of Minority Health, 2021a).
- In 2017, tuberculosis was 35 times more common in Asian Americans than among non-Hispanic Whites (U.S. Department of Health and Human Services, Office of Minority Health, 2021b).
- Native Hawaiians and Pacific Islanders have higher rates of smoking, alcohol consumption, and obesity in comparison to other populations (U.S. Department of Health and Human Services, Office of Minority Health, 2021c).
- In 2017, American Indian and Alaska Native adults were almost three times more likely to have diabetes than non-Hispanic White adults. They were also 2.5 times more likely to die from diabetes (U.S. Department of Health and Human Services, Office of Minority Health, 2020).

In 2020, the health disparities were illuminated due to the COVID-19 pandemic. These disparities exist by geography and race and ethnicity. For example, the Navajo Nation reported the highest per capita COVID-19 rate in the United States, with a rate of 2,304 cases per 100,000 people compared with the United States, with a rate of 605 cases per 100,000 at the end of 2020 (Johns Hopkins Coronavirus Resource Center, 2021). In Memphis, Tennessee, data reveal that most COVID-19 testing occurs in the predominantly White and well-off suburbs, not the majority–African American, lower-income neighborhoods (Farmer, 2020). The mortality rate was 40% greater in cities and towns "with higher poverty, higher household crowding, higher percentage of populations of color, and higher racialized economic segregation" than in those with the lowest levels of those measures (Chen et al., 2020). Disparities also exist by race and ethnicity (**Table 1.2**).

TABLE 1.2 COVID-19 and Race/Ethnicity as of September 9, 2021

Rate Ratios Compared to White, Non-Hispanics Persons	American Indian or Alaska Native, Non-Hispanic Persons	Asian, Non-Hispanic Persons	Black or African American, Non-Hispanic Persons	Hispanic or Latino Persons
Cases	1.7x	0.7x	1.1x	1.9x
Hospitalization	3.5x	1.0x	2.8x	2.8x
Death	2.4x	1.0x	2.0x	2.3x

Source: CDC (2022)

DID YOU KNOW?

April is National Minority Health month. The purpose is to raise awareness of health disparities. Public health agencies across the national engage in activities to raise awareness about the health disparities that exist around issues such as alcohol and drug addiction and infectious diseases.

Causes of Health Disparities

Health disparities exist due to both voluntary and involuntary factors. Voluntary factors related to health behaviors, such as smoking and diet, can be avoided. Factors such as genetics, living and working in unhealthy conditions, limited or no access to health care, and language barriers are often viewed as involuntary factors, because they are not within that person's control.

Most experts agree that the causes of health disparities are multiple and complex; no single factor explains why disparities exist across such a wide range of health measures. Access to health care and the quality of health care are important factors, but they do not explain why some groups experience greater risks for poor health in the first place.

Socioeconomic status (SES) is one of the most important predictors of health. Socioeconomic status is typically measured by educational attainment, income, wealth, occupation, or a combination of these factors. In general, the higher one's SES, the better one's health. A strong correlation between SES, lifestyle, and health has been shown (SES is linked to lifestyle, and lifestyle is linked to physical and psychological health (Wang & Geng, 2019). Lifestyle, which is strongly correlated with SES, plays a mediating role in the relationship between SES and health (Wang & Geng, 2019).

SES is related to health disparities, and racial and ethnic minorities are disproportionately found in lower socioeconomic levels. An important exception is the "Hispanic epidemiologic paradox." This refers to the fact that new Hispanic immigrants are found to have generally better health than U.S.-born individuals of the same SES. Latinos in the United States also typically live longer than Whites (Kelly, 2016). While not totally understood, these epidemiological findings have interested scholars, mostly because Latinos, on average, have lower SES than Whites. Lower SES is typically associated with higher death rates and worse health outcomes (Kelly, 2016).

Another way to frame the causes of health disparities is via the factors affecting health that were identified in the 1974 Lalonde report, "A New Perspective on the Health of Canadians." This report probably was the first acknowledgment by a major industrialized country that health is determined by more than biological factors. The report led to the development of the "health field" concept, which identified four health fields that were interdependently responsible for individual health:

1. *Environment.* All matters related to health external to the human body and over which the individual has little or no control. Includes the physical and social environment.

2. *Human biology.* All aspects of health, physical and mental, developed within the human body as a result of organic makeup.
3. *Lifestyle.* The aggregation of personal decisions over which the individual has control. Self-imposed risks created by unhealthy lifestyle choices can be said to contribute to, or cause, illness or death.
4. *Health care organization.* The quantity, quality, arrangement, nature, and relationships of people and resources in the provision of health care.

These four domains were later refined to include five intersecting domains:

1. Environmental exposures
2. Genetics
3. Behavior (lifestyle) choices
4. Social circumstances
5. Medical care (Institute of Medicine [IOM], 2001)

All five domains are integrated and affected by one another. For example, people who have more education usually have higher incomes (social circumstances), are more likely to live in neighborhoods with fewer environmental health risks (environmental exposures), and have money to purchase healthier foods (lifestyle). Let's look at each of these domains in more detail.

Environmental Exposures

Environmental conditions are believed to play an important role in producing and maintaining health disparities. The environment influences our health in many ways, including through exposures to physical, chemical, and biological risk factors and through related changes in our behavior in response to those factors. In general, Whites and minorities do not have the same exposure to environmental health threats because they live in different neighborhoods. Residential segregation still exists, but it is improving. Since 1990, more than 90% of U.S. metro areas have seen a decline in racial stratification, signaling a trend toward a more integrated America. Houston and Atlanta, for example, have undergone rapid demographic changes, while cities like Detroit and Chicago still have large areas dominated by a single racial group (Williams & Emamdjomeh, 2018). Over the past 30 years, suburbs have increasingly become the most racial and ethnically diverse areas in the country (Williams & Emamdjomeh, 2018).

"The effects of residential segregation are often stark: Blacks and Hispanics who live in highly segregated and isolated neighborhoods have lower housing quality, higher concentrations of poverty, and less access to good jobs and education. As a consequence, they experience greater stress and have a higher risk of illness and death" (Schwartz, 2018).

Minorities tend to live in poorer areas, and these disadvantaged neighborhoods are exposed to greater health hazards, including tobacco and alcohol advertisements, toxic waste incinerators, and air pollution. It has been known for a long time that Black and Hispanic Americans tend to live in areas with more pollution compared to where White Americans live. Because pollution exposure can cause a range of health problems, this inequity could contribute to unequal health outcomes (Lambert, 2019). Economic stress within a community may exacerbate tensions between social groups, magnify workplace stressors, induce maladaptive coping behaviors such as smoking and alcohol use, and translate into individual stress, all of which makes individuals more vulnerable to illness (e.g., depression, high blood pressure). Factors associated with living in poor neighborhoods—crime, noise, traffic, litter, crowding, and physical deterioration—also can cause stress.

Some health issues related to where one lives include the following (Cooper, 2014):

- Two to three times as many fast-food outlets are located in segregated Black neighborhoods than in White neighborhoods of comparable socioeconomic status, contributing to higher Black consumption of fatty, salty meals and in turn widening racial disparities in obesity and diabetes.
- Black neighborhoods contain two to three times fewer supermarkets than comparable White neighborhoods, creating the kind of "food deserts" that make it difficult for residents who depend on public transportation to purchase the fresh fruits and vegetables that make for a healthy diet.
- Fewer African Americans have ready access to places to work off excess weight that can gradually cause death. A study limited to New York, Maryland, and North Carolina found that Black neighborhoods were three times more likely to lack recreational facilities where residents could exercise and relieve stress.
- Because of "the deliberate placement of polluting factories and toxic waste dumps in minority neighborhoods," exposure to air pollutants and toxins is five to 20 times higher than in White neighborhoods with the same income levels.
- Regardless of their socioeconomic status, African Americans who live in segregated communities receive unequal medical care because the hospitals serving them have less technology, such as imaging equipment, and fewer specialists, like those in heart surgery and cancer.

Genetics

Genetics have been linked to many diseases, including diabetes, cancer, sickle-cell anemia, obesity, cystic fibrosis, hemophilia, Tay-Sachs disease, schizophrenia, and Down syndrome. There are over 6,000 genetic disorders, many of which are fatal or severely debilitating (Ben-Senior, 2018). Some genetic disorders are a result of a single mutated gene, and other disorders are complex, multifactorial, or polygenic mutations. (*Multifactorial* means that the disease or disorder is likely to be associated with the effects of multiple genes in combination with lifestyle and environmental factors.) Examples of multifactorial disorders are cancer, heart disease, and diabetes. Although numerous studies have linked genetics to health, social and cultural factors play a role as well. For example, smoking may trigger a genetic predisposition to lung cancer, but that gene may not have been expressed if the person did not smoke.

There are concerns about relating genetics and health disparities, because race is not truly biologically determined, so the relationship between genetics and race is not clear-cut. There are more genetic differences within races than among them, and racial categories do not capture biological distinctiveness. Another problem with linking genetics to race is that many people have a mixed gene pool due to interracial marriages and partnerships. Also, it is difficult at times to determine which diseases are related to genetics and which are related to other factors, such as lifestyle and the environment.

Sometimes disease is caused by a combination of factors. For example, African Americans have been shown to have higher rates of hypertension than Whites, but is that difference due to genetics? African Americans tend to consume less potassium than Whites and have stress related to discrimination, which could be the cause of their higher rates of hypertension. Health disparities also can be related to the level of exposure to environmental hazards, such as toxins and carcinogens, that some racial groups are exposed to more than others. Therefore, it is difficult to link health disparities to genetics alone because a variety of factors may be involved. Genetics does play a role in health, however, and some clear links have been made, such as people with lighter skin tones being more prone to skin cancer.

Lifestyle

Health behaviors are influenced by many factors, including SES, where one lives, culture, and stress. For example, research suggests that lesbian, gay, bisexual, and transgenders have high rates of substance addiction, which is linked to societal stigma, discrimination, and denial of their civil and human rights (CDC, n.d.).

Other lifestyle differences are among rural and urban populations. A CDC report found that only one in four rural adults practices at least four of five health-related behaviors that can prevent chronic disease such as not smoking, maintaining a normal body weight, being physically active, not drinking alcohol or drinking in moderation, and getting sufficient sleep (CDC, 2018). Many lifestyle differences exist among racial and ethnic groups as well. For example, the rate of past month (35.9%) and past year (54.3%) alcohol use among American Indians is significantly higher than other ethnic groups (Editorial Staff, 2020).

Social Circumstances

Social circumstances include factors such as SES, education level, stress, discrimination, marriage and partnerships, and family roles. SES is made up of a combination of variables, including occupation, education, income, wealth, place of residence, and poverty.

These variables do not have a direct effect on health, but they do have an indirect effect. For example, low SES does not cause disease, but poor nutrition, limited access to health care, and substandard housing certainly do, and these are just a few of the many indirect effects. Discrimination also does not cause poor health directly, but it can lead to depression and high blood pressure.

One variable of social circumstances, poverty, can be measured in many ways. One approach is to measure the number of people who are recipients of federal aid programs, such as food stamps, public housing, and Head Start. Another method is through labor statistics, but the most common way is through the federal government's measure of poverty based on income. The federal government's definition of poverty is based on a threshold defined by income, and it is updated annually. So how is poverty related to ethnicity?

Poverty is higher among certain racial and ethnic groups. According to 2018 U.S. Census data, the highest poverty rate by race is found among American Indians (25.4%), with Blacks (20.8%) having the second highest poverty rate, and Hispanics (of any race) having the third highest poverty rate (17.6%). Both Whites and Asians had a poverty rate of 10.1% (PovertyUSA, 2020). Poverty is a contributing factor to health disparities, because poverty affects many factors, including where people live and their access to health care. What may not be surprising is that low SES groups more often act in ways that harm their health than do high SES groups. It is perplexing that some of these unhealthy behaviors are adopted despite the monetary and health costs. For example, smoking cigarettes and alcohol consumption require that the person spend money on these items. Pampel et al. (2010) noted some important facts related to socioeconomic factors in health behaviors. One example is access to health aids. Adopting many healthy behaviors does not require money, but having more money to pay for tobacco cessation aids, joining fitness clubs and weight loss programs, and buying more expensive fruits, vegetables, and lean meats can help people achieve better health.

Medical Care

The shortfalls for minorities in the health care system in the United States can be categorized into three general areas: (a) lack of access to care, (b) lower quality of care, and (c) limited providers with the same ethnic background.

Lack of Access to Medical Care

Research has shown that without access to timely and effective preventive care, people may be at risk for potentially avoidable conditions, such as asthma, diabetes, and immunizable conditions (National Center for Health Statistics, 2006). Access to health care is also important for prompt treatment and follow-up to illness and injury.

Access to health care is a problem for many Americans due to lack of health care insurance. In 2019, 28.9 million nonelderly individuals were uninsured, an increase of more than 1 million from 2018 (Tolbert et al., 2020). In 2019, 7.8% of Whites, 11.4% of Blacks, 20% of Hispanics, 7.2% of Asians, 21.7% of American Indians/Alaska Natives, and 12.7% of Native Hawaiians and Other Pacific Islanders were uninsured (Tolbert et al., 2020).

The Patient Protection and Affordable Care Act (ACA), passed in 2010, was designed to increase the quality and affordability of health insurance, and hence lower the rate of uninsured. The ACA went into effect on January 1, 2014. Following the ACA, the number of uninsured nonelderly Americans declined by 20 million, dropping to an historic low in 2016. However, beginning in 2017, the number of uninsured nonelderly Americans increased for 3 straight years, growing by 2.2 million from 26.7 million in 2016 to 28.9 million in 2019, and the uninsured rate increased from 10.0% in 2016 to 10.9% in 2019 (Tolbert et al., 2020). Some of this change may be due to a Congressional change in the ACA eliminating the financial sanctions for not obtaining insurance. It is not yet clear how significantly the COVID-19 pandemic and related economic recession may have impacted affordability and access to health care insurance.

Lower Quality of Care

Despite improvements, differences persist in health care quality among racial and ethnic minority groups. People in low-income families also experience poorer quality care. Disparities in quality of care are common. Consider the following examples:

- Blacks, American Indians and Alaska Natives (AI/ANs), and Native Hawaiians/Pacific Islanders received worse care than Whites for about 40% of quality measures.
- Disparities were improving for only four measures for Blacks, two measures for AI/ANs, and one measure for NHPIs.
- Hispanics received worse care than Whites for about 35% of quality measures.
- From 2000 to 2017, disparities were improving for five measures for Hispanics.
- Asians received worse care than Whites for 27% of quality measures but better care than Whites for 28% of quality measures. Disparities were improving for only two measures for Asians (Agency for Healthcare Research and Quality, 2018).

Compared with non-Hispanic White Veteran Health Administration (VHA) users, VHA users of racial and ethnic minority groups had better access to care for 3% of measures, similar access to care for 58% of measures, and worse access to care for 39% of measures (Agency for Healthcare Research and Quality, 2020).

Legal Protections for Minorities

Many laws have been passed to help reduce discrimination, including in the health care arena. The Civil Rights Act of 1964 was passed by Congress and signed into law by President Lyndon Baines Johnson. Title VI of the Civil Rights Act prohibits federally funded programs or activities from discriminating on the basis of race, color, or national origin. Federal agencies are responsible for enforcement of this law. In areas involving discrimination in health care, the Office for Civil Rights (OCR) of the Department of Health and Human Services (HHS), is responsible for enforcement. Title VI of the act is the operative section that informs nondiscrimination in health care. It has three key elements:

1. It established a national priority against discrimination in the use of federal funds.
2. It authorized federal agencies to establish standards of nondiscrimination.
3. It provided for enforcement by withholding funds or by any other means authorized by law.

Since the Civil Rights Act of 1964 was passed, numerous other statutes and regulations have been created to address discrimination against ethnic minorities in health care, including the **Hill–Burton Act**. The Hill-Burton Act has been amended a number of times since its inception. The amendment entitled "Community Service Assurance under Title IV of the U.S. Public Health Service Act" requires facilities to provide services to persons living within the service area without discrimination based on race, national origin, color, creed, or any other reason not related to the person's need for services. The subsequent HHS regulations set forth the requirements with which a Hill-Burton facility must comply (HHS, OCR, 2006):

- A person residing in the Hill-Burton facility's service area has the right to medical treatment at the facility without regard to race, color, national origin, or creed.
- A Hill-Burton facility must post notices informing the public of its community service obligations in English and Spanish. If 10% or more of the households in the service area usually speak a language other than English or Spanish, the facility must translate the notice into that language and post it as well.
- A Hill-Burton facility may not deny emergency services to any person residing in the facility's service area on the grounds that the person is unable to pay for those services.
- A Hill-Burton facility may not adopt patient admission policies that have the effect of excluding persons on grounds of race, color, national origin, creed, or any other ground unrelated to the patient's need for the service or the availability of the needed service.

Title VI and HHS services regulations require recipients of federal financial assistance from HHS to take reasonable steps to provide meaningful access to limited English proficiency (LEP) persons. Federal financial assistance includes grants, training, use of equipment, donations of surplus property, and other assistance. Recipients of HHS assistance may include hospitals, nursing homes, home health agencies, managed care organizations, universities, and other entities with health or social service research programs. It also may include state Medicaid agencies; state, county, and local welfare agencies; programs for families, youth, and children; Head Start programs; public and private contractors, subcontractors, and vendors; and physicians and other providers who receive federal financial assistance from HHS (HHS, OCR, n.d.a.). Interpreters, who assist in communication between patients and providers, must meet specified qualifications and ideally be certified. Failure to use qualified interpreters can have serious negative consequences for both practitioners and patients.

Recipients are required to take reasonable steps to ensure meaningful access to their programs and activities by LEP persons. The obligation to provide meaningful access is fact dependent and starts with an individualized assessment that balances four factors: (a) the number or proportion of LEP persons eligible to be served or likely to be encountered by the program or grantee; (b) the frequency with which LEP individuals come into contact with the program; (c) the nature and importance of the program, activity, or service provided by the recipient to its beneficiaries; and (d) the resources available to the grantee/recipient and the costs of interpretation/translation services. There is no "one-size-fits-all" solution for Title VI compliance with respect to LEP persons, and what constitutes "reasonable steps" for large providers may not be reasonable where small providers are concerned (HHS, OCR, n.d.a.).

If, after completing the four-factor analysis, a recipient determines that it should provide language assistance services, a recipient may develop an implementation plan to address the identified needs of the LEP populations it serves. Recipients have considerable flexibility in developing this plan. The guidance provides five steps that may be helpful in designing such a plan: (1) identifying LEP individuals who need language assistance; (2) language assistance measures (such as how staff can obtain services or respond to LEP callers); (3) training staff; (4) providing notice to LEP persons (such as posting signs); and (5) monitoring and updating the LEP plan (HHS, OCR, n.d.a.).

In 2015, the Supreme Court declared same-sex marriage legal in all 50 states. This decision will support providing same-sex households with the same rights and privileges to health care, health insurance, and survivor benefits that are allowed to opposite-sex households. The medical and social science literature suggest that legal and social recognition of same-sex marriage has had positive effects on the health status of this at-risk community.

Some states also have laws to protect sexual minorities. An example is the California Gender Recognition Act (SB 179), signed into law on October 15, 2017. The bill allows Californians to apply to change their gender markers and creates a nonbinary gender category (the letter "x" or "nb") on California birth certificates, drivers' licenses, identity cards, and gender-change court orders. The law enables transgender, intersex, and nonbinary people to have full recognition in California. Oregon has a similar law.

Culturally and Linguistically Appropriate Services

In compliance with Title VI and the LEP regulations, the HHS Office of Minority Health (OMH) has developed "National Standards for Culturally and Linguistically Appropriate Services in Health Care (CLAS)." In promulgating these standards, OMH provided its rationale for preparing the standards and recommendations for their use. The CLAS standards are intended to advance health equity, improve quality, and help eliminate health care disparities by providing a blueprint for individuals and health and health care organizations to implement culturally and linguistically appropriate services. Adoption of these standards is expected to help advance better health and health care in the United States. The CLAS standards are listed in **Table 1.3**.

TABLE 1.3 National CLAS Standards

Principal Standard
1. Provide effective, equitable, understandable, and respectful quality care and services that are responsive to diverse cultural health beliefs and practices, preferred languages, health literacy, and other communication needs.
Governance, Leadership and Workforce
2. Advance and sustain organizational governance and leadership that promotes CLAS and health equity through policy, practices, and allocated resources.
3. Recruit, promote, and support a culturally and linguistically diverse governance, leadership, and workforce that are responsive to the population in the service area.
4. Educate and train governance, leadership, and workforce in culturally and linguistically appropriate policies and practices on an ongoing basis.
Communication and Language Assistance
5. Offer language assistance to individuals who have limited English proficiency and/or other communication needs, at no cost to them, to facilitate timely access to all health care and services.
6. Inform all individuals of the availability of language assistance services clearly and in their preferred language, verbally and in writing.
7. Ensure the competence of individuals providing language assistance, recognizing that the use of untrained individuals and/or minors as interpreters should be avoided.
8. Provide easy-to-understand print and multimedia materials and signage in the languages commonly used by the populations in the service area.
Engagement, Continuous Improvement, and Accountability
9. Establish culturally and linguistically appropriate goals, policies, and management accountability, and infuse them throughout the organization's planning and operations.
10. Conduct ongoing assessments of the organization's CLAS-related activities and integrate CLAS-related measures into measurement and continuous quality improvement activities.
11. Collect and maintain accurate and reliable demographic data to monitor and evaluate the impact of CLAS on health equity and outcomes and to inform service delivery.
12. Conduct regular assessments of community health assets and needs and use the results to plan and implement services that respond to the cultural and linguistic diversity of populations in the service area.

(continued)

TABLE 1.3 National CLAS Standards (*Continued*)

13. Partner with the community to design, implement, and evaluate policies, practices, and services to ensure cultural and linguistic appropriateness.
14. Create conflict and grievance resolution processes that are culturally and linguistically appropriate to identify, prevent, and resolve conflicts or complaints.
15. Communicate the organization's progress in implementing and sustaining CLAS to all stakeholders, constituents, and the general public.

Source: U.S. Department of Health and Human Services, "National Culturally and Linguistically Appropriate Services Standards" https://thinkculturalhealth.hhs.gov/clas/standards.

It is worth noting that both federal and state governments have begun addressing the need for cultural competence through various standards and legislation. States are requiring cultural competence education in medical and nursing schools, and legislation in many states includes requiring cultural competence training for health care providers to receive licensure or relicensure. **Figure 1.4** highlights the states that require, are proposing to implement, and do not require cultural competence training.

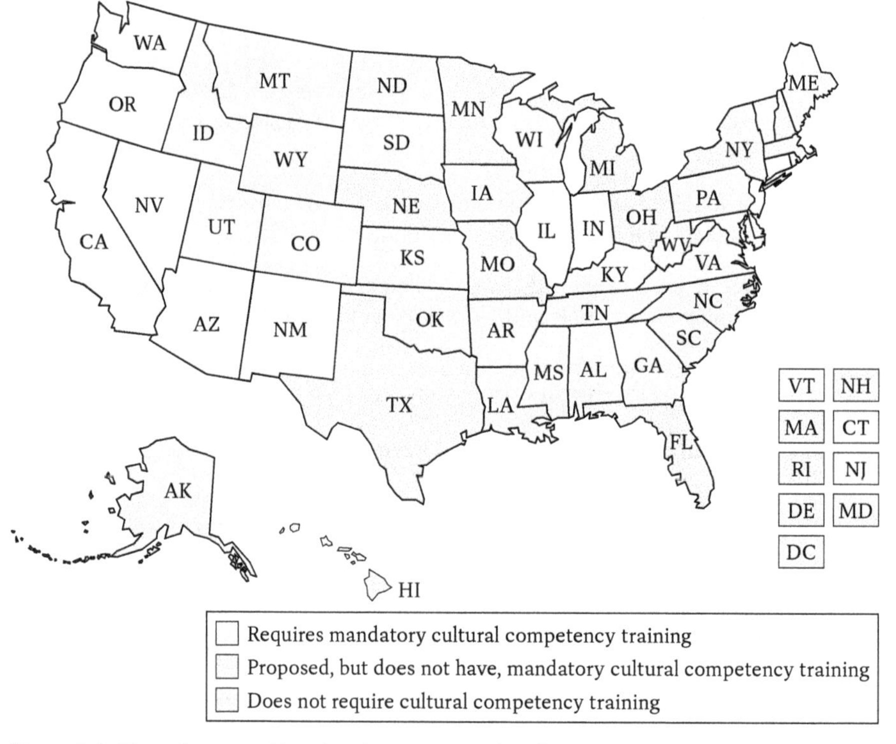

Figure 1.4 Map of states with cultural competence legislation.

Personal Health Decisions

Perhaps the area where law and cultural health issues intersect the most is in the area of personal health care decisions. How an individual approaches health care decisions is informed by personal experiences as well as family, religious, and cultural influences. Different cultures approach how to undergo treatment, when to treat, and when to stop treatment differently. Even more important, who will make such decisions for a patient may differ from culture to culture.

Therefore, it is important to understand the legal construct that affects health care decisions. The laws of all the states reflect an individual's constitutional right to privacy and autonomy to make personal decisions free from outside influence. Consequently, the right to make health care decisions is personal to the patient involved, and no one else has the right to interfere. In cultures where family input is sought for such decisions, or a surrogate decision-maker is used, this legal principle could create decision-making conflicts. Competent individuals can appoint someone else to make decisions for them, thus removing the conflict.

The more problematic situation is when the patient is unable to make his or her wishes known because of the patient's medical condition. In that situation, it is important to have documents prepared in advance that name who will make decisions for the person and what decisions are to be made that are consistent with the person's cultural beliefs. Health care powers of attorney are documents that appoint who will make decisions for the person if he or she is unable to decide. A living will documents desires a person has about end-of-life decisions, and it can, and should, include instructions respecting the person's cultural beliefs. Many states have combined these two documents into one advance health care document that covers all the various decisions. Whatever format is utilized in a particular state, the importance of having these documents remains.

Ethical Considerations

Ethics point to standards or codes of behavior expected by the group to which the individual belongs. Ethics are different from morals in that **morality** refers to personal character and what the individual believes is right or wrong conduct. For example, a nurse's moral code may consider murder to be wrong, but the nurse has an ethical obligation to provide services for a murderer if the murderer is a patient in the medical facility.

The legal system is a set of rules and regulations that are binding on the members of a society and that set out what behavior is acceptable. They are subject to review and change as the society changes. The relationship between law and ethics significantly affects health care decisions and cultural influences. The ethical principles with the most impact on cultural issues in health care are autonomy, nonmaleficence, beneficence, and justice.

Autonomy is the ethical principle that embodies the right of self-determination. It is the right to choose what happens to one's self and to make one's own decisions. It is embodied in the concept of informed consent in health care, which is the right to be informed about recommended treatment prior to consent. Autonomy requires that certain conditions exist, including understanding; an absence of controlling influences, which is traditionally understood as liberty; and agency, which is the ability to act intentionally (Beauchamp & Childress, 2001).

For this ethical principle to be achieved, the health care provider must respect and guard the patient's right to self-determination. This includes informing patients in a manner that considers both cultural and language barriers to understanding. The CLAS standards are an attempt to respect the ethical concept of autonomy. **Respect** takes into account individuals' rights to make determinations about their health and to live or die with the consequences. Respect for others does not allow cultural, gender, religious, or racial differences to interfere with that individual right. Respect is evident when the cultural heritage and practices of patients are considered in treatment even when the provider does not share that value.

In respect for autonomy, not only is the right to choose is respected, but a right not to choose should be respected as well. Valuing a patient's right to defer decision-making to another person, or not to be informed about the extent of his or her condition, is as essential to the principle of autonomy as ensuring that a patient who desires autonomy is fully informed about his or her treatment options.

Associated with respecting patient autonomy are two principles that should be followed by the caregiver: veracity and fidelity. **Veracity** involves being truthful and providing necessary information in an honest way. **Fidelity** entails keeping one's promises or commitments. It requires not promising what one cannot do or control. Both these principles are necessary for patients to be truly informed about their care so that they can make autonomous decisions.

Beneficence is the principle that requires doing good or removing harm. It is often intertwined with nonmaleficence, but it is a distinct ethical construct. Beneficence is at work when balancing the risk, benefit, harm, and effectiveness of treatment. When harm is found, positive actions are required to remove or limit it. This ethical principle was at work when segregated hospitals were outlawed by the Civil Rights Act.

Nonmaleficence is the principle that states that one should do no harm. Although simple in concept, it is often difficult in practice. In health care, actions can often cause harm, and very few treatment modalities are completely without risk of harm. Thus, the practitioner must weigh the risks and benefits of any treatment.

However, it is the unknown harm that should be addressed in the cultural context. Practitioners should be aware that patients from cultures other than their own may perceive situations as harmful that are not readily apparent to them. For example, physical examination of a female by a male practitioner is considered unacceptable in some cultures and can lead to serious consequences for the female patient. Making arrangements for a female examiner would evidence the ethical concept of nonmaleficence.

Justice is the ethical principle that holds that people should be treated equally and fairly. Justice requires that people not be treated differently because of their culture or ethnic background. Justice is also at issue when the allocation and distribution of limited health resources are discussed. Ensuring that health resources are available to all without regard to race or ethnicity is the theory of distributive justice. It is this ethical principle that is breached when care is denied or withheld on racial or ethnic grounds.

The fair opportunity rule of justice states that no one should receive social benefits based on undeserved advantages or be denied benefits on the basis of disadvantages (Beauchamp & Childress, 2001). Although this may seem fairly straightforward, it becomes difficult to manage when applied to the variances of social inequalities. The rule states that discrimination is not ethically justifiable on the basis of social status or ethnicity.

Summary

One of the great attributes of the United States is its diverse landscape. Immigrants (voluntary and forced) who have come to the United States and natives of this country have experienced different levels of cultural adaptation to blend into dominant society. Some have retained their strong cultural ties to create a society of rich and diverse cultures filled with various beliefs, traditions, languages, and societal norms. Understanding and respecting this diverse landscape is a goal for the nation, specifically for the health care industry. Health care providers need to be knowledgeable about and sensitive to cultural differences to provide effective care and education. Laws have been established to address inequalities.

This chapter provides a description of the foundations of multicultural health and the key terms and concepts associated with it, such as *culture*, *race*, *assimilation*, and *cultural relativism*. You should now have a general appreciation of how culture affects health, the breadth and depth of health disparities and their related causes, as well as the legal protections provided to people in the United States.

Review

1. What is the focus of multicultural health, and why is it important?
2. Is race a biological or a social construct? Why is race important?
3. What is the difference between ethnicity and culture? What is the difference between race and ethnicity?
4. Explain cultural ethnocentricity and cultural relativism.
5. Explain the differences between the concepts of acculturation, assimilation, and being bicultural.
6. Does the level of acculturation have a positive or negative effect on health? Explain.
7. Explain what health disparities are and their causes.
8. Describe the key intentions of the Civil Rights Act and the Hill-Burton Act.

9. Explain the ethical principles related to health care decision-making and how they influence health care services.

Activity

Conduct research to identify a legal case related to health and culture. Write a paper explaining the situation, the court's decision, the reason behind the decision, and your reaction to the outcome.

Case Study 1

The Spirit Catches You and You Fall Down is a book written by Anne Fadiman. The author writes about Lia Lee, a Hmong child who has epilepsy and lived in Merced, California. Lia was an infant when her parents, Foua and Nao Kao, took her to the emergency room due to seizures. Lia's parents and the doctors all wanted the best for Lia, but they had vast differences of opinion about what caused Lia's illness and how it should be treated.

While the medical field in the United States typically views illness from the perspective of mind and body being separate, the Hmong culture sees it differently. They view it from a spiritual perspective. The doctors saw Lia's condition as being caused by a biological reason; her parents saw the cause as her soul wandering. The doctors treated Lia with medication. Lia's parents took her to a shaman and clan leader and used animal sacrifice and amulets to help her heal and bring her soul back.

Believing that Lia's parents were endangering her life by not giving her the medication, the doctors contacted child protective services (CPS). Lia was removed from her home and placed in foster care, which was devastating to her parents as they loved her very much and wanted the best for Lia.

As shown in this case, health and culture are interrelated and can at times compete with each other. Health care providers should respect cultural values and be cognizant of cultural issues when providing care to diverse patients.

Issues to consider about this case:

1. Were Lia's parents noncompliant with her care plan? Why?
2. Was the call to CPS in Lia's best interest?
3. What responsibility does a health care provider have in this situation?
4. Explain the impact of the parents' beliefs about Lia's illness.
5. Were Lia's parents right or wrong in the decisions they made about her health?

Case Study 2

Alex grew up on the docks in Brooklyn, New York, in a poor family. Alex loved school and did very well in his classes. His grades and Scholastic Aptitude Test scores were very high. Several colleges offered him a scholarship. He accepted one from an Ivy League university. After earning top grades in the undergraduate program, the university offered Alex another scholarship to medical school. Alex completed his training with honors.

After completing his training he interviewed for a faculty position. The interview went well, but Alex was not offered the position, even though he was well qualified. When he spoke to Human Resources personnel, he was informed that while he was obviously intelligent and well educated, he did not come across that way.

Alex has maintained his New York street accent and is proud of it. He has been told that he should "speak proper English" in order to get ahead and not come across as uneducated. Alex wants to be true to his roots, so he maintains his accent.

Issues to consider about this case:

1. Based on the information provided, did the hiring university discriminate against Alex based on his accent? If so, do they have a valid reason as students may not see him as educated or qualified?
2. If you were Alex, what would you have said to the person in Human Resources?
3. If you were Alex's friend, what would you suggest he do on his next interview?

References

Agency for Healthcare Research and Quality. (2018). *National healthcare and disparities report.* https://www.ahrq.gov/sites/default/files/wysiwyg/research/findings/nhqrdr/2018qdr-final-es.pdf

Agency for Healthcare Research and Quality. (2020, November). *Chartbook on healthcare for veterans.* https://www.ahrq.gov/sites/default/files/wysiwyg/research/findings/nhqrdr/chartbooks/veterans/2020qdr-chartbook-veterans.pdf

Beauchamp, T., & Childress, J. (2001). *Principles of biomedical ethics* (5th ed.). Oxford University Press.

Ben-Senior, L. (2018, May 22). *10 most common genetic diseases.* Lab Roots. https://www.labroots.com/trending/infographics/8833/10-common-genetic-diseases#:~:text=There%20are%20over%206%2C000%20genetic,Chromosomal%20changes%20and%20mitochondrial%20mutations

Berchick, E. R., Hood, E., & Barnett, J. C. (2018, September 12). *Health insurance coverage in the United States: 2017.* U.S. Census Bureau. https://www.census.gov/library/publications/2018/demo/p60-264.html

Berry, J. W. (1997). Immigration, acculturation, and adaptation. *Applied Psychology: An International Review.* 46:5–68.

Centers for Disease Control and Prevention. (n.d.). *Lesbian, gay, bisexual, and transgender health.* https://www.healthypeople.gov/2020/topics-objectives/topic/lesbian-gay-bisexual-and-transgender-health

Centers for Disease Control and Prevention. (2017, August 2). *About rural health.* https://www.cdc.gov/ruralhealth/about.html

Centers for Disease Control and Prevention. (2018, January 10). *Health behaviors in rural America.* https://www.cdc.gov/ruralhealth/Health-Behaviors.html

Centers for Disease Control and Prevention. (2021, August 31). *Culture and language.* https://www.cdc.gov/healthliteracy/culture.html

Centers for Disease Control and Prevention. (2022). *Risk for COVID-19 infection, hospitalization, and death by race/ethnicity.* https://www.cdc.gov/coronavirus/2019-ncov/covid-data/investigations-discovery/hospitalization-death-by-race-ethnicity.html

Centers for Disease Control and Prevention, Division of Community Health. (2013). *A practitioner's guide for advancing health equity: Community strategies for preventing chronic disease.* U.S. Department of Health and Human Services.

Chen, J. T., Waterman, P. D., & Krieger, N. (2020, May). *COVID-19 and the unequal surge in mortality rates in Massachusetts, by city/town and ZIP code measures of poverty, household crowding, race/ethnicity, and racialized economic segregation* [Working paper]. Harvard Center for Population and Development Studies.

Cooper, K. J. (2014, September 21). *Residential segregation contributes to health disparities for people of color.*

Davis, B. A. (2020, February 25). *Discrimination: A social determinant of health inequities.* Health Affairs. https://www.healthaffairs.org/do/10.1377/hblog20200220.518458/full/

Editorial Staff. (January 2, 2020). *Risks of alcoholism among Native Americans.* American Addiction Centers. https://americanaddictioncenters.org/alcoholism-treatment/native-americans

Fadiman, A. (1998). The Spirit Catches You and You Fall Down. Farrar, Straus & Giroux.

Farmer, B. (2020, April 1). *Racial disparities emerge in Tennessee's testing for COVID-19.* WPLN. https://wpln.org/post/racial-disparities-emerge-in-tennessees-testing-for-covid-19/

González Castro, F. (2007). Is acculturation really detrimental to health? *American Journal of Public Health*, 97(7), 1162. http://www.ncbi.nlm.nih.gov/pmc/articles/PMC1913069/

Institute of Medicine. (2001). *Health and behavior: The interplay of biological, behavioral, and societal influences.* National Academies Press.

Johns Hopkins Coronavirus Resource Center. (2021). *COVID-19 dashboard.* https://coronavirus.jhu.edu/map.html

Juckett, G. (2005). Cross-cultural medicine. *American Family Physician, 72*, 2267–2274.

Kelly. R. B. (2016, May 26). *Q&A: Does the "Hispanic paradox" still exist?* Princeton University. https://www.princeton.edu/news/2016/05/24/qa-does-hispanic-paradox-still-exist

Lalonde, M. (1974). *A new perspective on the health of Canadians.* http://www.phac-aspc.gc.ca/ph-sp/pdf/perspect-eng.pdf

Lambert, J. (2019, March 11). *Study finds racial gap between who causes air pollution and who breathes it.* NPR. https://www.npr.org/sections/health-shots/2019/03/11/702348935/study-finds-racial-gap-between-who-causes-air-pollution-and-who-breathes-it

National Center for Health Statistics. (2006). Health, United States, 2006. https://www.cdc.gov/nchs/data/hus/hus06.pdf

Office of Disease Prevention and Health Promotion. (2020, October 8). *Healthy People 2030 framework.* https://www.healthypeople.gov/2020/About-Healthy-People/Development-Healthy-People-2030/Framework

Pampel, F. C., Krueger, P. M., & Denney, J. T. (2010). Socioeconomic disparities in health behaviors. *Annual Review of Sociology, 36*, 349–370.

PovertyUSA. (2020). *Facts.* https://www.povertyusa.org/facts

Schwartz, D. F. (2018, April 3). What's the connection between residential segregation and health? *Culture of Health.* https://www.rwjf.org/en/blog/2016/03/whats-the-connection-between-residential-segregation-and-health.html

Stephenson, M. (2000). Development and validation of the Stephenson Multigroup Acculturation (SMAS). *Psychological assessment, 12*(1), 77.

Tolbert, J., Orgera, K., & Damico, A. (2020, November 6). *Key facts about the uninsured population.* KFF. https://www.kff.org/uninsured/issue-brief/key-facts-about-the-uninsured-population/

Tylor, E. B. (1924). *Primitive culture: Researches into the development of mythology, philosophy, religion, language, art, and custom* (7th ed.). Brentano. (Original work published 1871)

U.S. Census Bureau. (n.d.). *Quick facts.* https://www.census.gov/quickfacts/fact/table/US/PST045219

U.S. Census Bureau. (2011, March). *Overview of race and Hispanic origin: 2010.* http://www.census.gov/prod/cen2010/briefs/c2010br-02.pdf

U.S. Census Bureau. (2020, March 7). United States Census 2020. https://www2.census.gov/programs-surveys/decennial/2020/technical-documentation/questionnaires-and-instructions/questionnaires/2020-informational-questionnaire.pdf

U.S. Department of Health and Human Services, Office for Civil Rights. (n.d.a.). *Guidance to federal financial assistance recipients regarding Title VI and the prohibition against national origin discrimination affecting limited English proficient persons—summary.* http://www.hhs.gov/ocr/civilrights/resources/laws/summaryguidance.html

U.S. Department of Health and Human Services, Office for Civil Rights. (2006, June). *Your rights under Title VI of the Civil Rights Act of 1964.*

U.S. Department of Health and Human Services, Office of Minority Health. (n.d.b.). *CLAS & the CLAS standards.*

U.S. Department of Health and Human Services, Office of Minority Health. (2019, November 8). *Minority population profiles.* https://www.minorityhealth.hhs.gov/omh/browse.aspx?lvl=2&lvlid=26

U.S. Department of Health and Human Services, Office of Minority Health. (April 2020). *Diabetes and American Indians/Alaska Natives.* https://minorityhealth.hhs.gov/omh/browse.aspx?lvl=4&lvlid=33

U.S. Department of Health and Human Services, Office of Minority Health. (2021a). *Cancer and Hispanic Americans.* https://minorityhealth.hhs.gov/omh/browse.aspx?lvl=4&lvlid=61

U.S. Department of Health and Human Services, Office of Minority Health. (2021b). *Profile: Asian Americans.* https://www.minorityhealth.hhs.gov/omh/browse.aspx?lvl=3&lvlid=63

U.S. Department of Health and Human Services, Office of Minority Health. (2021c). *Profile: Native Hawaiians/Pacific Islanders.* https://minorityhealth.hhs.gov/omh/browse.aspx?lvl=3&lvlid=65

Wang, J., & Geng, L. (2019). Effects of socioeconomic status on physical and psychological health: Lifestyle as a mediator. International Journal of Environmental Research and Public Health, *16*(2), 281.

Williams, A., & Emamdjomeh, A. (2018, May 10). America is more diverse than ever—but still segregated. *The Washington Post.* https://www.washingtonpost.com/graphics/2018/national/segregation-us-cities/

Williams, D. R., Lavizzo-Mourey, R., & Warren, R. C. (1994). *The concept of race and health status in America.* http://www.pubmedcentral.nih.gov/picrender.fcgi?artid=1402239&blobtype=pdf

CREDITS

Fig. 1.1: Source: https://www2.census.gov/programs-surveys/decennial/2020/technical-documentation/questionnaires-and-instructions/questionnaires/2020-informational-questionnaire.pdf.

Fig. 1.2: Source: https://www2.census.gov/programs-surveys/decennial/2020/technical-documentation/questionnaires-and-instructions/questionnaires/2020-informational-questionnaire.pdf.

Fig. 1.4: Source: Adapted from https://thinkculturalhealth.hhs.gov/clas/clas-tracking-map.

Fig. 1.4a: Copyright © 2016 Depositphotos/pyty.

CHAPTER 2

Theories and Models Related to Multicultural Health

Inadequate attention has been given to the range of variation in social, cultural, and health characteristics within and between racial or ethnic minority populations.

—WILLIAMS ET AL. (1994, P. 26)

KEY CONCEPTS AND TERMS

Ayurvedic system
Biomedical (allopathic) medicine
Germ theory
Holistic medicine
Humoral system
Naturalistic theories of disease
Personalistic belief system
Vitalistic system

LEARNING OBJECTIVES

After reading this chapter, you should be able to do the following:

1. Explain three overarching theories of the causes of illness and provide examples of each.
2. Explain the differences between the biomedical and holistic systems of care.
3. Explain two models of cultural competence.

"Being cold will give you a cold," "cracking your knuckles will give you arthritis," and "feed a fever, starve a cold" are three examples of beliefs in the United States about how illness can occur and be cured. People from different cultures hold their own beliefs about the causes and cures of illness, and these beliefs influence their behavior and where and when they decide to seek care. Many others factors also affect our health care experience, such as how we communicate about health, whether we believe we have control over our own health, and how health care decisions are made. These factors can be so deeply ingrained that they are almost invisible. Because of this invisibility, health care professionals can overlook these key differences and forget that not all people who reside within the United States have the same beliefs about health and illness. Therefore, it is essential to bring these issues to light, which is the purpose of this chapter.

This chapter begins with a discussion of theories about how illness occurs and then presents models of care for when illness does occur. The chapter ends with a focus on cultural competence and ways to improve cultural competence.

Theories of Health and Illness

Theories about health and illness address the beliefs people hold about how to maintain health and the causes of illness. These ideas, beliefs, and attitudes are socially constructed and are deeply ingrained in people's cultural experience, and they can have a profound effect on medical care. Where and when people seek care are rooted in their cultural belief system (Carteret, 2011). Their beliefs influence prevention efforts, delay or prevent medical care, and complicate the care given (Carteret, 2011). Cultural differences impact a patient's compliance, their ability to understand medical recommendations, and attitudes about medical care (EuroMed Info, 2020). Culture impacts how patients cope and manage an illness, the meaning of a diagnosis, and the outcomes of medical treatment (EuroMed Info, 2020).

Ideas about health maintenance vary among cultures and include ideologies such as consuming a well-balanced diet, wearing amulets, rewards for good behavior, and prayer. Illness causation ideologies include breach of taboo, soul loss, exposure to germs, upset in the hot-cold balance of the body, or a weakening of the body's immune system. Treatment methods range from medications and surgeries to witchcraft and returning the soul to the ill person. In the Western world, the human body is thought of as a machine; when the machine breaks, illness occurs. Eastern philosophies generally view health as a state of balance between the physical and social environments as well as the supernatural environment (Carteret, 2011).

Theories of health and illness serve to create a context of meaning within which patients can make sense of their bodily experience. They assist the patient in framing the illness in a meaningful and logical manner. A meaningful context for illness usually reflects core cultural values and helps the patient bring order to the chaotic world of serious illness and regain some sense of control in a frightening situation. Theories of illness shape how people receive and respond to prevention programs, treatment, and health education messages.

Theories of illness are often divided into three broad categories: personalistic, naturalistic, and biomedical (allopathic). In a personalistic system, illness is believed to be caused by the intentional intervention of an agent who may be a supernatural being (a deity or ancestral spirits) or a human being with special powers (a witch or sorcerer). The sick person's illness is considered a direct result of the harmful influence of these agents and is often linked to the ill person's behavior. In naturalistic causation, illness is explained in terms of a disturbed natural equilibrium. When the body is in balance with the natural environment, a state of health is achieved. When the balance no longer exists, illness occurs. In the biomedical theory, illness is identified and cured using scientific evidence. The cause of illness is physiological in nature.

Many people's beliefs systems are a combination of these three theories. The theories are used by people to understand and respond to the illness. Through communication, patients and providers can work together and combine the theories to try to achieve a positive outcome for the patient.

Personalistic Theories

In the **personalistic belief system**, illness is believed to be caused by the person's misbehavior. The behavior could be related to violations of social or religious norms. As a result of moral or spiritual failings, the person may have punishment invoked in the form of illness by a supernatural being or a human with special powers. The supernatural being may be a dead ancestor or a deity (Carteret, 2011). A dead ancestor may retaliate for not carrying out proper rituals of respect for the dead ancestor. The deity may retaliate for breaching a religious taboo. Bad luck or karma also may cause illness.

Illness also can be caused by people who have the power to make others ill, such as witches, practitioners of voodoo, and sorcerers. These malevolent human beings manipulate secret rituals and charms to cause illness in their enemies.

Recovery from the illness involves healers using supernatural means to understand what is wrong with their patients and return them to health. These supernatural means usually involve rituals or symbolisms used by healers, such as shamans, who are trained in the healing methods. American Indians and people from Latin America and Asia often hold the personalistic belief system (Carteret, 2011). Preventing personalistic illness includes avoiding situations that can provoke jealousy or envy, wearing certain amulets, adhering to social norms and moral behaviors, adhering to food taboos and restrictions, and performing certain rituals. Several personalistic beliefs and practices are reviewed in later chapters.

DID YOU KNOW?

Osteopathic medicine is a form of medical care based on the philosophy that all body systems are interrelated and dependent on one another for good health. In 1874, Dr. Andrew Taylor Still, who recognized the importance of treating illness within the context of the whole body, developed the philosophy of osteopathic medicine. In 1892, Dr. Still opened the first school of osteopathic medicine in Kirksville, Missouri. Physicians licensed as doctors of osteopathic medicine (DOs) must pass a national or state medical board examination to obtain a license to practice medicine (American College of Osteopathic Medicine, 2020).

Osteopathic physicians utilize the same tools available through modern medicine, including prescription medicine and surgery. In addition, DOs use osteopathic manipulative medicine (OMM) in their regimen of patient care when appropriate. "OMM is a set of manual medicine techniques that may be used to diagnose illness and injury, relieve pain, restore range of motion, and enhance the body's capacity to heal" (American College of Osteopathic Medicine, 2020).

Naturalistic Theories

Naturalistic theories of disease tend to view health as a state of harmony between the person and his or her environment; when this balance is upset, illness will result. The naturalistic explanation assumes that illness is due to impersonal, mechanistic causes in nature that potentially can be understood and cured by returning the patient to a balanced state. Humoral, Ayurvedic, and vitalistic are three of the widely practiced approaches to curing natural illness or to explain what causes illness. Preventing naturalistic illness includes methods such as proper hygiene, a balanced diet, and meditation. These types of illness are treated by practitioners such as physicians, nurses, acupuncturists, and chiropractors. Methods include dietary changes, massage, medication, exercise, and physical adjustments.

Humoral

Humoral pathology was developed and became the basis of both ancient Greek and Roman medicine. It is part of the mainstream medical system in Latin America and Asia.

The humoral system is an ancient belief system based on the idea that our bodies have four important fluids, or humors: blood, phlegm, black bile, and yellow bile. These four fluids are related to seasons, internal organs, physical qualities (hot-cold; wet-dry), and human temperaments (see **Table 2.1**). Each humor is thought to have its own "complexion." For example, blood is hot and wet, and yellow bile is hot and dry. Different kinds of illnesses, medicines, foods, and most natural objects also have specific complexions.

TABLE 2.1 Humor and Related Organ and Complexion

Humor (Fluid)	Associated Internal Organ	Associated Season	Associated Element	Normal Complexion	Temperament
Blood	Liver	Spring	Air	Hot and wet	Sanguine (cheer fully confident; optimistic)
Phlegm	Brain and lungs	Winter	Water	Cold and wet	Phlegmatic (calm, sluggish; apathetic)
Black bile	Spleen	Fall	Earth	Cold and dry	Melancholic (in low spirits; gloomy)
Yellow bile	Gallbladder	Summer	Fire	Hot and dry	Choleric (easily angered)

Curing an illness involves discovering the complexion imbalance and rectifying it. A hot injury or illness must be treated with a cold remedy and vice versa. In the 19th century there was a radical transition from the humoral theory to the germ theory of disease, which involved new concepts, rules, and classifications, as well as the abandonment of old ones.

Ayurvedic

Ayurvedic is an ancient naturalistic approach to health that is used in India and other parts of the world. The term *ayurveda* is taken from the Sanskrit words *ayus*, meaning life or life span, and *veda*, meaning knowledge. In the Ayurvedic system, illness is caused by an energy imbalance. The belief system has a long history and embraces the ideology that disease is a result of an imbalance in vital energies, which distinguish living and nonliving matter. In ayurvedic medicine the vital force is called the *prana*.

Ayurveda suggests that three primary principles govern every human body. These principles, called *doshas*, are derived from the five elements: earth, air, water, fire, and space. Doshas regulate all actions of the body. Most people have a predominant dosha, and each dosha type has typical attributes or characteristics. The Ayurveda system of medicine uses a genetically determined concept, *prakriti*, to categorize the population into several subgroups based on phenotypic characters such as appearance, temperament, and habits. This system is useful in predicting an individual's susceptibility to a particular disease, prognosis for that illness and selection of therapy, and variations in platelet aggregation (Bhalerao et al., 2012).

When the doshas are balanced, we experience good health, vitality, ease, strength, flexibility, and emotional well-being. When the doshas fall out of balance, we experience energy loss, discomfort, pain, mental or emotional instability, and, ultimately, disease. Ayurvedic ways to restore balance include breathing exercises, rubbing the skin with herbal oil, meditation, yoga, mantras, massage, and herbs. These modalities are energetic ways to balance the chakras.

The system links the body's *chakras*, or energy centers associated with organs of the body, with primal forces, such as *prana* (breath of life), *agni* (spirit of light or fire), and *soma* (manifestation of harmony). Each and every cell has a chakra, but like the doshas, one or more can often be found to be more dominant than some of the others. When the life force withdraws, the physical body dies; if the life force becomes blocked or compromised, illness or disease is the likely result. Two ways in which the life force enters the body are through breath and through the chakra system.

Breath sustains all life, and when we breathe we take in life-force energy and move the energy to the entire body via the respiratory and circulatory system. The chakra system is another way in which that energy force enters the body. *Chakra* means "wheels of life," and these invisible "wheels" pull in this vital life force. Our physical bodies contain seven major chakras between the base of the spine and the top of the head as well as many minor chakras (see **Figure 2.1**). Each chakra is associated with a major gland or organ and plays an important role in our emotional well-being. As we become older or ill, these chakras may slow down or become blocked, reducing the amount of life force taken into the body, which compromises health and vitality. Our life force also may become depleted due to prolonged stress, poor health habits, or unexpressed emotions.

Vitalistic

In China a system similar to Ayurveda was developed. The vitalistic system can be defined as the concept that bodily functions are due to a vital principle or "life force" that is

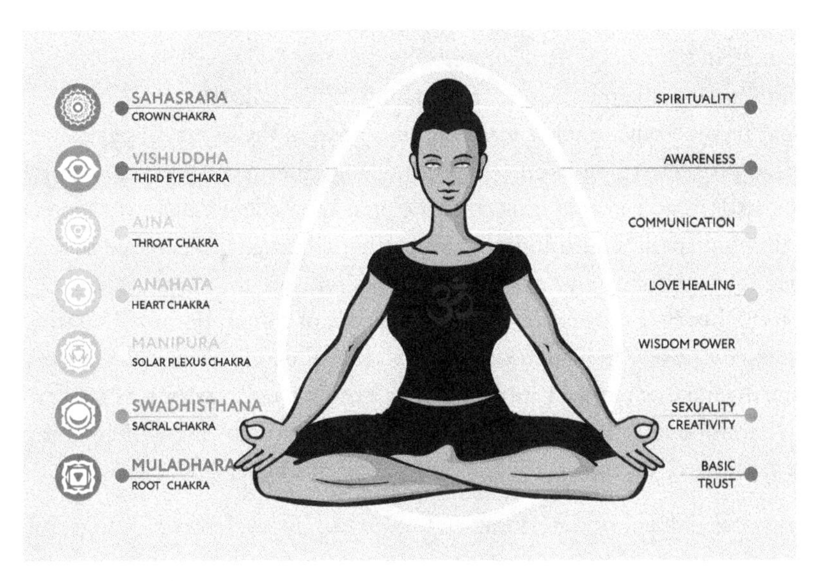

Figure 2.1 Chakra system.

distinct from physical forces explainable by the laws of chemistry and physics and is not detectable by scientific instrumentation. The system is built on the belief that an imbalance in vital energies causes disease.

The imbalance is related to the polar opposites, *yin* (female, dark, cold) and *yang* (male, light, hot), in which one combines the interaction of body fluids and energy channels, or meridians. This vitalistic belief system is widespread in China, South Asia, and Southeast Asia. In the Chinese system, the vital force is called the *chi*; in the ayurvedic system it is the prana. When vital forces within the body flow in a harmonious pattern, a positive state of health is maintained. Illness results when this smooth flow of energy is disrupted, and therapeutic measures are aimed at restoring a normal flow of energy in the body. In China the ancient art of acupuncture is based on this understanding of the body. Acupuncture needles help restore a proper flow of energy within the body.

Biomedical Theory

Biomedical medicine (also known as **allopathic medicine**) is based on the mechanical view, or machine view, of the body: When the machine breaks illness occurs. Spirituality is generally kept separate from health and healing matters. Spirituality is usually viewed as a nonscientific approach to health and healing. Mental health problems are generally viewed as disorders of the mind, and physicians tend to treat these disorders by affecting brain physiology with pharmaceuticals or with counseling or behavior modification.

Allopathic medicine is the type of medicine most familiar to Westerners today. Allopathy is a biologically based approach to healing. For instance, if a patient has high blood pressure, an allopathic physician might give him or her a drug that lowers blood pressure. A core assumption of the value system of allopathic medicine is that diagnosis and treatment should be based on scientific data. The system is built on a molecular understanding of the mechanisms underlying disease, and this lays the foundation for all medical application, diagnosis, and treatment (Carteret, 2011).

Allopathic medicine quickly rose to dominance in the West, in part due to successful scientific progress in developing specific drugs that treat disease. The discovery of antibiotics also triggered rapid growth of the pharmaceutical industry. Pharmacy evolved as an enabling discipline to allopathic medicine, helping it to achieve and maintain its dominance through many successful treatments and cures.

The germ theory of disease is a core component of contemporary allopathic medicine. **Germ theory** proposes that microorganisms are the cause of many diseases. Although highly controversial when first introduced, it is now a cornerstone of modern medicine and has led to innovations and concepts such as antibiotics and hygienic practices.

Typical causes of illness, according to the allopathic belief, are as follows (O'Neil, 2005):

- Organic breakdown or deterioration (e.g., tooth decay, heart failure, senility)
- Obstruction (e.g., kidney stones, arterial blockage due to plaque buildup)
- Injury (e.g., broken bones, bullet wounds)
- Imbalance (e.g., too much or too little of specific hormones and salts in the blood)
- Malnutrition (e.g., too much or too little food, not enough proteins, vitamins, or minerals)
- Parasites (e.g., bacteria, viruses, amoebas, worms)

WHAT DO YOU THINK?

What are your personal beliefs about how health is maintained and illness occurs? Do you hold any beliefs such as that a glass of milk will help you fall asleep? Where does that belief come from? Is it valid? How do your beliefs affect your behavior?

Pathways to Care

The theory of illness with which a person identifies has an impact on where he, she, or they seeks care. Within the United States there are two general systems of care to choose from: the allopathic (biomedical) approach and the holistic approach. The allopathic approach is often viewed as being scientific and focuses more on the physical components of illness than on the social aspects. Holistic medicine is viewed by some as unscientific, and it is based on a psychosocial model of health care. A comparison of these two approaches is shown in **Table 2.2**. People select one health care delivery system over the other for a variety of reasons, and this decision-making process includes considerations such as culture, access to care, health beliefs, and affordability, but many people use both.

TABLE 2.2 Two Health Paradigms

Allopathic	Holistic
Focuses on measurements; symptoms	Focuses on experience; causes and patterns
Disease as entity; pain avoiding	Disease as process; pain reading
General classified diagnosis	Specific individual needs
Health as commodity	Health as process
Technical tools	Integrated therapies
Remedial, combative, reactive	Preventive, corrective, proactive
Crisis oriented; occasional intervention	Lifestyle oriented; sustained maintenance
Radical, defensive	Natural, ecological
Medicine as counteragent	Medicine as coagent
Side effects: chemicals, surgery, radiation, replacement	Low risk: conservative, organic, purification, manipulation, correction
Emphasis on cure	Emphasis on healing
Speed, comfort, convenience	Restoration, regeneration, transformation
Practitioner as authority; pacifying	Practitioner as educator; activating
Patient as passive recipient	Patient as source of healing
Mechanical, analytical, biophysical	Systemic, multidimensional, body–mind–spirit
Best for infectious diseases, trauma, structural damage, organ failure, acute conditions	Best for degeneration, chronic stress and life-style disorders, toxemia, glandular conditions, weakness, systemic imbalances, immunity

Source: Adapted from Lonny J. Brown, ***Self-Actuated Healing (More Crystals and New Age)***. Copyright © 1989 by Naturegraph & Keven Brown Publications.

Allopathic Medicine

In the Western world, the theoretical construct about the cause of illness is biomedicine. In biomedicine, the body is viewed as a machine, and a core assumption of biomedicine is that scientific data should be the basis of diagnosis and treatment. The approach is built on the ideology that illness occurs when the human biological system goes out of balance and that microorganisms are the cause of many diseases.

Care in the biomedical system is provided by a variety of types of professionals with diverse expertise and levels of training. Allopathic physicians include doctors of medicine (MDs) and doctors of osteopathic medicine (DOs). Numerous allied health professionals, such as nurses, respiratory therapists, physical therapists, physician assistants, health educators, and radiologists, also practice allopathic medicine.

Holistic Medicine

The holistic approach (also called alternative medicine or complementary medicine) has a long history and has been rapidly gaining popularity worldwide. **Holistic medicine** is an approach to maintaining and resuming health that takes the body, mind, and spiritual being into consideration. Holistic medicine uses a variety of therapies, such as massage, prayer, herbal remedies, and reiki. More detail about these therapies is provided in Chapter 4.

Holistic providers have vast differences in their levels of training. These differences include length of training, certification and licensing requirements, and required experience. For example, people who study ayurvedic medicine in India often have four or more years of training, and in the United States it is often much less. Because of this broad range of training and educational requirements, it is essential to inquire about education and experience when seeking a provider. Providers include professionals such as homeopaths, naturopaths, acupuncturists, and hypnotherapists.

Cultural Competence

Cultural competence occurs when an individual or organization has the ability to function effectively within the cultural context of beliefs, behaviors, and needs of the patients or community it serves. The CDC (2020) defined cultural competence as "a set of congruent behaviors, attitudes, and policies that come together in a system, agency, or among professionals that enables effective work in cross-cultural situations." Cultural competence requires a set of skills and knowledge that all health care professionals and organizations should strive to acquire. The ability to be culturally competent is on a continuum, with cultural destructiveness on one end of the continuum and cultural proficiency at the other end, as illustrated in **Figure 2.2**.

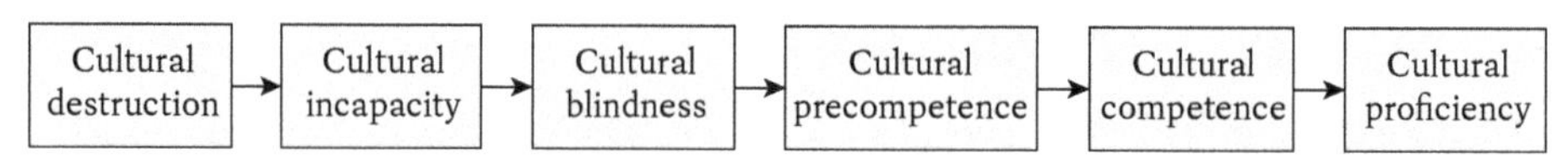

Figure 2.2 Cultural competence continuum.

Being culturally competent does not mean that people need to know everything about every culture, because that is not possible. What it does mean is that people are respectful and sensitive to cultural differences and can work with clients' cultural beliefs and practices. To be culturally competent, one needs to understand his or her own worldviews and those of the person or community in which he, she, or they serves while avoiding stereotyping, judgment, and misapplication of scientific knowledge. Becoming culturally competent is a process that health care professionals should continue to strive to achieve. Models have been developed to assist individuals and organizations in achieving this goal.

Cultural Competence Models

Models are tools that assist with understanding the causes of behaviors, predicting behaviors, and evaluating interventions. Cultural competence models help the learner understand the different components of cultural competence, guide their interactions with people of different cultural groups, and help them identify areas in which they may need to increase their education.

The Process of Cultural Competence in the Delivery of Health Care Services

Josepha Campinha-Bacote (2009) developed a model of cultural competence that is based on five constructs:

1. *Cultural awareness.* The process of conducting a self-examination of one's own biases toward other cultures and an in-depth exploration of one's cultural and professional background.
2. *Cultural knowledge.* The process in which the health care professional seeks and obtains a sound information base regarding the worldviews of different cultural and ethnic groups as well as biological variations, diseases and health conditions, and variations in drug metabolism found among ethnic groups (biocultural ecology).
3. *Cultural skill.* The ability to conduct a cultural assessment to collect relevant cultural data regarding the client's presenting problem as well as accurately conducting a culturally based physical assessment.
4. *Cultural encounter.* The process that encourages the health care professional to directly engage in face-to-face cultural interactions and other types of encounters with clients from culturally diverse backgrounds to modify existing beliefs about a cultural group and to prevent possible stereotyping.
5. *Cultural desire.* The motivation of the health care professional to "want to" rather than to "have to" engage in the process of becoming culturally aware, culturally knowledgeable, culturally skillful, and to seek cultural encounters.

The Purnell Model for Cultural Competence

The Purnell model for cultural competence started as an organizing framework in 1991 when Dr. Larry Purnell discovered the need for both students and staff to have a framework for learning about their cultures and the cultures of their patients and families. The purposes of the model are to provide a framework for health care providers to learn concepts and characteristics of culture and to define circumstances that affect a person's cultural worldview in the context of historic perspectives (Purnell, 2005).

The model (illustrated in **Figure 2.3**) is a circle in which an outlying rim represents global society, a second rim represents community, a third rim represents family, and an inner rim represents the person. **Table 2.3** lists the four rings with their related definitions. The interior of the circle is divided into 12 pie-shaped wedges that depict cultural domains and their concepts. The dark center of the circle represents unknown phenomena. Along the bottom of the model is a jagged line that represents the nonlinear concept of cultural consciousness. The 12 cultural domains (constructs) provide the organizing framework of the model. Health care providers can use this same process to understand their own cultural beliefs, attitudes, values, practices, and behaviors.

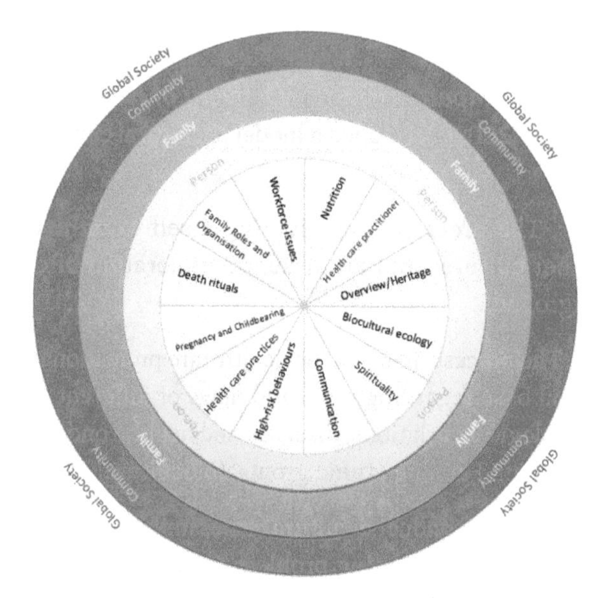

Figure 2.3 The Purnell model for cultural competence.

TABLE 2.3 The Rings of the Purnell Model for Cultural Competence

Ring	Definition
Global society	World communications and politics; conflicts and warfare; natural disasters and famines; international exchanges in business, commerce, and information technology; advances in the health sciences; space exploration; and the increased ability for people to travel around the world and to interact with diverse societies
Community	A group of people who have a common interest or identity and live in a specified locality
Family	Two or more people who are emotionally involved with each other and who may or may not be blood relatives
Person	A biopsychosociocultural human being who is constantly adapting

Source: Dr. Larry Purnell, University of Delaware

Sunrise Model

The sunrise model (**Figure 2.4**) was developed by Madeleine Leininger. The model represents a culture care theory structure. It describes the relationship between anthropological and nursing beliefs and principles (Leininger, 1991). Leininger believed that

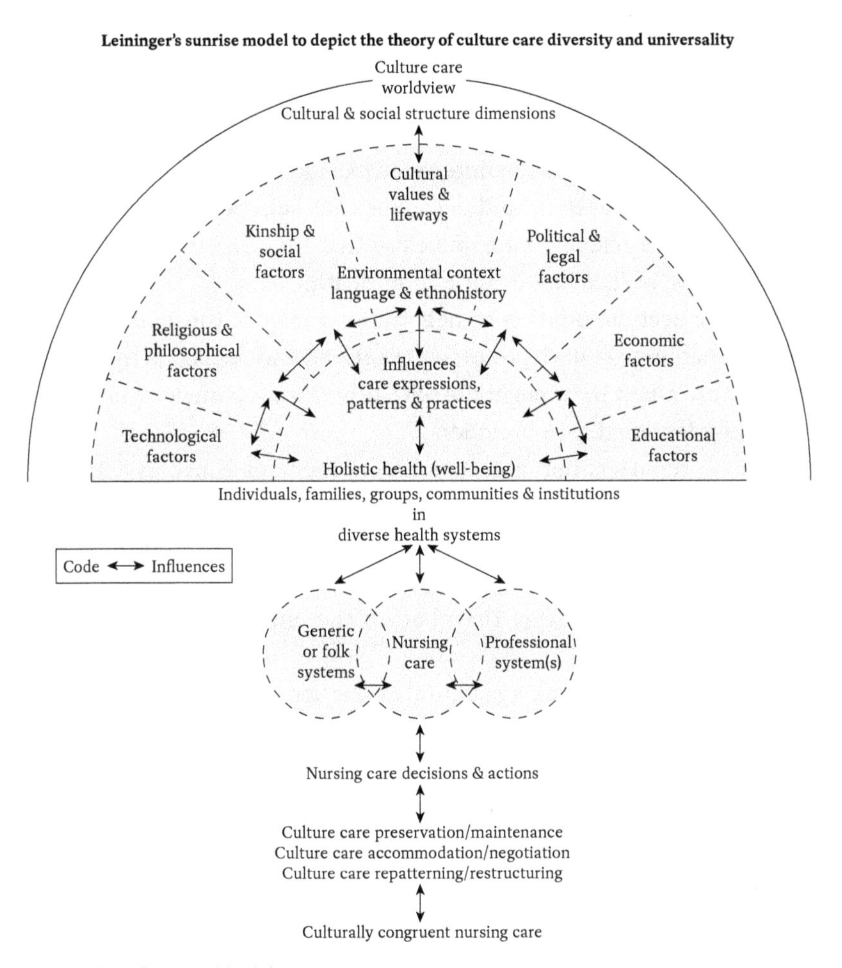

Figure 2.4 Sunrise Model

knowing and understanding different cultures was needed to provide meaningful and efficacious nursing care services. Therefore, the model focuses on the fact that different cultures have different caring behaviors and different health and illness values, beliefs, and patterns of behaviors.

The cultural care worldview flows into knowledge about individuals, families, groups, communities, and institutions in diverse health care systems. This knowledge provides culturally specific meanings and expressions in relation to care and health. The next focus is on the generic or folk system, nursing care, and professional systems. This information enables the recognition of similarities and differences or cultural care universality and cultural care diversity. Culture care universality refers to the common, similar, or dominant uniform care meanings, pattern, values, lifeways, or symbols that are manifest among many cultures and reflect assistive, supportive, facilitative, or enabling ways to assist people (Gonzalo, 2019). "Culture care diversity indicates the variabilities and/or differences in meanings, patterns, values, lifeways, or symbols of care within or between collectives that are related to assistive, supportive, or enabling human care expressions" (Gonzalo, 2019).

Included next in the model are nursing care decisions and actions that include cultural care preservation or maintenance, cultural care accommodation or negotiation, and cultural care repatterning or restructuring.

Cultural care preservation or maintenance includes assistive, supporting, facilitative, or enabling professional actions and decisions that help people of a particular culture retain and/or preserve relevant care values so that they can maintain their well-being, recover from illness, or face handicaps and/or death.

Cultural care accommodation or negotiation includes those assistive, supportive, facilitative, or enabling creative professional actions and decisions that help people of a designated culture adapt to or negotiate with others for a beneficial or satisfying health outcome with professional care providers.

Culture care repatterning or restructuring includes those assistive, supporting, facilitative, or enabling professional actions and decisions that help clients reorder, change, or greatly modify their lifeways for new, different, and beneficial health care patterns while respecting the client's cultural values and beliefs and still providing a beneficial or healthier lifeway than before the changes were coestablished with the clients.

The model is useful with making cultural evaluations of patients. It provides a systemic approach to identifying values, beliefs, behaviors, and community customs. It includes various dimensions of culture such as religion, economics, kinship/social, technological, educational, legal, political, and philosophical factors. Leininger's (2002) model also assists health care professionals with avoiding stereotyping patients.

Promoting Cultural Competence

Promoting cultural competence within organizations is increasingly becoming a higher priority in the health care industry. The rationale for this includes the existence of health disparities, existing differences in access to care and quality of care among minorities, concerns about providing quality of care and legal actions, and credentialing. Ways to promote and assess your own level of cultural competence and that of your organization are the focus of this section.

Implementing cultural competence programs is a nonlinear, multilevel, complex process. The paths to progression are varied. Areas for promoting cultural competence are related to policies, human resource development, and services. Two tools are used to assess cultural competence: one at an individual level and the other at an organizational level. These types of assessments are a good place to start, and they will help you identify areas in need of improvement.

Individual Assessment of Cultural Competence

As a member of the organization, the knowledge you have of yourself and others is important and is reflected in the ways you communicate and interact. The individual assessment instruments in **Box 2.1** and **Box 2.2** were developed to assist you in reflecting on and examining your journey toward cultural competence.

BOX 2.1 Multicultural Self-Awareness

To more effectively help others explore and understand the significance of their cultural identity on their life, take a moment to explore the various aspects of your own cultural identity.

What aspects of my cultural identity do I identify with or value most?

Why do I identify with or value these aspects of my identity?

What messages did I receive about my or my family's cultural identity growing up (directly or indirectly)?

How does this influence my view of the world and the people in it (positively or negatively)?

How does this influence my view of my clients?

Source: Fisher, 2018

BOX 2.2 Multicultural Countertransference Challenge

Take a moment to explore the ways in which your own past personal and professional experiences may influence your views, perspectives and interactions with individuals from various cultural backgrounds.

Are there any individuals from particular cultural backgrounds who make me feel angry, resentful, anxious, or uncomfortable (even before I interact with them)?

What past experiences have I had that may be contributing to these feelings?

What are the legitimate reasons for my feelings?

In what ways can I change my perspective in light of my increasing cultural empathy and understanding of people from various backgrounds?

Source: Fisher, 2018

Organizational Assessment of Cultural Competence

Box 2.3 offers a means of assessing an organization's cultural competence. Some suggestions for achieving a culturally competent organization include the following:

- Maximize diversity among the workforce.

(continued)

BOX 2.3 Multiculturally Competent Service System Assessment Guide (*Continued*)

Instructions: Rate your organization on each item in Sections I through VIII using the following scale:

1	**2**	**3**	**4**	**5**
Not at all		To a moderate degree		To a great degree

Suggested Rating Interpretations:
#1 and #2: "Priority Concerns"; #3: "Needs Improvement"; #4 and #5: "Adequate"

When you have rated all items and assessed each section, please follow the instructions in Section IX to make an assessment of your program or agency and then formulate a culturally competent plan that addresses the need you feel is a priority.

I. *Agency demographic data (assessment)*

A culturally competent agency uses basic demographic information to assess and determine the cultural and linguistic needs of the service area.

_____ Have you identified the demographic composition of the program's service area (from recent census data, local planning documents, statement of need, etc.) which should include ethnicity, race, and primary language spoken as reported by the individuals?

_____ Have you identified the demographic composition of the persons served?

_____ Have you identified the staff composition (ethnicity, race, language capabilities) in relation to the demographic composition of your service area?

_____ Have you compared the demographic composition of the staff with the client demographics?

II. *Policies, procedures and governance*

A culturally competent agency has a board of directors, advisory committee, or policy-making group that is proportionally representative of the staff, client/consumers, and community.

_____ Has your organization appointed executives, managers, and administrators who take responsibility for, and have authority over, the development, implementation, and monitoring of the cultural competence plan?

_____ Has your organization's director appointed a standing committee to advise management on matters pertaining to multicultural services?

_____ Does your organization have a mission statement that commits to cultural competence and reflects compliance with all federal and state statutes, as well as any current Connecticut Commission on Human Rights and Opportunities nondiscriminatory policies and affirmative action policies?

_____ Does your organization have culturally appropriate policies and procedures communicated orally and/or written in the principal language of the client/consumer to address confidentiality, individual patient rights and grievance procedures, medication fact sheets, legal assistance, etc. as needed and appropriately?

(continued)

BOX 2.3 Multiculturally Competent Service System Assessment Guide (*Continued*)

III. *Services/programs*

A culturally competent agency offers services that are culturally competent and in a language that ensures client/consumer comprehension.

A. *Linguistic and communication support*

_____ Has the program arranged to provide materials and services in the language(s) of limited English-speaking clients/consumer (e.g., bilingual staff, in-house interpreters, or a contract with outside interpreter agency and/or telephone interpreters)?

_____ Do medical records indicate the preferred languages of service recipients?

_____ Is there a protocol to handle client/consumer/family complaints in languages other than English?

_____ Are the forms that client/consumers sign written in their preferred language?

_____ Are the persons answering the telephones, during and after-hours, able to communicate in the languages of the speakers?

_____ Does the organization provide information about programs, policies, covered services, and procedures for accessing and utilizing services in the primary language(s) of client/consumers and families?

_____ Does the organization have signs regarding language assistance posted at key locations?

_____ Are there special protocols for addressing language issues at the emergency room, treatment rooms, intake, etc.?

_____ Are cultural and linguistic supports available for clients/consumers throughout different service offerings along the service continuum?

B. *Treatment/rehabilitation planning*

_____ Does the program consider the client/consumer's culture, ethnicity and language in treatment planning (assessment of needs, diagnosis, interventions, discharge planning, etc.)?

_____ Does the program involve client/consumers and family members in all phases of treatment, assessment, and discharge planning?

_____ Has the organization identified community resources (community councils, ethnic cultural social entities, spiritual leaders, faith communities, voluntary associations, etc.) that can exchange information and services with staff, client/consumers, and family members?

_____ Have you identified natural community healers, spiritual healers, clergy, etc., when appropriate, in the development and/or implementation of the service plan?

_____ Have you identified natural supports (relatives, traditional healers, spiritual resources, etc.) for purposes of reintegrating the individual into the community?

(*continued*)

BOX 2.3 Multiculturally Competent Service System Assessment Guide (*Continued*)

_____ Have you used community resources and natural supports to reintegrate the individual into the community?

C. ***Cultural assessments***

_____ Is the client/consumer's culture/ethnicity taken into account when formulating a diagnosis or assessment?

_____ Are culturally relevant assessment tools utilized to augment the assessment/ diagnosis process?

_____ Is the client/consumer's level of acculturation identified, described, and incorporated as part of cultural assessment?

_____ Is the client/consumer's ethnicity/culture identified, described, and incorporated as part of cultural assessment?

D. ***Cultural accommodations***

_____ Are culturally appropriate, educative approaches, such as films, slide presentations, or video tapes, utilized for preparation and orientation of client/consumer family members to your program?

_____ Does your program incorporate aspects of each client/consumer's ethnic/cultural heritage into the design of specialized interventions or services?

_____ Does your program have ethnic/culture-specific group formats available for engagement, treatment, and/or rehabilitation?

_____ Is there provider collaboration with natural community healers, spiritual healers, clergy, etc., where appropriate, in the development and/or implementation of the service plan?

E. ***Program accessibility***

_____ Do persons from different cultural and linguistic backgrounds have timely and convenient access to your services?

_____ Are services located close to the neighborhoods where persons from different cultures and linguistic backgrounds reside?

_____ Are your services readily accessible by public transportation?

_____ Do your programs provide needed supports to families of clients/consumers (e.g., meeting rooms for extended families, child support, drop-in services)?

_____ Do you have services available during evenings and weekends?

IV. ***Care management***

_____ Does the level and length of care meet the needs for clients/consumers from different cultural backgrounds?

_____ Is the type of care for clients/consumers from different backgrounds consistently and effectively managed according to their identified cultural needs?

(*continued*)

BOX 2.3 Multiculturally Competent Service System Assessment Guide (*Continued*)

_____ Is the management of the services for people from different groups compatible with their ethnic/cultural background?

V. *Continuity of care*

_____ Do you have letters of agreement with culturally oriented community services and organizations?

_____ Do you have integrated, planned, transitional arrangements between one service modality and another?

_____ Do you have arrangements, financial or otherwise, for securing concrete services needed by clients/consumers (e.g., housing, income, employment, medical, dental, other emergency personal support needs)?

VI. *Human resources development*

A culturally competent agency implements staff training and development in cultural competence at all levels and across all disciplines, for leadership and governing entities as well as for management, supervisory, treatment, and support staff.

_____ Are the principles of cultural competence (e.g., cultural awareness, language training, skills training in working with diverse populations) included in staff orientation and ongoing training programs?

_____ Is the program making use of other programs or organizations that specialize in serving persons with diverse cultural and linguistic backgrounds as a resource for staff education and training?

_____ Is the program maximizing recruitment and retention efforts for staff who reflect the cultural and linguistic diversity of populations needing services?

_____ Has the staff's training needs in cultural competence been assessed?

_____ Has the staff attended training programs on cultural competence in the past two years? Describe: ____

____

VII. *Quality monitoring and improvement*

A culturally competent agency has a quality monitoring and improvement program that ensures access to culturally competent care.

_____ Does the quality improvement (QI) plan address the cultural/ethnic and language needs?

_____ Are client/consumers and families asked whether ethnicity/culture and language are appropriately addressed in order to receive culturally competent services in the organization?

_____ Does the organization maintain copies of minutes, recommendations, and accomplishments of its multicultural advisory committee?

(*continued*)

BOX 2.3 Multiculturally Competent Service System Assessment Guide (*Continued*)

_____ Is there a process for continually monitoring, evaluating, and rewarding the cultural competence of staff?

VIII. Information/management system

_____ Does the organization monitor, survey, or otherwise access, the QI utilization patterns, Against Medical Advice (AMA) rates, etc., based on the culture/ethnicity and language?

_____ Are client/consumer satisfaction surveys available in different languages in proportion to the demographic data?

_____ Are there data collection systems developed and maintained to track clients/consumers by demographics, utilization and outcomes across levels of care, transfers, referrals, readmissions, etc.?

IX. Formulating a culturally competent plan based on the assessment of your program or agency

Focus on the following critical areas of concern as you develop goals for a culturally competent plan for your agency's service system.

Access: Degree to which services to persons are quickly and readily available.

Engagement: The skill and environment to promote a positive personal impact on the quality of the client's commitment to be in treatment.

Retention: The result of quality service that helps maintain a client in treatment with continued commitment.

Based on an assessment of your agency, determine whether, in your initial plan, you need to direct efforts of developing cultural competency toward one, or a combination, of the above critical areas. **Then, structure your agency's cultural competence plan using the following instructions:**

1. Based on the results of this assessment, summarize and describe your organization's perceived **strengths** in providing **services to persons from different cultural groups**. Please provide specific examples. Attach supporting documentation (e.g., Data, Policies, Procedures, etc.)
2. Based on your assessment, summarize and describe your organization's primary areas considered either **"Priority Concerns" (#1 and/or #2)**, or **"Needs Improvement" (#3)** in providing services to persons from different cultural groups.
3. Based on your organization's **strengths** and **needs**, **prioritize** both the organizational goals and objectives addressed in your **cultural competence plan**. Describe clearly what you will do to provide services to persons who are culturally and linguistically different.
4. Using the developed goals and objectives, please describe in detail the plans, activities, and/or strategies you will implement to assist your organization in meeting each of the goals and objectives indicated.

Source: "Multiculturally Competent Service System Assessment Guide," *Assessment Guidelines for Developing a Multiculturally Competent Service System for an Organization or Program*, pp. 3-7.

- Involve community representatives in the organization's planning and quality improvement meetings.
- Establish a cultural competence board to help guide the implementation of culturally sensitive prevention and treatment efforts.
- Provide ongoing training to staff members.
- Develop health materials for the target population written at the appropriate literacy level, in a variety of languages and with culturally appropriate images—this includes materials such as educational brochures, consent forms, signage, postprocedural directions, and advance directives.
- Make on-site interpretation services available when possible, and be sure that all appropriate staff members are educated about how to use telephone interpretation services.
- Assess customer satisfaction and clinical outcomes regularly.
- Consider the health disparities that exist in your community when planning outreach efforts.

When an individual, organization, or system has implemented change to progress toward cultural competence, the change process should be measured. This is important because it can indicate the progress that has been made and identify areas that are in need of improvement. The measurement process itself can be a catalyst for change.

Summary

We all have probably heard an abundance of stories about how illness can occur and how it can be cured. Some of these are ancient and are believed to be true, regardless of whether controversial evidence exists. These beliefs influence who we ask for medical advice and when. This is part of our worldview, which is our perception of how the world works. Health care professionals need to take these issues into consideration, and that is a step toward the progression of cultural competence.

Several concepts that one needs to consider when working with people from different cultures have been identified in this chapter. These concepts include different beliefs about how illness occurs, which affects how, where, and when people seek medical care. Health care professionals should assess the person's worldview and tailor their approach and communication to successfully prevent and treat illness. Because of these differences, health care professionals need to become culturally competent. The concept of cultural competence and what that means has been discussed, and two tools to assess the level of cultural competence among individuals and organizations are included to assist with assessing cultural competence at both the individual and organizational levels.

Review

1. Explain three overarching theories about the causes of illness.
2. Explain the two overarching systems of care in the United States and their differences.
3. Explain the components of the process of cultural competence in the delivery of health care services model.
4. Explain the components of the Purnell model for cultural competence.
5. List ways to improve cultural competence within an organization.

Activity

Write a research paper on three types of holistic healers (e.g., shamans, medicine men, acupuncturists). Include information about their training, approaches to healing, and evidence-based patient outcomes.

Case Study 1

Public health workers are offering free measles vaccinations to children. The worker is speaking with the parents of a child and explaining why the vaccination is important. The parents express concerns that the vaccine will interfere with God's plan, and they refuse to have the child vaccinated.

1. What are the parents' beliefs about how health is maintained?
2. How do the theories of health and illness discussed in this chapter apply to this case study?
3. Using one of the models described in this chapter, what approach, if any, should the public health workers take to help protect the child by assisting the parents with understanding the need for the vaccination?

Case Study 2

Juan has been diagnosed with COVID-19. He is 32 years of age and has no other health problems. Juan is married with four children, works with his father and two brothers, and has close relations with extended family members. Juan has a slight fever and mild cough. The hospital physician stated that he can go home but that he needs to be in quarantine for 2 weeks to not spread the disease. He was also prescribed two medications. Juan refuses to stop working and be in quarantine. He states that he needs to work and be with his family. Juan is of Mexican decent, where providing for the family and close family ties are of high importance. He also does not want to take the medication. Juan shared that he has been under a lot of stress and when his body returns to be in balance the fever and cough will go away.

1. How can Juan's priorities be leveraged to support the doctor's recommendations?
2. How do the theories of health and illness discussed in this chapter apply to this case study?
3. Using the one of the models described in this chapter, what approach, if any, should the physician take to help Juan recover from COVID-19 and protect his family by limiting his contact with them?

References

American College of Osteopathic Medicine. (2020). *The history of osteopathic medicine.* http://www.aacom.org/about/osteomed/Pages/History.aspx

Bhalerao, S., Deshpande, T., & Thatte, U. (2012). Prakriti (Ayurvedic concept of constitution) and variations in platelet aggregation. *BMC Complementary & Alternative Medicine,* 12–248.

Brown, L. J. (1989). *Self-actuated healing (more crystals and new age).* Naturegraph.

Campinha-Bacote, J. (2009). *The process of cultural competence in the delivery of healthcare services.*

Carteret, M. (2011, February 21). *Culturally-based beliefs about illness causation.* http://www.dimensionsofculture.com/2011/02/culturally-based-beliefs-about-illness-causation/

Centers for Disease Control and Prevention. (2020, October 21). *Cultural competence in health and human services.* https://npin.cdc.gov/pages/cultural-competence

EuroMed Info. (2020). *How culture influences health beliefs.* https://www.euromedinfo.eu/how-culture-influences-health-beliefs.html/

Fisher, Lambers. (2018). *Multicultural awareness and diversity: Essential cultural self-assessment worksheet collection.* https://www.lambersfisher.com/uploads/1/2/2/6/122652082/pesi-multicultural-worksheets.pdf

Gonzalo, A. (2019, September 11). *Madeleine Leininger: Transcultural nursing theory.* Nurseslabs. https://nurseslabs.com/madeleine-leininger-transcultural-nursing-theory/

Leininger, M. (2002). Culture care theory: A major contribution to advance transcultural nursing knowledge and practices. *Journal of Transcultural Nursing, 13,* 189-192.

Leininger, M. M. (Ed.). (1991). *Culture care diversity and universality: A theory of nursing.* National League for Nursing Press.

O'Neil, D. (2005). *Explanations of illness.*

Purnell, L. (2005). The Purnell model for cultural competence. *Journal of Multicultural Nursing & Health, 11*(2), 7–15.

Substance Abuse and Mental Health Services Administration (SAMHSA). (2014). Improving cultural competence. Center for Substance Abuse Treatment. https://www.ncbi.nlm.nih.gov/books/NBK248429/

Williams, D. R., Lavizzo-Mourey, R., & Warrren, R. C. (1994). The concept of race and health status in America. *Public Health Reports, 109*(1), 26–41.

CREDITS

CHAPTER 3

Worldview and Health

After all, when you come right down to it, how many people speak the same language even when they speak the same language?

—RUSSELL HOBAN

Nothing is so conducive to good health as the regularity of life without haste and without worry which the rational practice of religion brings in its train.

—JAMES J. WALSH

To prevent disease or to cure it, the power of truth, of divine Spirit, must break down the dream of the material senses.

—MARY BAKER EDDY

KEY CONCEPTS AND TERMS

Advance directive
Ahimsa
Animal sacrifice
Biomedical worldview
Collectivism
Durable power of attorney
Euthanasia
Fate versus free will
Individualism
Karma
Living will
Mind–body integration
Proxemics
Religion
Rituals
Shrines
Spirituality
Temporal relationships
Worldview

LEARNING OBJECTIVES

After reading this chapter, you should be able to do the following:

1. Explain what worldview means and how it is related to culture.
2. Describe how worldview is related to health behaviors and decisions, how health is perceived, and how problems are expressed.
3. Explain the difference between spirituality and religion.
4. Describe ways religion can have positive and negative effects on physical and mental health.
5. Describe religious differences in birthing and death rituals.

A person's worldview is closely linked to his or her cultural and religious background, and it has profound implications for health care. Worldview influences lifestyle, and it is imperative that health care professionals understand its impact on health care decisions, involve patients in decisions and actions, and accommodate patients' beliefs to provide congruent care.

This chapter begins with a discussion of worldview and how it is related to health care. Then we move into more specific ways that worldview affects medical decisions and how people perceive and respond to illness. The chapter ends with a discussion on religion, spirituality, rituals, and health.

Worldview

A **worldview** is a set of cultural assumptions and beliefs that express how people see, interpret, and explain their experience (Tilbert, 2010). It helps us make sense of our lives. Worldview includes our relationships with nature, our social relationships, our ethical reasoning, and cosmology (study of the universe and humanity's place) (Purnell, 2013). It even affects our view of aesthetics. For example, most of us know that sun exposure contributes to skin cancer, but some cultures view tans as looking healthy whereas others see very white skin as beautiful, which is why skin lightening is done.

Culture fits within the larger structure of worldviews. Worldviews are the beliefs and assumptions by which an individual can make sense of experiences, and these are what culture is built on. Cultural groups have varied views of the world, and when they clash, people may find the behavior of others offensive or confusing. Because worldviews contain and shape cultures, working effectively across cultures requires some understanding of the soil from which cultures grow—the seedbed called worldviews.

A person's worldview is closely linked with their cultural and religious background and has profound health care implications. For example, people with chronic diseases who believe in fatalism (predetermined fate) may not adhere to treatment, because they believe that medical intervention cannot affect their outcomes. Worldview is an equally important concept for educating health professionals about their own beliefs and assumptions that may influence the care they deliver. The medical profession consists of its own beliefs and assumptions just as do the cultures of the patients. Some of the major components of worldview that affect health care professionals are discussed in the following sections.

Temporal Relationships

Temporal relationships refer to people's worldview in terms of time. These perceptions of time vary among cultures. In the West, time tends to be seen as quantitative elements of past, present, and future and is measured in units that reflect the march of progress. It is logical and sequential. In the East, time feels like it has unlimited continuity, and it does not have a defined boundary. Birth and death are not such absolute ends, because the universe continues, and humans, though changing form, continue as part of it.

Some cultures are present oriented, and others focus on the past or future. Time perspective affects our health behaviors and expectations of health care behavior. Present-focused people may not willing to make sacrifices now for the future health benefits and engage in behaviors to satisfy their immediate desire regardless of the long-term consequences. Present-oriented cultures, including Native Americans and African Americans, may see living in the moment as the priority and are less willing to forgo immediate pleasures for future benefits. Future-oriented individuals may be willing to make sacrifices now knowing that their current health behaviors impact their future health status. Cultures that are past oriented tend to value elders and honor traditions. For example, the Asian culture is generally past oriented, and they value and perform traditional healing practices, such as acupuncture and herbal remedies.

Another component of time related to health care is expectations related to punctuality. Some cultures are very punctual, and people in these groups (e.g., people with a Polish culture) will arrive for appointments on time. Others are less rigid and will arrive around the time of the appointment. Some clinics who serve cultures who have less rigidity around time have stopped making appointments and changed to seeing patients on a first-come, first-served basis.

Space (Proxemics)

Another variable across cultures is perception of space, or **proxemics**, which includes interpersonal distance and boundaries. Violating these boundaries can lead to conflict, stress, anxiety, miscommunication, or discomfort. If someone is accustomed to standing or sitting very close when they are talking with another, that person may see the other's attempt to create more space as evidence of coldness, condescension, or a lack of interest. Those who are accustomed to more personal space may view attempts to get closer as pushy, disrespectful, or aggressive. Research indicates that cultures that live in crowded areas, such as in a heavily populated city, are more tolerant of closeness and proximity to others when compared to members of other cultures who are not tolerant to closeness and instead prefer to be in and live in less crowded and congested areas. This distance and space tolerance may influence and impact on a person's tolerance of crowded areas and being in close proximity (Burke, 2020).

Social Organization and Family Relationships

Social organization refers to patterns of social interactions. Examples include how people interact and communicate, the kinship system, marriage residency patterns, division of labor, who has access to specific goods and knowledge, social hierarchy, religion, and economic systems. Examples of social organization that have an impact in health care include individualism versus collectivism, fate versus free will, communication, and family relationships.

Individualism Versus Collectivism

Individualism and collectivism are contrasting perspectives and values (see **Table 3.1**). In individualism each person is seen as a social unit, and each person has primary responsibility for him- or herself. In the United States the overarching culture values of individualism, autonomy, and independence are rewarded and respected. Other individualistic cultures include Germany, Canada, and Sweden (Purnell, 2013). If someone is successful, it is primarily because of their personal qualities.

TABLE 3.1 Individualism Versus Collectivism

Individualism	Collectivism
Focus on self rather than group	Focus on group rather than self
Guilt	Shame
Self-respect	Saving face
Behavior primarily regulated by likes and dislikes	Behavior primarily regulated by group norms
Conflict more acceptable	Conflict avoidance; emphasis on harmony and hierarchy
Person is basic unit of analysis and reality	Group is basic unit of analysis and reality
Focus on being unique	Focus on fitting in
Direct	Indirect
Achievement is a product of personal qualities	Achievement is a product of society
Priority given to promotion of own goals	Priority given to promotion of goals of others

In collectivism, people are socialized to view themselves as part of a larger group, such as a family, a community, or a tribe. The group is the social unit, and dependence and connections within the group are valued. An individual's identity is determined by his or her relationship and position within the group. People make decisions based on what is good for the group rather than on what is good for themselves. Saving face is valued, as is showing respect for others. The needs and goals of the individual are subordinate to those of the larger group and should be sacrificed when the collective good so requires. Collectivists believe that achievement is a product of society. Examples of collectivist cultures include the Amish, Chinese, Mexicans, and Vietnamese (Purnell, 2013).

Why are these two opposing views important in health care? People from individualistic cultures make their health care decisions independently, whereas individuals in collectivist cultures involve their families in the decision-making process.

In collectivist cultures, illness is considered a family event rather than an individual occurrence. Knowledge transmission, personal responsibility, shame and guilt, help-seeking behaviors, competitiveness, and communication are affected by this aspect of worldview (Purnell, 2013). In individualistic cultures, direct questioning, sharing personal issues, and asking personal questions are typical. In a collectivist culture, disagreeing or saying no to a health care professional is considered rude; therefore, when a health care professional asks if the patient understands, the patient may answer yes even though understanding has not really occurred. In addition, disabilities, mental health issues, and other health problems that are stigmatized may be kept hidden to save face, and treatment may be delayed and care provided in the home (Purnell, 2013).

In the United States, legal documents, such as advance directives and durable powers of attorney, are strategies to prolong autonomy in situations in which patients can no longer represent themselves. Other cultures de-emphasize autonomy, perceiving it as isolating rather than empowering. Their belief is that communities and families, not individuals alone, are affected by life-threatening illnesses and that they should be involved in making medical decisions.

Fate Versus Free Will

"Fate and free will" refer to the degree to which people believe they are the masters of their own lives (**free will**) or believe they are subject to events outside their control (**fate**). Basically, fate and free will refer to the beliefs people hold about their ability to change and maneuver the course of their lives and relationships. This concept also is called *locus of control*. People who believe that they have control over their health have an internal locus of control (free will belief), and people who believe that it is outside of their control (fate belief) have an external locus of control. In some ethnic groups, factors outside medical intervention, such as a divine plan and personal coping skills, may be more important for health and survival than medical intervention and health behaviors.

Health care professionals need to consider this aspect of social organization. For example, when health outreach workers in India attempted to provide children with free polio vaccinations, they found that many parents refused the immunization because they believed Allah would take care of their children's health. Providing preventive care and treatment can be challenging when people believe that fate will determine their health and that their health behaviors will not change what the master plan is for them.

Communication

Communication is an interactive process that involves sending and receiving information, emotions, thoughts, and ideas through verbal and nonverbal means. It is the basis of human interaction. Effective communication enables health care professionals to accurately exchange information, establish relationships, and understand the person's needs and concerns. Effective communication is important in all facets of life, but in health care it can be the deciding factor between life and death.

Intercultural communication is sensitive to exchanging information across cultural boundaries in a way that preserves mutual respect and minimizes miscommunication and conflict. If communication is hindered, patients who utilize traditional remedies may be reluctant to inform their biomedical providers about them, leading to potentially dangerous interactions between medications and the undisclosed traditional remedies.

In addition to better health outcomes, effective communication can lead to higher patient satisfaction, continued care, and better adherence to treatment recommendations while reducing conflict and errors, lost opportunities for encouraging health behavior changes, misinterpretations of treatment plans, damaged relationships (including a loss of trust) between provider and patient or community member, and legal actions. All these reasons illustrate why culturally competent communication is a vital component of health care.

Verbal Communication

As indicated in the quotation of Hoban at the beginning of this chapter, even people who speak the same language do not necessarily communicate even when using the same words. For example, in some age groups the word *fox* means attractive, but someone from a different generation may think of the animal. People in the United States whose first language is English have a difficult time communicating, so imagine how difficult it must be to communicate with people when English is not their first language. The limitations of language to convey experience—even between people who speak the same language—are extremely obvious when we cannot explain something as important as the intensity of pain we feel or the unrelenting worry and frustration pain sometimes causes. To further complicate communications, not all cultures describe health problems in the same way, and words from their language may not be easily translated to English and vice versa. For example, words used to describe pain typically include *sharp, throbbing, stabbing, or aching.* But in many tribal cultures, stories or symbols are essential in relating one's worldview, so very different words are used to describe pain. Clinicians might be baffled by patients explaining their pain using natural symbols like lightning, trees with deep spreading roots, spider webs, or the tones of drums and flutes (Carteret, 2010a).

In addition to the risks of everyday language breeding possibilities for miscommunication, health care has a language of its own with specialized terminology that can increase the chances of communication mishaps. Health care providers should avoid jargon and select words that people will understand without making them feel like you are talking down to them. Ask the receiver to summarize what you said to check for understanding, and look for nonverbal cues that indicate when miscommunication has occurred. A few cultural communication differences are described in the following paragraphs.

In some cultures, asking questions of health care providers is not an acceptable behavior. Patients from these cultures may be less likely to ask even clarifying questions and, subsequently, may not understand their condition or be able to follow their treatment plan, potentially resulting in a lower quality of care or even medical error.

In some cultures patients do not want doctors to inform them about their health problem. This nondisclosure may be because of the belief that the discussion about illness may eliminate or reduce the patient's hope or induce depression or anxiety. An example is that family members in the Asian culture may wish to avoid discussing (sometimes withholding) information from a patient with a terminal illness or impending death. The discussion of death in the Chinese culture is usually considered forbidden and offensive. The Chinese do not discuss death with health care providers. They feel discussing death can lead to hopelessness; instead, the silence regarding the patient's condition is designed to maintain hope and alleviate undue stress on the patient. African, Asian, Chinese, East Indian, Hispanic, Indonesian, Japanese, Native American, and Vietnamese families may request providers not to disclose a terminal diagnosis as they want to avoid emotional suffering and preserve hope (Givler et al., 2020). Reluctance to discuss the patient's condition, especially making life-sustaining treatment decisions, often leads to a lack of preparation for advance directives (Saccomano & Abbatiello, 2014). Discussing the illness may raise concerns about making the person worse or that it is disrespectful. This issue also is a concern with regard to consent forms. The patient may believe that discussing the possible death or side effects of a medical procedure or medication may make it self-fulfilling and actually happen. Not discussing possible or eminent death may be viewed as doctors protecting patients from the emotional and physical harm caused by directly addressing death and end-of-life care. For example, cultures that value beneficence (physicians' obligation to promote patient welfare) by encouraging the patient's hope, even in the face of terminal illness. Emotional reaction to news of serious illness may be considered directly harmful to health. It is thought that a patient who is already in pain should not have to struggle with depression or stress as well.

Nonverbal Communication

Communication is more than just words, and much information is conveyed nonverbally. Our system of nonverbal communication includes gestures, touch, posture, body language, objects, silence, spatial relations, emotional expression, eye contact, and physical appearance. Our sense of what nonverbal behavior is appropriate is derived from our culture. Differences in nonverbal communication may lead to misunderstandings, misinterpretations about the person's character, damaged relationships, conflict, or escalate an existing conflict.

Nonverbal communication can be received in three general ways: (a) the nonverbal message may exist in both cultures but not have the same meaning, (b) the nonverbal message exists in the sender's culture but not in the receiver's culture, or (c) the nonverbal message exists in both cultures and has the same meaning. Here are some examples of nonverbal communications that have different meanings in various parts of the world:

- In Asian cultures smiling is used to show pleasure, and it also is used to cover emotional pain or embarrassment. When a patient is asked if he, she, or they understands the treatment plan, if the person does not understand he, she, or they may smile to cover embarrassment.
- The "ring" or "okay" gesture has different meanings in different countries. In the United States and other English-speaking countries, the ring or okay gesture means

"everything is okay." In Japan it can mean money; in some Mediterranean countries it is used to infer that a man is gay; in Indonesia it means zero.

- In the United States, getting someone to come toward you by motioning with your index finger is common or acceptable; however, in the Philippines, Korea, and parts of Latin America, as well as other countries, the same gesture is considered rude.
- In some cultures, direct eye contact is an indication of honesty, listening, and respect. People from some other cultures consider direct eye contact rude and feel as though they are being disrespected or challenged; therefore, they may avoid direct eye contact.
- Touch has variations of meanings among cultures as well. For some, casual touching is seen as a sexual overture and should be avoided. People of the same sex (especially men) or opposite sex do not generally touch one another. In other cultures, especially among collectivist ones, same genders can touch without having a sexual connotation. Health care providers should ask permission before touching someone (Purnell, 2013).

WHAT DO YOU THINK?

Reflect on your own worldview and how it differs from others. What are the philosophical reasons for how your worldview differs from others? How do these beliefs affect relationships and possibly lead to conflict? Consider the following questions:

- How comfortable are you with being touched?
- What is your perspective of time?
- What does it mean to you when people are late?
- How do you make health care decisions?
- How do you view illness?

Worldview and Health Decisions

Medical decisions such as abortion, the use of birth control, permission to allow blood transfusion, utilization of chemotherapy, advance directives, and euthanasia are difficult and life altering. In this section the focus is on two areas of medical decisions: beginning-of-life and end-of-life decisions.

Beginning-of-Life Decisions

The beginning-of-life decisions include choices related to pregnancy, abortion, birth control use, fertility practices, birthing, and the postpartum period. Some of these decisions have deep ties to religious beliefs.

Birth Control

Decisions surrounding the use of birth control center around the view about the purpose of sexual intercourse. Is it for procreation or other reasons? The use of birth control is prohibited by some religions for reasons such as that men are not permitted to waste "their seed" or that it is a violation of the design built into the human race by God. Other religions permit the use of hormonal birth control methods such as pills, patches, injections, and implants, but they do not allow the use of birth control methods that block or destroy sperm, such as condoms and vasectomies. Condom use may be permitted to protect one from sexually transmitted infections, and birth control may be allowed when a woman needs a rest between pregnancies, when pregnancy poses a risk to the mother or baby, or when the man cannot financially support another child.

Abortion

A central issue surrounding abortion is related to the core question about when life begins. Does it begin when the egg is fertilized, when the soul enters the fetus, when consciousness occurs, when the embryo becomes embedded in the uterine wall, when the fetus moves, or when the birth occurs? The answer to this question depends on who you ask, and the answer one gives will shape his or her views on the morality of abortion. Some religions prohibit abortion, because it is viewed as murder, because it brings bad karma, or because it is an act of violence regardless of when or why the abortion takes place.

Many religions approve of abortion under certain circumstances, such as when

- the health of the mother is at risk if the pregnancy is continued,
- the child may be born with a disability that will cause suffering, or
- in cases of rape or incest.

End-of-Life Decisions

In "The Parable of the Mustard Seed," the Buddha teaches a lesson that is valid for all cultures: Human beings receive no exemption from mortality. Deep in the throes of grief after the death of her son, a woman seeks wisdom from the Buddha, who says that he does indeed have an answer to her queries. Before giving it, however, he insists that she must first collect a mustard seed from every house that has not been touched by death. She canvasses her entire community but fails to collect a single seed. Returning to the Buddha, she understands that, like all other living beings, we are destined to die.

Death is inevitable, but how people respond to death has cultural ties. In some cultures it is appropriate to cry, sob, and wail loudly, whereas mourning in other cultures requires controlling grief and being stoic in public. Variations in burial practices also are culturally determined.

Although death is inevitable, modern life-extending technologies have changed the process. Organ transplantation, respirators, surgical procedures, and feeding tubes enable life to be prolonged. Other technologies, such as lethal injections, may hasten death. Using these technologies is a complex choice. In some situations, prolonging life in these ways may be contradictory to another fundamental human value—going against God's will. Human beings struggle with not overstepping these boundaries or playing God with life and death. Individual wishes may be subsumed by the will of other family members or the dictates of their religion.

Decisions surrounding continuing treatment, discontinuing treatment, or hastening death are difficult and agonizing. As individuals and their families face these controversial questions, and as many states consider revising their laws about end-of-life choices, religious traditions and values can offer guidance and insight, if not solutions, for some.

In the remainder of this section the more controversial and general decisions are addressed, but there are many other end-of-life decisions to consider, such as burial versus cremation, timing of the burial, length of the mourning process, appropriate dress and behavior before and during the service and after the burial, and permission to conduct an autopsy.

Organ Transplants

Organ transplantation is the removal of tissues of the human body from a person who has recently died or from a living donor for the purpose of transplanting or grafting them into other persons. Cultural and religious views regarding organ transplantation are changing. Some religions that previously prohibited organ donation are now altering their views and seeing it as an act of compassion, but others continue to prohibit organ donation. Religions that prohibit organ transplants do so because of their beliefs regarding life after death and resurrection. Some religions will consent to an organ donation if they are certain that it is for the health and welfare of the transplant recipient, but if the outcome is questionable, then the donation is not encouraged.

Euthanasia

Euthanasia is a Greek term that means "good death." Also called mercy killing, it is the act or practice of ending the life of an individual who is suffering from a terminal illness or an incurable condition by lethal injection or the suspension of extraordinary medical treatment. The person who is suffering from the painful and incurable disease or incapacitating physical disorder is painlessly put to death. Because there is no specific provision for it in most legal systems, it is usually regarded as a crime: suicide (if performed by the patient) or murder (if performed by another person, which includes physician-assisted suicide).

Murder and suicide are against the belief systems of most religions, so in those systems it would be considered morally wrong. In some religions, such as Hinduism, suicide is acceptable if it is done by fasting because it is nonviolent. Other reasons for religious opposition are the concern for patients who may be in vulnerable positions because of their illness or their lack of social and economic resources. There is fear that patients who cannot afford expensive treatment, for example, will be pressured to accept euthanasia. There also is great concern about the moral nature of the doctor's professional self. For Christian scientists, Hinduism, Jehovah's Witnesses, Mormons, Muslim, and Seventh-day Adventists, it is considered contrary to the church's teachings to perform euthanasia and use drugs that may hasten death (Givler et al., 2020).

Karma and rebirth are other considerations for not supporting euthanasia. The philosophical concept of karma is the total effect of a person's actions and conduct during the successive phases of the person's existence, which is regarded as determining the person's destiny. Karma extends beyond one's present life to all past and future lives as well. In Hinduism and Buddhism, human beings are believed to be captured in endless cycles of rebirth and reincarnation. In both traditions, all living creatures (humans, animals, and plants) represent manifestations of the laws of karmic rebirth. To honor these laws, one must show great respect for the preservation of life and the noninjury of conscious beings. Acts that are destructive of life are morally condemned by the principle of **ahimsa**, which is the conceptual equivalent of the Western principle of the sanctity of life. Religions may permit physicians to hasten death in the very few jurisdictions that allow it through legal injection but not by withholding care.

On the other side of the issue, most religions also consider acts of compassion and concern about the dignity of the dying person to be part of humanity. Concern for the welfare of others as one is dying is seen as a sign of spiritual enlightenment. A person can decide to forgo treatment to avoid imposing a heavy burden of caregiving on family or friends. He or she may also stop treatment to relieve loved ones of the emotional or economic distress of prolonged dying.

These two different perspectives lead to the dilemma of whether euthanasia is an act of compassion or murder. Different cultures and religions answer the question differently, and debate exists within religions. This personal and difficult decision obviously needs to be made on an individual basis, but health care professionals should be aware of the conflicting perspectives and the rationale behind them.

Advance Directives and End-of-Life Care

Advance directives are legal documents that enable people to convey their decisions about end-of-life care ahead of time. Advance directives include the living will and durable power of attorney, and they provide a way for patients to communicate their wishes to their family, friends, and health care professionals and to avoid confusion later in the event that the person becomes unable to communicate.

A **living will** is a set of instructions that documents a person's wishes about medical care intended to sustain life. People can accept or refuse medical care, and many types of life-sustaining care should be taken into consideration when drafting a living will:

- The use of life-sustaining equipment, such as dialysis and breathing machines
- Resuscitation if breathing or heartbeat stops

- Artificial hydration and nutrition (tube feeding)
- Withholding food and fluids
- Organ or tissue donation
- Comfort care

A **durable power of attorney** for health care is a document that names your health care representative who can speak for you when you cannot. This is someone you trust to make health care decisions if you are unable to do so.

Studies have documented ethnic differences in advance directive completion, with lower rates in minority groups (Portanova et al., 2017). Using data from 2000 to 2012, researchers noted that 46% of decedents had completed an advance directive (Whites 51.7%, Hispanics 18.0%, Blacks 15.0%). Blacks had 75% lower odds of completing an advance directive, and Hispanics had 70% lower odds than Whites (Portanova et al., 2017).

This difference is likely attributable to several factors, including cultural differences in family-centered decision-making, distrust of the health care system, religion, and poor communication between health care professionals and patients. Collectivist groups, such as Hispanics, may be reluctant to formally appoint a specific family member to be in charge because of concerns about isolating this person or offending other relatives. Instead, a consensual decision-making approach seems to be more acceptable in this population. Among Asian Americans, aggressive treatment for elderly family members is likely to be frowned upon because family members should have love and respect for their parents and ancestors and because of their high respect for the elderly. Numerous studies have shown that Blacks are more likely than Whites to pursue aggressive care at the end of life (Portanova et al., 2017).

Studies investigating racial and ethnic differences in advance directive completion have found that age, income, medical diagnoses, and religion influence completion rates (Portanova et al., 2017). Examples include that older adults are more likely to complete advance directives than younger adults and lower income has been associated with lower rates of advance directive completion. Religious beliefs may also influence advance directive completion rates and end-of-life care preferences. Some religious individuals, for example, prefer aggressive care regardless of their prognosis because of their belief in God's will (Portanova et al., 2017).

Religion also has an impact on do-not-resuscitate orders. In the Jewish religion, life is extremely valuable, and no one has the right to shorten it. The only exception is when physiologic resuscitation is not possible or the patient is imminently dying or at the point of death. Most Christians believe that the patient has the right to reject trying to be revived. Muslims must take the necessary measures to prevent premature death. However, treatments that prolong life for patients who, physicians are certain, do not have a great chance of survival, can be discontinued or not initiated (Cheraghi et al., 2016).

DID YOU KNOW?

The ability to take medical histories and diagnose current symptoms may be adversely affected by the patient's comfort with modesty. Cultural values surrounding modesty are more than one's comfort level with covering the intimate body parts. By definition, modesty is about respect. A provider who takes cultural modesty into consideration shows respect and caring in the highest degree. Modesty in many cultures often means showing good manners via verbal communication, dress, or behavior.

> In societies that place a high value on modesty, it is important for both sexes, but particularly emphasized for women. A woman's sexual purity and chastity honors her entire family. American women may view this as more discriminatory than protective. It is important not to assume that women in high-modesty cultures are forced to accept the restrictions placed on them by men. In fact, for many women in these cultures modesty is an attribute to be admired and attained. Women often impose modesty on themselves and other women as a way of keeping boundaries of privacy and respect. (Carteret, 2010b)

Worldview and Response to Illness

Worldview has an impact on how people perceive and respond to illness. The dominant values and standards regarding pain and illness affect the behaviors of the individual. When people with a **biomedical worldview** of the mind and body being separate was shared by providers and most patients, this shared belief often contributed to substantial patient stress and alienation. In contrast, in a study conducted in Puerto Rico, providers and patients often shared a view of **mind–body integration** in illness and valued treatments that addressed chronic pain as a biopsychosocial experience. Culture also impacts on the ways which some cultures cope with stress. Some cultures cope with stress by openly expressing their feelings; other cultures avoid thinking about and expressing their feelings when confronted with stress. These cultures suppress their feelings. For example, members of the Asian culture tend to suppress their feelings and discussions about their true feelings rather than expressing their feelings; and, on the other hand, African Americans actively confront their stress and, more often than other cultural groups, tend to resolve their stress and distress on their own, often drawing on spiritual influences to assist them during stressful times (Burke, 2020).

The level of stigma plays a role in how people respond to illness as well. Mental health issues, tuberculosis, HIV, and other illnesses create a sense of embarrassment and shame in some cultures. As a result, people may not seek care or delay seeking care. If the person is diagnosed with a stigmatized illness, it can affect how the family responds. For example, the person may be "hidden" from the public, the family may be embarrassed by the ill family member and distance themselves from the patient, or the patient may be shunned.

In some cultures chronic illness and disability are viewed as forms of punishment, and the patient is viewed as being evil.

How people express and communicate about the illness has cultural roots. Most people experience pain sensations similarly, yet studies show there are important differences in the way people express their pain and expect others to respond to their discomfort. Stoic and emotive are two categories in which patients' culturally based responses to pain are often divided. Stoic patients are less expressive of their pain, tend to "grin and bear it," and socially withdraw. Native American, Asian, Black, and Hispanic are very stoic regarding pain and may maintain a neutral facial expression despite being in severe pain (Givler et al., 2020). Emotive patients are more likely to verbalize their expressions of pain, prefer to have people around, and expect others to react to their pain to validate their discomfort. There are also culturally based attitudes about using pain medication. Some patients might not take pain medications due to being fearful of harmful effects, including addiction (Givler et al., 2020). A summary of pain and end-of life issues as they related to culture is in **Box 3.1**.

BOX 3.1 A Summary of Pain and End-of-Life Issues

African American Culture

Death: Tend to display grief openly. Family and relatives usually present.

Pain: May avoid the use of pain medicine due to fear of addiction. Pain scales are often helpful.

Palliative care: Generally accepting of end-of-life care if educated on appropriate forms of pain management.

Amish Culture

Death: Death carries a lot of spiritual meaning.

Pain: Very high pain tolerance.

Palliative care: May accept palliative care.

Arab Culture

Death: May avoid discussions of impending death.

Pain: Very expressive.

Palliative Care: Usually not willing to accept do-not-resuscitate (DNR) orders.

Cuban Culture

Death: Everything possible should be done.

Pain: May be stoic regarding pain, and thus reluctant to accept pain medication.

Palliative care: May be reluctant to accept palliative care.

East Asian Culture

Death: Reluctant to talk about death.

(continued)

BOX 3.1 A Summary of Pain and End-of-Life Issues (*Continued*)

Pain: May be stoic; look for nonverbal signs.

Palliative care: May believe dying at home may bring bad luck. Will accept palliative care.

East Indian Culture

Death: Death should be discussed with family first, who may not inform the patients.

Pain: Will accept pain medicine for severe pain.

Palliative care: May accept palliative care.

Filipino Culture

Death: A loud grieving process is typical. May avoid discussing.

Pain: Often expressed as "cold" or "hot."

Palliative care: Will accept palliative care and pain control.

Egyptian Culture

Death: Avoid discussions of death.

Pain: Will accept pain medications but require being alert near death.

Palliative care: May accept care but no euthanasia.

Iranian Culture

Death: Avoid discussions with the patient.

Pain: Tend to express pain loudly.

Palliative care: May accept pain medications.

Jamaican Culture

Death: May be very emotional with crying and mourning.

Pain: Highly variable.

Palliative: Will seek health care but may believe in a possible cure despite terminal illness. Generally, accept end-of-life care.

Japanese Culture

Death: May avoid discussion.

Pain: May be very stoic.

Palliative: May take assistance, often at home.

Ghanaian Culture

Death: Telling a patient they are going to die is unacceptable. It is more culturally acceptable to say, "It is time to put your home in order."

Pain: Often described as emotional or spiritual.

(*continued*)

BOX 3.1 A Summary of Pain and End-of-Life Issues (*Continued*)

Palliative care: Usually, they prefer to die at home with little or no medical assistance.

Gypsy Roma Culture

Death: May involve wailing and calling out to God.

Pain: Accepting of pain medicine.

Palliative care: May not be accepting of institutional care.

Haitian Culture

Death: May be very vocal regarding pain

Pain: Acceptable of pain medicine.

Palliative care: Usually, they die at home.

Hispanic Culture

Death: A large number of family members may be present. The family may not want to inform the patient of the end stage of a terminal illness.

Pain: May not complain of pain and may only provide nonverbal clues.

Palliative care: May have reservations regarding accepting end-of-life care.

Indonesian Culture

Death: Grief may be filled with emotion.

Pain: May request no pain medicine near death.

Palliative care: Commonly wish to die at home.

Kenyan Culture

Death: Generally, desire life to be preserved at all costs.

Pain: Usually, they avoid pain medicine.

Palliative care: Commonly wish to die at home.

Korean Culture

Death: Mourning and crying.

Pain: May be stoic. May accept pain medicine as well as herbal.

Palliative care: Usually, they prefer to die at home.

Libyan Culture

Death: Tend to be very emotional.

Pain: May accept pain medicine up until nearing death when they prefer to be alert.

Palliative care: May accept palliative care.

Native American Culture

Death: May avoid contact with dying. Verbal grieving may include wailing.

(*continued*)

BOX 3.1 A Summary of Pain and End-of-Life Issues (*Continued*)

Pain: May be undertreated and only expressed privately to family or friends.

Palliative care: May not be willing to discuss terminal status as it is thought to hasten death.

Native Hawaiian Culture

Death: Tend to celebrate life rather than death.

Pain: May only accept treatment for severe pain. Nonverbal cues may be the only way to appreciate pain levels.

Palliative care: May prefer to have family present when discussing an unfavorable prognosis. Accepting of palliative care.

South African Culture

Death: Avoid the discussion as they believe talking about it will make it happen.

Pain: Accept pain medicine.

Palliative care: Usually, die at home with limited involvement of health professionals.

Vietnamese

Death: Will have a tough time discussing death and DNR. These subjects stir deep emotions.

Pain: May be very stoic.

Palliative care: Will probably accept palliative care and pain medicine.

Source: Copyright © by Amy Givler, Harshil Bhatt, and Patricia A. Maani-Fogelman (CC BY 4.0) at https://www.ncbi.nlm.nih.gov/books/NBK493154/.

The family structure and child-rearing practices also influence the expression and communication of illness and pain. Stoicism in European American culture has a long history. For many generations, children, especially boys, would be reprimanded for crying like babies but applauded for keeping a stiff upper lip. In general, people made as little fuss as possible over injuries and illness. Children socialized in this manner will grow up to be "easy patients" who behave in ways consistent with the values of the Western medical system. In other cultures a child's crying immediately elicits the greatest sympathy, concern, and aid. In such cultures, children's health is fretted over constantly—even a sneeze can be seen as illness. This predisposes children to become more anxious about their health in general, and as adults they may need greater reassurance from caregivers even when their symptoms are minor. In general, when people are ill, they revert to childhood behavior. If complaining brought them attention as children, they will likely complain out of habit as adults—even if the desired results are not provided by their caregivers (Carteret, 2010a). Some families and cultures value and honor their elders and others do not to the same extent; and still more culturally bound dynamics can include who makes the decisions and decision-making overall. For example, some families elicit and seek the help and support of those outside of the family unit to aid their decision-making, and others restrict discussions and decision-making to one person/persons, only the nuclear family members, or only the members of the extended family in collaboration with the nuclear family (Burke, 2020).

Patients from Asian cultures are often stoic in the face of pain because self-restraint is a strong cultural value. Complaining is viewed as having poor social skills. In traditional Asian cultures, preserving harmony in interactions with others is very important, so an individual should never draw personal attention, especially in negative ways. Though an individual may feel sadness or pain, it is not customary to make this obvious. This translates to communications with doctors and nurses, who have high status in Asian cultures. People of high status should not be bothered with complaints and should not be questioned (Carteret, 2010a).

Worldview, Religion, and Rituals

Spirituality, religion, and health have been related in all population groups since the beginning of recorded history (Koenig, 2012). In earlier times, physicians were often clergy, and for hundreds of years religious organizations were responsible for licensing physicians (Koenig, 2012). Belief in the ability of the supernatural to heal surfaced in shamanism thousands of years ago. Recorded history describing spiritual healing includes Egyptian belief in the healing power of a particular holy site and Greek and Roman temples built to the healing gods. These types of practices are still known today. Shamanic traditions continue today in Africa, Central and South America, and among some Native American tribes, and Christians continue to make pilgrimages to holy sites that are believed to heal, such as the Sanctuary of Our Lady of Lourdes in France.

Spirituality is often described as a belief in a higher power, something beyond the human experience. For many people, spirituality is a means of living with, confronting, or otherwise addressing universally mysterious events and occurrences. These events include birth, death, health, personal challenges, and tragedies. Scientific research has determined that spiritual practices positively influence health and increase longevity. However, there is disagreement as to the mechanism of these benefits.

Closely related but distinctive is religion, which is the acceptance of the specific beliefs and practices of an organized religion. Religion is generally an organized approach to practicing a form of spiritual belief in and respect for a supernatural power or powers, which is regarded as a creator or a governing framework of the universe and is supported by personal or institutionalized systems grounded in belief and worship.

Although many people find spirituality in the form of religious practice, religion and spirituality are conceptually different. A person may be spiritual without being religious, or may be both. Research has shown that both spirituality and religious beliefs have positive effects on health.

Those who practice Eastern religions seek to refine the life force within themselves, and they attempt to find meaning and purpose in life through these efforts. Practitioners of Western Christianity may focus more on faith and belief in external guidance and salvation from a supreme being, a god, or gods.

Although much human conduct is related to spiritualism that goes beyond practicing formal religious teachings, these two concepts flow universally throughout all cultures. However, most of the research has focused on health and religion, as opposed to health and spirituality, primarily because religion is associated with behaviors that can be quantified (e.g., how often one prays or attends a place of worship), it can be categorized by type of religion, and there is more agreement about its meaning. Religion has a significant role in the United States and in the health. It has an impact on social lives and health behaviors and, hence, on physical and mental well-being.

Religion and rituals overlap, but not all rituals are related to religion. Rituals such as baptism and the burning of ghost money when a person dies (a tradition in China) are related to religious practices, but other rituals are not tied to religion, such as drinking tea at 3 o'clock in the afternoon every day.

Religion in the United States

Spiritualism was part of the Indigenous populations when the Europeans first arrived in what would become the United States. The conquering Spanish brought their Catholic priests not only for their own guidance but also to impose Christian beliefs on the natives. To a large extent the United States was established by people of strong religious beliefs, including Protestants from Europe seeking a place to practice their beliefs free from religious conflict with other European religions, including Catholicism.

Religion and race/ethnicity are linked, but it is important not to assume a person's religion is based on his or her ethnicity. It also is not safe to assume that a person strictly adheres to the practices of a religion. Adherence to religious practices exists on a continuum, with some strictly adhering to all the guidelines and others having looser ties.

Religion and Health Behaviors

Lifestyle represents the single most prominent influence on our health today. As a result, the United States is seeing the need for more emphasis on prevention and behavior modification. People with religious ties of any kind have been shown to engage in healthier behavioral patterns, and these positive lifestyle choices lead to improved health and longer lives. Why do people with stronger religious ties have better health? The answer includes several possible factors, such as proscribed behaviors, closer social relationships, and improved coping mechanisms.

Health behaviors encouraged or proscribed by particular religions are one possible explanation for how religion can positively affect health. Some religions prohibit tobacco, alcohol, caffeine, certain sexual practices, and premarital sex, and some encourage vegetarianism. Social relationships are another potential explanatory factor for the connection between religion and improved health indicators. Social ties can provide both support and a sense of connectedness. Many churches and temples offer workshops, health fairs, and craft fairs, which provide social interactions. Social relationships are also tied to coping mechanisms because they provide support in multiple forms during times of stress. For example, financial support may be provided to people who have incurred a tragedy, such as a disability, loss of job, or a house fire. Religious organizations also conduct fundraisers for families who have experienced a death or personal tragedy in the family. Churches and temples assist elders by providing transportation or taking food to the homebound. Friendships and a sense of purpose are also methods of support.

Dietary Practices

Dietary practices have a long history of being incorporated into religions around the world. Some religions prohibit followers from consuming certain foods and drinks all of the time or on certain holy days; require or encourage specific dietary and food preparation practices and/or fasting (going without food and/or drink for a specified time); or prohibit eating certain foods at the same meal, such as dairy and meat products. Other religions require certain methods of food preparation and have special rules about the use of pans, plates, utensils, and how the food is to be cooked. Foods and drinks also may be a part of religious celebrations or rituals.

The restriction of certain foods and beverages may have a positive impact on the health of those engaged in such practices. For example, restricting consumption of animal products, such as beef and pork or all animal products, may reduce the risk of health problems. Many religions, such as Hinduism and Buddhism, practice or promote vegetarianism, and these diets have been shown to have several health effects, such as the reduction of heart disease, cancer, obesity, and stroke. Some religions help prevent obesity through beliefs that gluttony is a sin, you should only take what you need, and self-discipline is necessary.

Religions may incorporate some element of fasting in their practices. In many religions, the general purpose for fasting is to become closer to God, show respect for the body (temple) that is a gift from God, understand and appreciate the suffering that the poor experience, acquire the discipline required to resist temptation, atone for sinful acts, and/or cleanse evil from within the body. Fasting may be recommended for specific times of the day; for a specified number of hours; on designated days of the week, month, or year; or on holy days.

During times of fasting, most but not all religions permit the consumption of water. Water restriction can lead to a risk of dehydration. Some fasters may not take their medication during the fast, which may put their health at risk. Prolonged fasting and/or restrictions from water and/or medications may pose health risks for some followers. Because of these health risks, certain groups are often excused from fasting. These groups include people with chronic diseases, frail elderly, pregnant and lactating women, people who engage in strenuous labor, young children, and people suffering from malnutrition.

DID YOU KNOW?

Most Hindus prefer to die at home. If that cannot occur, then certain rituals are to be performed at the hospital. Examples include assisting the patient with facing east and lighting a lamp near the patient's head. Often family and friends will be present, singing hymns or chanting mantras from sacred scriptures.

Holy ash or sandalwood paste is applied on the forehead after the patient dies. Members of the family may want the body to face south, as that symbolizes facing the god of death. A few drops of holy water are trickled into the mouth, and the incense near the head of the deceased remains burning.

Use of Stimulants and Depressants

In addition to foods, some religions prohibit or restrict the use of stimulants. A stimulant is a product (including medications), food, or drink that stimulates the nervous system and alters the recipient's physiology. Stimulants include substances that contain caffeine, including some teas, coffee, chocolate, and energy drinks. Caffeine is prohibited or restricted by many religions because of its addictive properties. A depressant slows down the nervous system. Alcohol is an example. Some religions prohibit the use of stimulants and depressants, but others use them during ceremonies. For example, Roman Catholics, Eastern Orthodox Christians, and certain Protestant denominations use wine as a sacramental product to represent the blood of Christ in communion services. Native Americans use tobacco and the hallucinogenic peyote as part of their spiritual ceremonies.

As a result of religion's effects on health behaviors, it is not surprising that religion has been shown to have positive effects on both physical and mental health. Over the last several decades, a notable body of empirical evidence has emerged that examines the relationship between religion or religious practices and a host of outcomes. Most of the outcomes have been positive, but it is important to note that religion does not always have favorable effects on health.

Religion has sometimes been used to justify hatred, aggression, and prejudice. Religion can be judgmental, alienating, and exclusive. Religious conflict is perhaps the greatest controllable threat to health and well-being in the modern era. Though raised as a Christian, during World War II, Adolph Hitler intentionally murdered 6 million Jews. Jews and Muslims repeatedly attack one another, keeping the Middle East in a constant state of tension over the last 50 years. Islamic extremists have declared war on Christian believers and used explosives on subways in Spain, crashed jetliners into high rises in New York, and used modern media to display multiple and serial beheadings while ostensibly practicing their religion. Threats of nuclear proliferation and potential use of nuclear weapons have been driven by religious conflict.

Religion also may have a negative impact on health through the failure to conform to community norms. Open criticism by other congregation members or clergy can increase stress in social relationships. Feelings of religious guilt and the failure to meet religious expectations or cope with religious fears can contribute to illness. In some cases, parents' reliance on religion instead of traditional medical care has led to children's deaths. Also, people may not participate in healthy behaviors because they believe that their health is in God's hands, so their behaviors will not change God's plan. This is referred to as a fatalistic attitude.

WHAT DO YOU THINK?

Health care professionals should take a patient's religion and spirituality into consideration, but to what extent should a health care professional's beliefs be taken into consideration? If pharmacists have religious beliefs against abortion, should they be required to fill prescriptions for the emergency contraceptive? If a pharmacist works in Oregon, where doctors are, by law, permitted to write life-ending prescriptions for dying patients, should a pharmacist who believes that such a practice is murder be required to fill that prescription? Should a faith-based hospital be able to prohibit providing an abortion? Would your answer be different if it were the only hospital in a large rural region, so women wanting an abortion would have to travel for 5 hours to reach a clinic? Should the rural hospital be able to prohibit providing an abortion if the life of the mother is threatened?

Rituals

A ritual is a set of actions that usually is structured and has a symbolic value or meaning. The performance of rituals is usually tied to religion or traditions, and their forms, purposes, and functions vary. These include compliance with religious obligations or ideals, satisfaction of spiritual or emotional needs of the practitioners, warding off evil, ensuring the favor of a divine being, maintaining or restoring health, as a demonstration of respect or submission, stating one's affiliation, obtaining social acceptance, or for the pleasure of the ritual itself. A ritual may be performed on certain occasions, at regular intervals, or at the discretion of individuals or communities. It may be performed by an individual, a small group, or the community, and it may occur in arbitrary places or specified locations. The ritual may be performed in private or public, or in front of specific people. The participants may be restricted to certain community members, with limitations related to age, gender, or type of activity (hunting and birthing rituals).

Rituals are related to numerous activities and events, such as birth, death, puberty, marriages, sporting events, club meetings, holidays, graduations, and presidential inaugurations. Handshaking, saying hello and goodbye, and taking your shoes off before entering a home are also rituals. These actions and their symbolism are neither arbitrarily chosen by the performers nor dictated by logic or necessity, but they either are prescribed and imposed on the performers by some external source or are inherited unconsciously from social traditions. Many have practical roots. Shaking hands originated as a gesture to assure each person that neither was carrying a weapon, and taking off shoes before entering a home helps keep it clean.

The biomedical system contains numerous rituals, including its own language filled with scientific terminology, jargon, and abbreviations (e.g., MRI, CAT scan). There are formal rules of behavior and communication, such as how physicians should be addressed and where the patient should sit. There are rituals such as hand washing, how to perform a physical examination, how to make a hospital bed, and how to document information in medical records. The values and expectations include being on time for your appointment and adhering to the treatment regimen. People who are unaccustomed to this culture and these rituals can experience difficulty with them, and this includes maneuvering through the complex health insurance system, which is laden with unfamiliar rituals and rules. This can be particularly challenging if English is the patient's second language and if the patient did not come from a place with a similar system, such as socialized medicine.

In addition to rituals within health care systems numerous rituals are related to health. These rituals are discussed here to help prompt people who are working in health care to ask about, be sensitive to, and not be surprised about these key differences.

Objects as Rituals

People wear various items to maintain their health. These may include amulets that may be worn on a necklace or strung around the neck, wrist, or waist. For example, people may place a bracelet on the wrist of a baby to ward off the evil eye. In addition to being worn, amulets may be placed in the home. For example, items such as written documents, statues, crosses, or horseshoes may be hung on the home to protect the family's health as well as other factors. It is important to ask about removing these objects first because removal may cause great stress and concern for the person.

Shrines

For centuries people have described certain places as being holy or magic, as having a concentrated power, or having the presence of spirit. Ancient legends, historic records, and contemporary reports tell of extraordinary, even miraculous, happenings at these places. Different sacred sites have the power to heal the body, enlighten the mind, increase creativity, develop psychic abilities, and awaken the soul to a knowing of its true purpose in life. Shrines are located at some of these sacred sites. A shrine was originally a container, usually made of precious materials, but it has come to mean a holy or sacred place. Shrines may be enclosures within temples, home altars, and sacred burial places. Secular meanings have developed by association, and some of the associations are related to health and healing. People visit numerous shrines that represent health to maintain or restore health. Some examples of these shrines are Our Lady of La Leche, Our Lady of San Juan, and St. Peregrine. These shrines can be associated with healing for a specific disease or condition or with healing in general.

Animal Sacrifice

Animal sacrifice is not only practiced for food consumption but also is believed to be needed for one to build and maintain a personal relationship with the spirit. It is also believed that it brings worshippers closer to their creator or spirit and makes them aware of the spirit in them. Sacrifices are performed for events such as birth, marriage, and death. They are also used for healing. Animals are killed in a way similar to a kosher slaughter. Animals are cooked and eaten following most rituals, except for some healing and death rituals in which the animal is not eaten because it is believed that the sickness is passed onto the dead animal.

Birthing Rituals

The birth of an infant is a life-altering event that is surrounded by many traditional and ancient rituals. These rituals are often related to protecting the health of the child, which includes protecting him or her from evil spirits. The rituals are related to events prior to, during, and after the birth. Because the rituals are so numerous, we have listed the general variations, but the list is not exhaustive.

Prior to birth:

- Food restrictions
- Wearing of amulets
- The fulfilling of food cravings
- Exposure to cold air
- Avoidance of loud noises or viewing certain types of people (i.e., deformed people)

During labor:

- How the placenta is discarded
- Silent birth (some cultures require that no words or sounds are spoken by the woman and/or family members)
- People present during labor
- Utilization of a midwife
- Place of delivery
- Medications used

After birth:

- Breastfeeding
- Amulets (placed on the baby, crib, or in the newborn's room)
- Female and male circumcision
- Baptism
- Animal sacrifice
- Cutting of child's lock of hair

- Bathing of baby
- Food restrictions
- When the naming of the baby occurs
- Rubbing the baby with oils or herbs
- Acceptance of postpartum depression
- Woman's and child's confinement period

Death Rituals

Responses to death vary widely across cultures. Although some cultures may perform the same or similar rituals, they may have different meanings among the cultures. The rituals, in part, are related to beliefs about the meaning of life and life after death. Is death the end of existence or a transition to another life? Rituals play a role in behaviors, such as how people discuss death, respond to death, handle the deceased's body, the behaviors that occur at the funeral, and the mourning process.

Some general variations include the following:

- The method of disposing of the body
- Open versus closed casket
- The length of the mourning process and appropriate behavior
- Dress, including colors, at the funeral ceremony and afterward
- Food restrictions or traditions
- Appropriate emotional responses
- The role of the family
- Use of prayer
- What is buried with the body
- Rituals engaged in before, during, and after the ceremony (e.g., burning of ghost money or candles, use of flowers)
- Animal sacrifice

Summary

Worldview is our perception of how the world works. It includes issues such as moral and ethical reasoning, social relationships, and communication. Health care professionals need to take a person's worldview into consideration because it affects behaviors, perceptions, communication, and decisions. Some decisions are made daily, such as whether to take a medication, but major health decisions, such as beginning- and end-of-life decisions, are also subject to patients' worldview.

Religion, which is a part of worldview, plays a major role in the lives of Americans. It shapes our health behaviors and has been shown to have an overall positive effect on health behaviors. Religion also guides people when making difficult and sometimes life-altering decisions. With technological advances, medical decisions can be complicated. Some people find the answers within their religion, but many people within religious sectors have differences in opinions. It is important for health care professionals not to assume someone's religion based on their ethnicity and not to assume that everyone strictly adheres to the religious practices.

In this chapter we have described how important worldview is in the lives of Americans and how it can influence health behaviors and decisions. In addition, some reasons people who are religious may have positive health habits and outcomes as well as the potential negative effects of religion were discussed. The chapter ended with a discussion about rituals that are related to health. Many of those rituals are tied to religious beliefs, and health care professionals should make efforts to adhere to these rituals.

Review

1. What does worldview mean? Provide examples of why it is important to consider worldview in health care.
2. Provide examples of differences in verbal and nonverbal communication methods among different cultures.
3. Explain some beginning- and end-of-life decisions related to worldview and culture.
4. Provide examples of how religion shapes health behaviors and the rationale behind them.
5. Explain some of the positive and negatives effects religion can have on health outcomes.
6. Provide examples of medical decisions that are made based on religion and the rationale behind them.
7. Explain issues that health care professionals should take into consideration related to beginning- and end-of-life transitions.

Activity

Select a religion that you are interested in learning more about. Write a three-page paper about the practices and beliefs of that religion that are related to health.

Case Study 1

A physician receives the pathology report from a recent endoscopy of her patient, a 78-year-old Japanese man. The report reveals adenocarcinoma of the stomach. The physician intends to disclose the diagnosis to the patient. However, as the provider approaches the patient's room, the patient's daughter stops her. The daughter demands to know the diagnosis and states that, if indeed it is cancer, her father should not be told. The daughter insists that she and her mother will decide what is best for her father. She argues that in her father's culture, family members make the decisions for the patient.

1. Is it the physician's duty to disclose the truth to her patient?
2. How can the physician–patient relationship be preserved while taking into consideration the wishes of family members?
3. What role should culture play in how a case is handled?

Source: Rosen et al. (2004)

Case Study 2

Uri is a child of Jewish decent. He is 9 years old. His life is centered around his community at the synagogue, the Jewish community, and his extended family. Uri has three siblings in a small home next to his grandparents' house. The family dinners are traditional Jewish meals and Yiddish prayer, and conversation is heard throughout the house.

When Uri was 2 years of age, he was diagnosed with fragile X syndrome, a genetic condition that causes a range of developmental problems, including learning disabilities and cognitive impairment. It is the leading cause of inherited intellectual disabilities like autism. There are behavioral, physical, intellectual, and mental health symptoms. Females have milder symptoms than males. Uri has been in and out of the hospital on a regular basis and struggles in school due to his condition.

When Uri's mother became pregnant when Uri was 5, her doctors strongly suggested that she go for genetic counseling and possibly testing. The reason is that Uri's condition is genetically related, and the doctors had concerns about her newborn having the same condition. Uri's parents discussed the doctor's recommendations with their rabbi. The parents decided not to have genetic testing based on the premise that the unborn child's health was in God's hands.

1. What are the various ways in which religious beliefs can affect the understanding of illness?
2. Do you believe that the Jewish belief system will affect Uri's treatment?
3. What are some of the main tenets of Judaism?

4. Do you believe that Uri's parents should have been required to have genetic testing done? Why or why not?

References

Burke, A. (2020, August 8). *Cultural awareness and influences on health: NCLEX-RN.* https://www.registerednursing.org/nclex/cultural-awareness-influences-health/

Carteret, M. (2010a, November 2). *Cultural aspects of pain management.* http://www.dimensionsofculture.com/2010/11/cultural-aspects-of-pain-management/

Carteret, M. (2010b, November 3). *Modesty in health care: A cross-cultural perspective.* http://www.dimensionsofculture.com/2010/11/modesty-in-health-care-a-cross-cultural-perspective/

Cheraghi, M., Bahramnezhad, F., Mehrdad, N., & Zendehdel, K. (2016). View of main religions of the world on: Don't attempt resuscitation order (DNR). *International Journal of Medical Reviews, 3*(1), 401–405. http://www.ijmedrev.com/article_63020.html

Cross Cultural Health Care. (2003). *Cross cultural health care-case studies.*

Givler, A., Bhatt, H., & Maani-Fogelman, P. A. (2020, December 1). *The importance of cultural competence in pain and palliative care.* StatPearls. https://www.ncbi.nlm.nih.gov/books/NBK493154/

Koenig, H. G. (2012). Religion, spirituality, and health: The research and clinical implications. *Psychiatry.* http://www.hindawi.com/journals/isrn/2012/278730/

Portanova, J., Ailshire, J., Perez, C., Rahman, A., & Enguidanos, S. (2017). Ethnic differences in advance directive completion and care preferences: What has changed in a decade? *Journal of the American Geriatrics Society, 65*(6), 1352–1357. https://doi.org/10.1111/jgs.14800

Purnell, L. D. (2013). *Transcultural health care.* F. A. Davis Company.

Rosen, J., Spatz, E. S., Gaaserud, A. M. J., Abramovitch, H., Weinreb, B., Wenger, N. S., & Margolis, C. Z. (2004). A new approach to developing cross cultural communication skills. *Medical Teacher, 26*(2), 126–132.

Saccomano, S. J., & Abbatiello, G. (2014, February 15). Cultural considerations at the end of life. *The Nurse Practitioner, 39*(2), 24–31. https://doi.org/10.1097/01.NPR.0000441908.16901.2e

Tilbert, J. C. (2010). The role of worldviews in health disparities education. *Journal of General Internal Medicine, 25*(2), 178–181. http://www.ncbi.nlm.nih.gov/pmc/articles/PMC2847101/

CHAPTER 4

Complementary and Alternative Medicine

Everyone has a doctor in him or her; we just have to help it in its work.
The natural healing force within each one of us is the greatest force in getting well.
Our food should be our medicine.
Our medicine should be our food.
—HIPPOCRATES

KEY CONCEPTS AND TERMS

Acupuncture
Alternative medicine
Complementary medicine
Doshas
Five elements
Hydrotherapy
Meditation
Meridians
Mindfulness meditation
Naturopathy
Prakriti
Qi
Qigong
Reiki
Tai chi
Transcendental meditation
Yin and yang
Yoga

After reading this chapter, you should be able to do the following:

1. Identify the difference between complementary and alternative medicine (CAM) practices.
2. Understand the various types of CAM practices.
3. Discuss the potential benefits and risks of CAM practices.
4. Appreciate the cultural influences on CAM practices.
5. Describe laws related to CAM.

It is not entirely clear when humans began to develop modalities to deal with pain, injury, and disease. However, we know that these practices have been in existence for ages. The various practices to treat disease and injury have been passed down through the centuries from person to person and family member to family member. The practices have been influenced by observation and experimentation, as well as religious, social, and cultural practices. Over time, the various forms of these practices have taken on the unique characteristics of the people and cultures that utilize them.

These practices have been termed *folk medicine* by the mainstream science-based medical professions. With the advent of the scientific approach to medicine, it might be assumed that the various traditional folk medicine practices would die out. However, that has not been the case. As new cultures immigrated to the United States, so did their traditional healing practices. Increased interest in these traditional practices has spurred research into their efficacy and recharacterized them as complementary and alternative medical practices.

Complementary medicine refers to using a nonmainstream approach *with* conventional medicine. **Alternative medicine** refers to using a nonmainstream approach *in place of* conventional medicine. CAM is a broad range of modalities outside the traditional Western medicine approach to care. The types of CAM are listed in **Box 4.1**. Folk medicine, or the use of traditional remedies, is considered a form of complementary and alternative medicine. Folk remedies include, but are not limited to long-existing practices, such as Chinese medicine, acupuncture, and naturopathy, to name a few. The history and utilization of CAM, along with culturally based CAM modalities and related laws, are the focus of this chapter.

BOX 4.1 Types of CAM

I. Traditional alternative medicine
- Acupuncture
- Ayurvedic medicine
- Homeopathy
- Naturopathy
- Chinese or Oriental medicine

II. Body
- Chiropractic and osteopathic medicine
- Massage
- Body movement therapies
- Tai chi
- Yoga

III. Diet and herbs
- Dietary supplements
- Herbal medicine
- Nutrition/diet

IV. External energy
- Qigong
- Electromagnetic therapy
- Reiki

V. Mind
- Meditation
- Biofeedback
- Hypnosis

VI. Senses
- Art, dance, and music
- Visualization and guided imagery

Source: Johns Hopkins Medicine (2020).

History of Complementary and Alternative Medicine

CAM predates the history of the United States. Prior to the latter part of the 19th century, medical care was provided by lay healers, naturopaths, homeopaths, midwives, and botanical healers as well as formally trained doctors. Nineteenth-century advances in science, such as germ theory, antisepsis, and anesthesia, spurred the trend to scientific medical education. Interest in whole foods and dietary supplements in the 1950s began a resurgence of interest in alternative medical practices. The traditional health practices of immigrant cultures exposed Americans to alternatives, and the counterculture movements of the 1960s renewed the interest in natural healing practices. In the 1970s, the holistic health approach began incorporating Eastern medical traditions with conventional Western medical practices (White House Commission on Complementary and Alternative Medicine Policy, 2002).

This resurgent public interest in modalities, characterized as folk medicine, has encouraged medical practitioners to investigate their efficacy and impact on conventional medical practices. Being aware of cultural differences in beliefs regarding disease and treatment is imperative to a modern medical practitioner because patients who engage in CAM practices may also seek help from Western medicine.

Use of Complementary and Alternative Medicine

The National Health Interview Survey (NHIS) is an annual study, conducted by the CDC's National Center for Health Statistics (NCHS), in which tens of thousands of Americans are interviewed about their health- and illness-related experiences. The complementary health approaches section of NHIS, developed by the NCHS and National Center for Complementary and Integrative Health (NCCIH), was administered in 2002, 2007, 2012 and 2017. The 2017 survey was less broad than the previous surveys and focused primarily on meditation, yoga, and chiropractic. Therefore, the 2012 results are presented here. Data from 34,525 adults aged 18 and over collected as part of the 2012 NHIS. **Figures 4.1–4.4** provide information on CAM usage among adults and children.

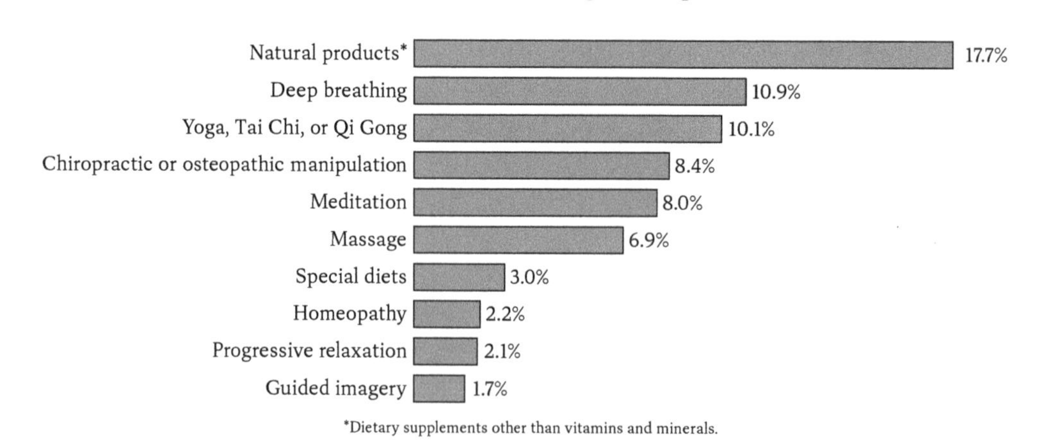

Figure 4.1 Ten most common CAM theories among adults, 2012.

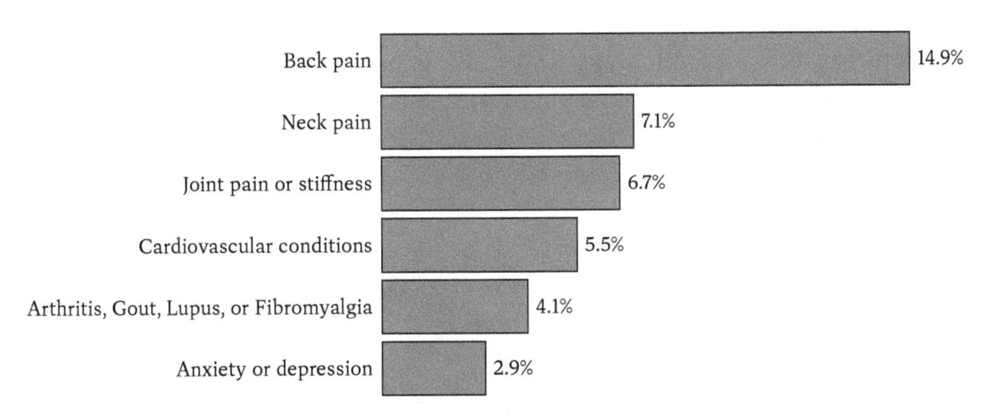

Figure 4.2 CAM use for diseases/conditions among adults, 2012.

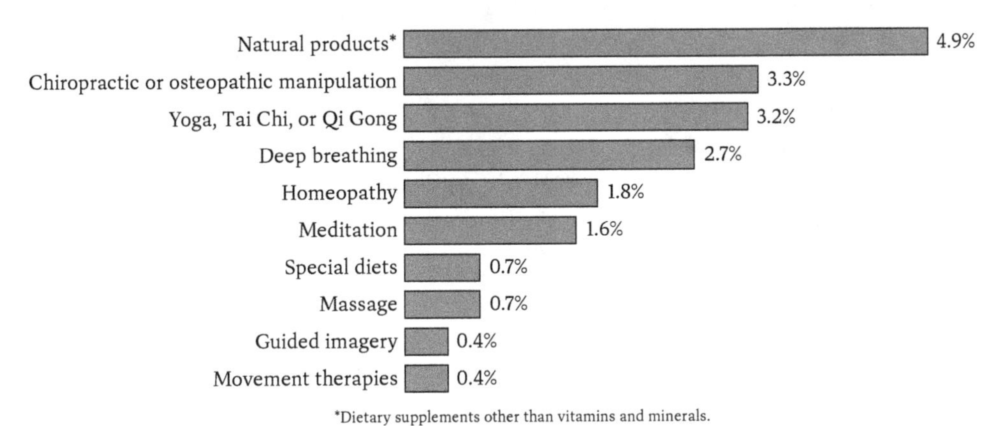

Figure 4.3 Ten most common therapies among children, 2012.

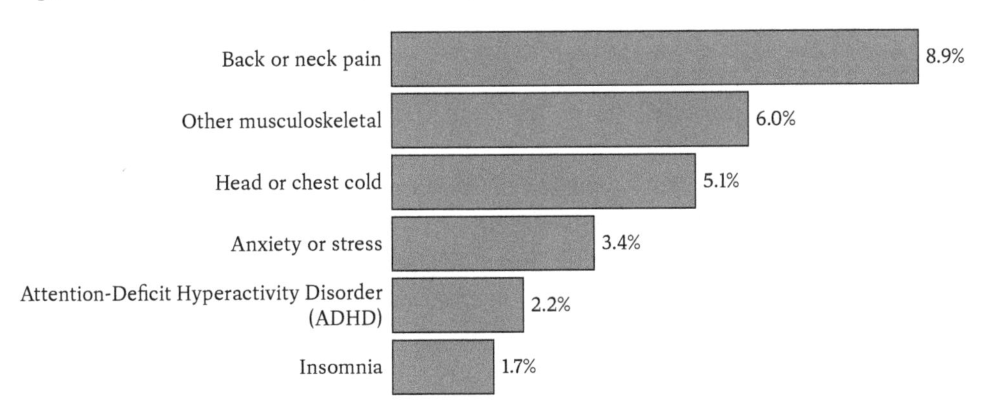

Figure 4.4 CAM use for diseases/conditions among children, 2012.

In 2012, the out-of-pocket amount that was spent in the United States on complementary health approaches was $30.2 billion (see **Figure 4.5**). Of that $30.2 billion, $28.3 billion was for adults and $1.9 billion was for children. Americans spent $14.7 billion out of pocket on visits to complementary practitioners such as chiropractors, acupuncturists, or massage therapists. That is almost 30% of what they spent out of pocket on services by conventional physicians. Americans spent $12.8 billion out of pocket on natural product supplements, which was about one quarter of what they spent out of pocket on prescription drugs.

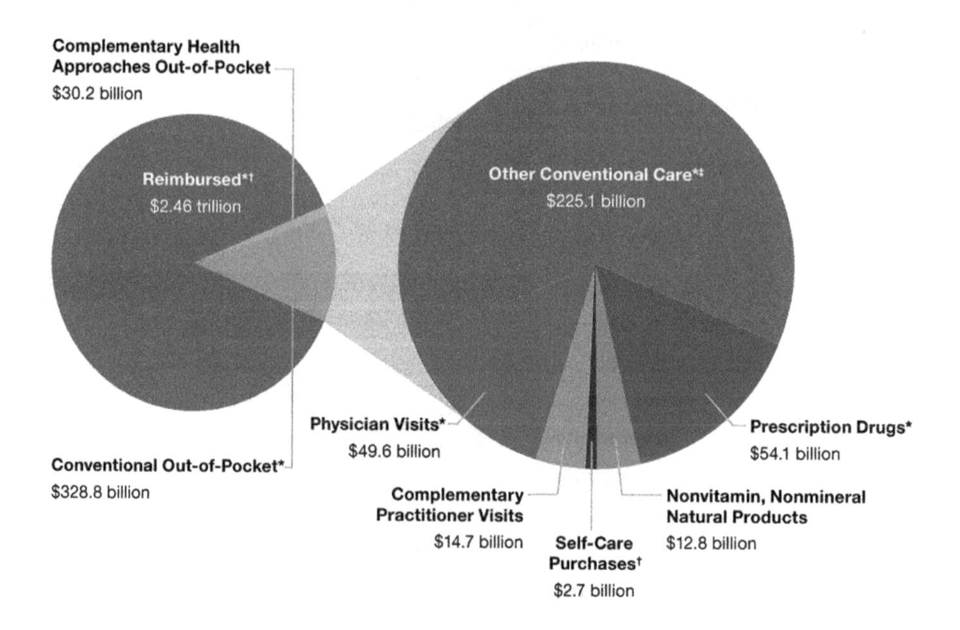

* National Health Expenditure Data for 2012. U.S. Department of Health and Human Services, Centers for Medicare and Medicaid Services Web site. Accessed at: https://www.cms.gov/Research-Statistics-Data-and-systems/Statistics-Trends-and-reports/NationalHealthExpendData/index.html on March 31, 2016.

† Self-care purchases includes, for example, homeopathic medicines and self-help materials such as books or CDs related to complementary health topics.

‡ Other conventional care includes dental care, nursing homes, home health care, nondrug medical products, hospital care, and other professional services.

Source: Nahin RL, Barnes PM, Stussman BJ. Expenditures on complementary health approaches: United States, 2012. National Health Statistics Reports. Hyattsville, MD: National Center for Health Statistics. 2016.

Figure 4.5 Out-of-pocket spending on CAM, 2012.

More current studies focus on the use of CAM by particular age groups or to treat a specific disease. An example is a study of 3,118 participants reporting a history of cancer (1,230 men and 1,888 women). One third (n = 1023) had used CAM in the past 12 months. The most commonly used CAM modality was herbal supplements (n = 363, 35.8%), followed by chiropractic or osteopathic manipulation (n = 256, 25.4%), massage (n = 129, 14.1%), and yoga/tai chi/qigong (n = 85, 7.6%) (Sanford et al., 2019).

The NCCIH is the lead federal agency for scientific research on the usefulness and safety of complementary and integrative health practices. To address the need for objective evidence as to the safety and efficacy of many of these approaches, NCCIH supports rigorous scientific investigation to better understand how these interventions work, for whom, and the optimal methods of practice and delivery.

The NCCIH released its most recent strategic plan in 2016. A new plan is released every 5 years. The plan presents a series of objectives to guide the NCCIH in determining priorities for future research in complementary and alternative medicine. The five strategic objectives are as follows:

1. Advance fundamental science and methods development
2. Improve care for hard-to-manage symptoms
3. Foster health promotion and disease prevention
4. Enhance the complementary and integrative health research workforce
5. Disseminate objective evidence-based information on complementary and integrative health interventions (National Center for Complementary and Alternative Medicine, 2021).

The top scientific priorities are as follows:

- Nonpharmacologic management of pain
- Neurobiological effects and mechanisms
- Innovative approaches for establishing biological signatures of natural products
- Disease prevention and health promotion across the life span
- Clinical trials utilizing innovative study designs to assess complementary health approaches and their integration into health care
- Communications strategies and tools to enhance scientific literacy and understanding of clinical research (NCCIH, 2021).

The NCCIH has made pain management a major emphasis in its research efforts. Pain is a major public health problem and is the most common reason Americans use complementary and integrative health practices. The 2012 NHIS (2021) data estimated that 126.1 million adults reported some pain in the previous 3 months, with 25.3 million adults (11.2%) suffering from daily (chronic) pain and 23.4 million (10.3%) reporting a lot of pain. In 2016, an estimated 20.4% of U.S. adults had chronic pain (Dahlhamer et al., 2018). Those with chronic pain were mostly among adults living in poverty, with less than a high school education, and with public health insurance (Dahlhamer et al., 2018). Conventional care often fails to manage chronic pain effectively, and other approaches to relieve or reduce pain and increase functional ability are needed (NCCIH, 2021). Research studies have shown that some complementary health modalities may reduce pain associated with some conditions; examples include massage, spinal manipulation, and yoga for chronic back pain and tai chi for fibromyalgia pain (NCCIH, 2021).

The NCCIH also seeks to identify strategies for promoting health and preventing disease. Behavioral risk factors, including an unhealthy diet, being overweight or obese, living a sedentary life, smoking or using tobacco products, and the excessive consumption of alcohol, are linked to increased rates of cardiovascular disease, cancer, and diabetes.

Preliminary evidence indicates that some complementary health approaches may be useful in encouraging improved self-care, an improved personal sense of well-being, and a greater commitment to a healthy lifestyle. For example, analysis of the 2012 NHIS data indicates that many people who practiced yoga reported that it motivated them to practice healthier behaviors, including eating better and exercising more regularly. While causal relationships between the practice of complementary approaches and healthy behaviors have not been established, further research is needed to explore, clarify, and examine their relationship (NCCIH, 2021).

Complementary and Alternative Health Care Modalities

The White House Commission on Complementary and Alternative Medicine Policy (2002) noted that the major CAM systems have common characteristics that include focusing on individual treatment, a holistic approach to care, promotion of self-care and self-healing, and addressing spiritual influences on health. The modalities of complementary and alternative medicine that are culturally related are explained in this chapter.

Ayurvedic Medicine

Ayurveda, a Sanskrit word meaning science of life, was originally described in the ancient Hindu texts called Vedas. This ancient practice is based on the theory that the five great elements—ether, air, fire, water, and earth—are the basis for all living systems. The five elements are in constant interaction and are constantly changing. The elements combine in pairs to form **doshas**, the three vital energies that regulate everything in nature (see **Table 4.1**).

TABLE 4.1 The Doshas

Vata. Composed of air and ether
Pita. Composed of fire and water
Kapha. Composed of water and earth

At the time of conception, the doshas combine in a unique way for each individual. This combination is known as **prakriti**. A person's physiology, personality, intellect, and weaknesses are governed by two dominant doshas. If the doshas become imbalanced, the flow of *prana* (life energy) and *agni* (digestion) become upset. It is these imbalances that result in illness.

Ayurvedic practitioners seek to balance the doshas through methods such as herbal remedies, yoga, meditation, and massage. For example, *Panchakarma* is a purification process used to remove impurities and restore balance to the doshas. Panchakarma is a set of therapeutic procedures that is intended to improve health and expand the life span. The specific treatments vary and may include using a special diet, emetics, herbal enemas, massage, herbs, and nose cleaning.

Yoga

Yoga is an ancient system of exercises and breathing techniques designed to encourage physical and spiritual well-being. It incorporates a number of guidelines for well-being, including good nutrition and hygiene. The physical practice of yoga consists of going through *asanas* (physical postures) to improve the physical body and calm the nerves. *Pranayamas* are breathing techniques and meditations designed to improve spiritual well-being.

Some yoga practitioners teach that centers of energy, known as *chakras*, are connected to the nerves and spinal cord. It is believed that certain asanas and meditations can positively influence the chakras, improving physical and mental health. The exercise and relaxation techniques utilized in yoga are practiced by many people every day.

Yoga has been shown to have many health benefits. These include increased strength, balance, and flexibility; decreased back pain; it also eases arthritis symptoms; improves sleep and heart health; increases energy; improves mood; manages stress; and improves self-care (Johns Hopkins Medicine, 2021). In the 2017 NHIS, non-Hispanic White adults were more likely to use yoga (17.1%) in the past 12 months compared with Hispanic (8.0%) and non-Hispanic Black (9.3%) adults (n = 26,742). In that same study, women were more than twice as likely to use yoga in the past 12 months (19.8%) compared with men (8.6%) (Clarke et al., 2018).

Traditional Chinese Medicine

Traditional Chinese medicine (TCM) is the term used for a group of ancient healing practices that date back some 2,000 years to 200 BCE. The concepts utilized have been adapted by the Koreans, Japanese, and Vietnamese into their own versions of treatment. The system includes, among other treatments, herbalism, acupuncture, qigong, and tai chi.

TCM is based on diagnosis from the pattern of symptoms rather than on endeavoring to identify a specific illness. It is believed that the cause of disease must be cured, not just its symptoms. TCM considers a person's body, mind, spirit, and emotions as part of one complete whole rather than individual parts that are to be treated separately. TCM is based on a number of interrelated theories: the theory of Qi, the theory of the five elements, the theory of yin and yang, and the meridian theory.

The Theory of Qi

Qi, pronounced "chee," is the vital life force that animates all things. Qi flows through the 12 meridians that run through the body. Physical, emotional, and mental harmony rely on the flow of qi. Qi has two parts, energy or power, and conscious intelligence. These parts are found in organ systems and allow them to perform their physical and energetic functions. Qi also can be described by how it functions. Qi creates all movement, protects the body, provides for harmonious transformation, such as water being turned into urine, keeps the organs and body parts in proper position, and warms the body. This theory holds that qi

- is spiritual in origin;
- makes up and moves through all living things;
- is available in infinite quantities, is positive in nature, and is important to all aspects of health;
- is present both inside the body and on its surface;
- flows throughout the body in specific channels; and
- has its flow disturbed by negative thoughts or feelings.

Qi deficiency can result in problems, what Western medicine calls chronic fatigue syndrome or a fever. Qi stagnation, where the energy cannot flow correctly, can result in what Western medicine calls pain.

The Five Elements Theory

The **five elements** are based on the perception of the relationships between all things. These patterns are grouped and named for the five elements: (a) wood, (b) fire, (c) earth, (d) metal, and (e) water. This theory states that the five organ systems are each tied to a particular element and to a broader group of phenomena that are associated with their elements, including the seasons, colors, emotions, and foods (see **Table 4.2**). This theory illustrates the interrelatedness of all things.

TABLE 4.2 The Characteristics of the Five Elements

	Fire	Earth	Metal	Water	Wood
Season	Summer	Indian summer	Autumn	Winter	Spring
Taste	Bitter	Sweet	Pungent	Salty	Sour
Emotion	Joy	Worry	Grief	Fear	Anger
Body	Heart	Spleen	Lungs	Kidneys	Liver
	Small intestine	Stomach	Large intestine	Bladder	Gallbladder
	Tongue	Mouth	Nose	Hair	Tendons
	Blood vessels	Muscles	Skin	Bones	Eye
Energy/control	Melts metal	Dries water	Cuts wood	Douses fire	Breaks earth
	Water douses it	Wood breaks it	Fire melts it	Earth dries it	Metal cuts it

The Yin and Yang Theory

The yin and yang theory holds that everything is made up of two polar energies. Neither can exist without the other, and they never separate. It is the principle of interconnectedness and interdependence. Yin and yang describe how things function in relation to one another and the important principle of harmony where things blend into a whole.

Yin is female and is associated with the moon and night, late afternoon, cold, rest, responsiveness, passivity, darkness, interiority, downwardness, inwardness, and decrease. Yang is male and is associated with the sun and daytime, early morning, heat, stimulation, movement, activity, excitement, vigor, light, exteriority, upwardness, outwardness, and increase (see **Figure 4.6**).

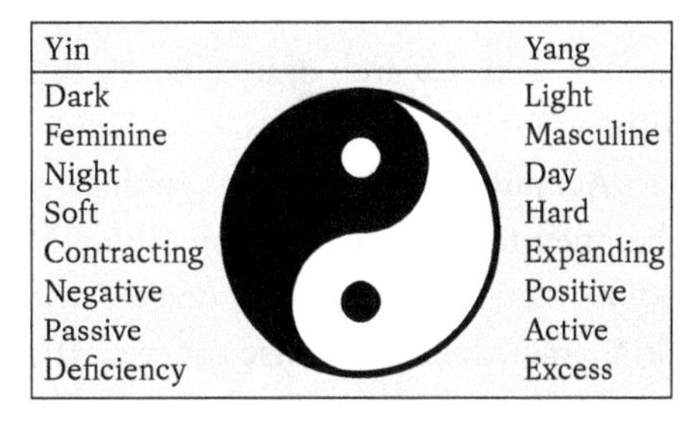

Figure 4.6 The symbol of yin and yang is a circle with two equal and opposite halves.

The Meridian Theory

Meridians are channels through which qi, blood, and information flow to all parts of the body (**Figure 4.7**). There are 12 meridians in the body; six are yin and six are yang. Although each meridian is attributed to, and named for, an organ or body function, the network of meridians connects the meridians to one another and all parts of the body, and they connect the body to the universe. When qi flows easily, the body is balanced and healthy. The meridians work to regulate the energy functions of the body and keep it balanced and in harmony.

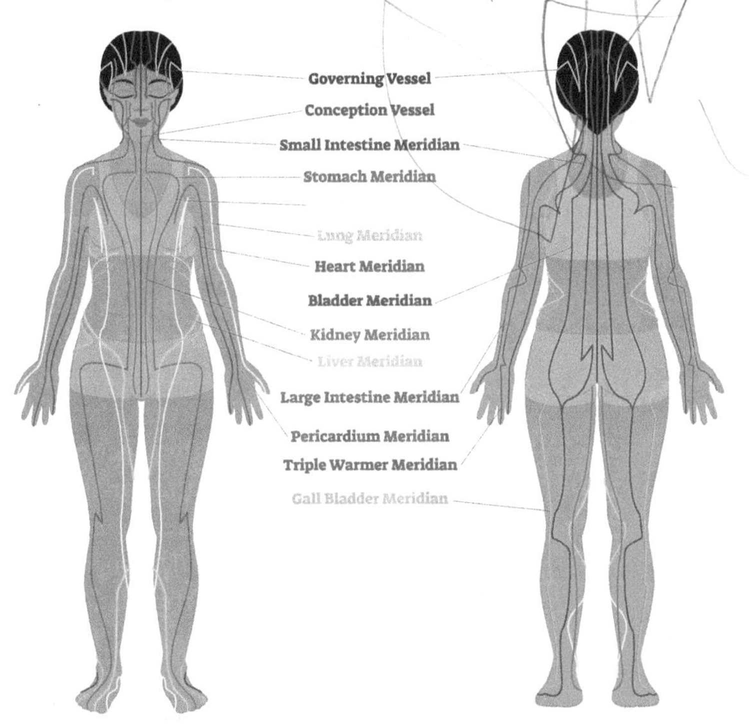

Figure 4.7 Meridians.

TCM encompasses many different treatment modalities. Some of the treatment options utilized include acupuncture, herbal therapies, and qigong.

Acupuncture

Acupuncture is one of the most researched and accepted complementary practices in the United States today. It is experiencing greater acceptance by traditional medical practitioners, and research of its efficacy in treating various conditions has been undertaken, although it has proven to be a difficult subject to study.

Acupuncture involves stimulating specific points along the meridians to achieve a therapeutic purpose. The usual practice involves inserting a needle into one of the acupoints along a meridian associated with that organ or function. Besides puncturing the skin, practitioners also use other methods, including pressure, heat, friction, or electrical stimulation of the needle.

The TCM theory is that acupuncture works by bringing healing energy, qi, to the affected part of the body through the meridians. The stimulation of the appropriate meridian can assist in bringing the affected organ into balance.

Chinese Herbal Therapies

Another significant aspect of traditional Chinese medicine is the use of herbal remedies. Like acupuncture, herbal remedies are used to bring balance back to the body. Herbs are classified according to the five elements and their yin and yang properties to determine how they will be used. Herbs are combined according to their properties to treat a particular disharmony. They are usually administered as teas, pills, powders, or creams. Safety and efficacy issues related to herbal remedies are discussed in the "Herbal Remedies" section of this chapter.

Qigong

The term **qigong** translates to "energy work." It is a part of TCM that involves movement, breathing, and meditation, and it is intended to improve the flow of qi throughout the body. Qigong is an ancient technique that is practiced by millions of people every day. It involves a number of basic postures that are involved in daily practice, and a master can tailor the techniques to address specific problems.

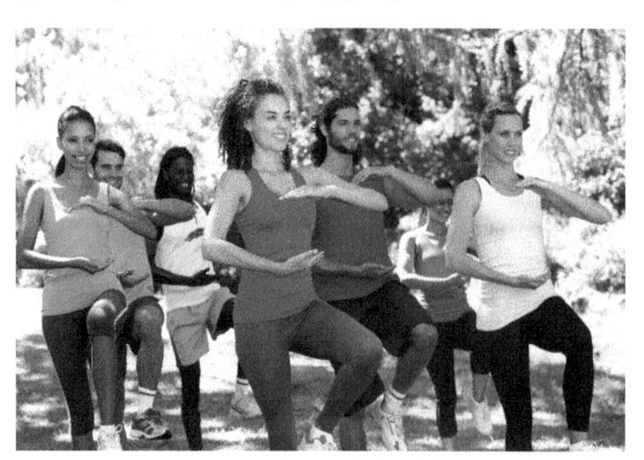
Image 4.1

The ancient noncombative martial art, **tai chi**, is a form of qigong. The purpose of tai chi is to improve the flow of qi through the body to encourage balance and harmony.

Naturopathy

Naturopathy, also known as naturopathic medicine, is a holistic system of medicine based on the healing power of nature. Naturopathy was influenced by Ayurvedic medicine, TCM, and Native American medicine. The system is built on the ancient belief in the healing power of nature and that natural organisms have the ability to heal themselves and maintain health. Such systems include hydrotherapy (water therapy). In 1902 naturopathy was introduced to the United States by Benjamin Lust, a German immigrant. Lust founded the American School of Naturopathy. The school emphasized the use of natural cures, proper bowel habits, and good hygiene as the tools for health. This was the first time that principles of a healthy diet, such as increasing fiber intake and reducing saturated fats, became popular (University of Maryland, 2011).

Naturopaths believe that the body strives to maintain a state of equilibrium, known as homeostasis, and unhealthy environments, diets, physical or emotional stress, and lack of sleep or fresh air can disrupt that balance (see **Table 4.3**). When homeostasis is upset, naturopaths utilize any number of treatments to return the body to balance. All treatments are designed to enhance the body's ability to heal itself. Modalities include diet, yoga, manipulation, massage, hydrotherapy, and natural herbs. Naturopathic practitioners take a holistic approach to treatment and focus on the cause of a disruption of homeostasis rather than treating only symptoms.

TABLE 4.3 The Six Key Principles of Naturopathy

1. The healing power of nature.
2. Do no harm.
3. Treat the whole person.
4. Identify and treat the causes.
5. Prevention.
6. The physician as teacher.

Source: Association of Accredited Naturopathic Medical Colleges (2020).

Herbal Remedies

Plants used for medicinal purposes are classified as medicinal herbs. Herbs have been used to treat diseases for centuries. Many conventional medications were originally developed from herbs. Naturopaths as well as other types of practitioners use herbs to restore homeostasis through treating the cause of diseases.

Herbal preparations use either whole plants or parts of plants. Many herbalists believe in synergy, the idea that whole plants are more effective than their individual parts. Herbal remedies are prepared in pill or liquid form for ingestion or as tinctures, creams, or ointments for external use.

In the United States, herbal products are not regulated by the U.S. Food and Drug Administration and are sometimes sold as dietary supplements. A dietary supplement is a product that contains a "dietary ingredient" intended to supplement the human diet. Dietary ingredients include vitamins; minerals; herbs or other botanicals; amino acids; and other substances such as enzymes, extracts, or concentrates. Dietary supplements, including probiotics, which contain potentially beneficial bacteria or yeasts, may be found in many forms such as tablets, capsules, soft gels, gel caps, liquids, or powders (Consumer Healthcare Products Association, 2021).

When considering using herbal remedies, it is important to consult a professional who is informed about the use of these remedies. Because a product is labeled "natural" does not mean it is safe or does not have harmful effects. Further, the product may not be recommended for a person's specific situation, such as pregnancy. It should be remembered that these remedies can act in the same way as many prescription or over-the-counter drugs and can cause side effects or interfere with the actions of other medications. As with any medication, herbal remedies are not without hazards, and their use must be properly monitored. Yet a 2013 Consumer Reports Survey found that only 28% of people taking dietary supplements and prescription drugs together checked with a pharmacist about potential interactions (when a substance such as a vitamin, mineral, herb, or another medication affects the activity of a drug) (Hendel, 2015).

Cannabis is an herbal remedy that is sold in many forms such as supplements, gummies, and in food. People often use the words *cannabis* and *marijuana* interchangeably, but they do not have the same meaning. The word *cannabis* refers to all products derived from the plant *Cannabis sativa*. The cannabis plant contains about 540 chemical substances. The word *marijuana* refers to parts of or products from the plant *Cannabis sativa* that contain substantial amounts of tetrahydrocannabinol (THC). THC is the substance that's primarily responsible for the effects of marijuana on a person's mental state. Some cannabis plants contain very little THC. Under U.S. law, these plants are considered "industrial hemp" rather than marijuana (NCCIH, 2019).

In China, cannabis seeds and oil have been found that date back to 6,000 BCE, and archeological traces suggest even earlier cultivation. Cannabis was not always considered alternative medicine on American soil. It was widely used by native tribes from coast to coast. Even George Washington grew cannabis and noted its medicinal qualities in agricultural ledgers.

Today, cannabis is gaining respect for its healing capabilities. Drugs containing cannabinoids may be helpful in treating certain rare forms of epilepsy, nausea and vomiting associated with cancer chemotherapy, and loss of appetite and weight loss associated with HIV/AIDS. In addition, some evidence suggests modest benefits of cannabis or cannabinoids for chronic pain and multiple sclerosis symptoms (NCCIH, 2019). It is now widely used to treat pain, nausea, anxiety, depression, muscle spasms, and seizures. The use of cannabis has been linked to some harmful effects. For example, there is an increased risk of motor vehicle crashes, and smoking cannabis during pregnancy has been linked to lower birth weight (NCCIH, 2019). Some people who use cannabis develop cannabis use disorder, which has symptoms such as craving, withdrawal, lack of control, and negative effects on personal and professional responsibilities (NCCIH, 2019). In addition to a general craving to use cannabis, withdrawal symptoms can include anxiety, sleep difficulties, decreased appetite, restlessness, depressed mood, aggression, irritability, nausea, sweating, headache, stomach pain, strange dreams, increased anger, and shakiness (Bansal, 2021).

Cannabis is not legal under federal law. The FDA has determined that products containing THC or CBD cannot be sold legally as dietary supplements. Foods to which THC or CBD has been added cannot be sold legally in interstate commerce. Whether they can be sold legally within a state depends on that state's laws and regulations. The states laws vary. For example, some permit the sale of marijuana for medicinal purposes only, while others have made it fully legal. Other variations include areas such as growing, possession, and the sale of the substance.

DID YOU KNOW?

Ephedra is a plant native to Central Asia and Mongolia. Ephedrine, the main ingredient in ephedra, is a compound that can powerfully stimulate the nervous system and heart. Ephedra has been used for more than 5,000 years in China and India to treat conditions such as colds, fever, flu, headaches, asthma, wheezing, and nasal congestion. More recently, ephedra was used as an ingredient in dietary supplements for weight loss, increased energy, and enhanced athletic performance.

In 2004, the FDA banned the U.S. sale of dietary supplements containing ephedra. The FDA found that these supplements had an unreasonable risk of injury or illness. This includes the risk of anxiety, cardiovascular complications, headache, seizures, and death (National Center for Complementary and Alternative Medicine, 2013).

Reiki

Reiki, pronounced "ray-kee," is a complementary health approach in which practitioners place their hands lightly on or just above a person, with the goal of facilitating the person's own healing response (see **Figure 4.8**). More high-quality research in this field is needed to determine its effectiveness. Reiki has not been clearly shown to be effective for any health-related purpose. It has been studied for a variety of conditions, including pain, anxiety, and depression, but most of the research has not been of high quality, and the results have been inconsistent (NCCIH, 2018). Reiki appears to be generally safe, and no serious side effects have been reported. There are many different forms of Reiki, and no special background is needed to receive training. Training programs and certification are available from Reiki organizations; however, these organizations are not regulated by any government agency.

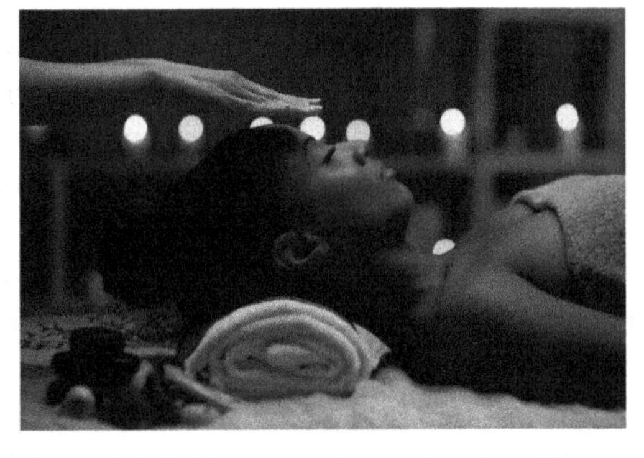

Figure 4.8 Reiki being performed by a practitioner.

The basis for modern-day Reiki practice may have started in Tibet more than 2,500 years ago. Reiki was rediscovered in the early 1900s by a Japanese man named Mikao Usui. During a lengthy period of travel and research, Usui found ancient texts that described Reiki and its power to heal by using the energy that flows through all living things. From his studies and meditations, he developed what came to be known as the Usui system of Reiki. Other systems of Reiki have been developed as well. The word *Reiki* comes from Japanese terms that translate as "universal life energy" (American Cancer Society, 2012).

Reiki is not used to diagnose or treat specific illnesses. Reiki is used to promote relaxation, decrease stress and anxiety, and increase a person's general sense of well-being. Therapy is delivered through the Reiki practitioner's hands, with the goal of raising the amount of universal life energy in and around the client. "Reiki practitioners intend to strengthen the flow of energy, which they say will decrease pain, ease muscle tension, speed healing, improve sleep, and generally enhance the body's ability to heal itself" (American Cancer Society, 2012).

A Reiki session is usually about an hour. The practitioners place their hands in 12 to 15 positions on or above parts of the patient's clothed body. Each hand position is sustained for 2 to 5 minutes. The hands are intended to be a conduit for universal life energy, balancing energy within and around the body. Some practitioners believe that the best results occur when patients have three Reiki sessions within a relatively short time, take a break, and then repeat the process.

WHAT DO YOU THINK?

Many of the CAM modalities do not have scientific evidence that they work yet are frequently used. Should a hospital offer these services if there is no scientific merit for their use? Is a hospital that does not offer CAM culturally insensitive? Does a hospital that does offer CAM give users the impression that the hospital believes in these practices and encourages their use?

Meditation

Meditation refers to a group of mental techniques intended to provide relaxation and mental harmony, quiet one's mind, and increase awareness. It has been a practice in many cultures for thousands of years. Meditative practices are found in Christian, Jewish, Buddhist, Hindu, and Islamic religious traditions. Although meditation found its origins in religious practices, it is currently utilized for nonreligious purposes, such as improved emotional and physical health. Meditation is utilized to decrease stress and anxiety, decrease pain, improve mood, and positively affect heart disease and the symptoms of physical illness. Some research suggests that practicing meditation may reduce blood pressure, symptoms of irritable bowel syndrome, anxiety and depression, and insomnia. Evidence about its effectiveness for pain and as a smoking-cessation treatment is uncertain (NCCIH, 2019).

Various techniques are used by different groups and religions. All techniques have some common factors, namely use of a quiet location, assuming a comfortable position, focusing one's attention by concentrating on one's breath or a mantra (word or sound), and having an open attitude by not allowing distractions to disrupt focus. There are two common types of meditation practices: mindfulness meditation and transcendental meditation.

Mindfulness meditation originated in the Buddhist traditions. It is the concept of increasing awareness and acceptance of the present. During meditation one observes thoughts and images in a nonjudgmental manner with the goal of learning to experience thoughts and feelings with greater balance and acceptance. This technique has been used to treat posttraumatic stress disorder, drug abuse, and chronic pain and to increase cognitive function in the elderly.

Transcendental meditation found its origins in the Indian Vedic tradition. This practice is designed to allow the practitioner to experience ever-finer levels of thought until the source of thought is experienced. A mantra (a sound uttered repeatedly) is used to focus the mind, and the choice of mantra is vital to success. Transcendental meditation enables the mind to reach a quiet state and strives to create a state of relaxed alertness. Transcendental meditation has been found to stimulate what is termed the "relaxation response," which is responsible for decreased blood pressure, muscular relaxation, decreased heart and respiratory rate, and a decrease in lactate levels, which are associated with anxiety.

Spiritual meditation includes centering prayer and contemplative meditation. Spiritual meditation is used in Eastern religions, such as Hinduism and Daoism, and in Christian faith. It is similar to prayer in that the person reflects on the silence around him or her and seeks a deeper connection with his or her God or Universe. Essential oils are commonly used to heighten the spiritual experience.

Research shows that a number of relaxation meditation techniques include four parts: a mental focus, passive attitude, decreased muscle tone, and a quiet environment (Freeman, 2004). One relaxation technique is described in **Table 4.4**.

TABLE 4.4 Relaxation Technique

1. Find a quiet place to sit.
2. Sit in a comfortable position with your feet on the floor, hands relaxed, and eyes closed.
3. Take three slow, deep breaths.
4. Begin to relax your muscles, starting with your toes and progressing upward to your feet and ankles, then lower legs, then upper legs, and so on, until you reach your face and head. Sometimes it is helpful to contract the muscles and then allow them to relax.
5. Breathe through your nose, concentrating on the breath going in and out. As you exhale, say a word in your mind like *calm* or *relax*.
6. Continue to concentrate on your breathing for 10 to 20 minutes. At the end of the time, sit quietly for a few minutes and gradually begin to arouse.

There is no failure in meditation. The benefit comes from maintaining a positive attitude and allowing relaxation to happen and ignoring distracting thoughts by gently pushing them from your mind when they appear.

Research has confirmed a myriad of health benefits associated with the practice of meditation. These include stress reduction, decreased anxiety, decreased depression, reduction in physical and psychological pain, improved memory, and increased efficiency. Physiological benefits include reduced blood pressure, heart rate, lactate, cortisol, and epinephrine; decreased metabolism, breathing pattern, oxygen utilization, and carbon dioxide elimination; and increased melatonin, among others (Sharma, 2015). The only situation in which meditation is considered unsafe is for people with serious mental disorders such as psychosis and schizophrenia. Otherwise, meditation has been determined to be a safe practice for almost everyone.

The 2017 NHIS shows that meditation is used by more often by non-Hispanic Whites than non-Hispanic Blacks and Hispanics (see **Figure 4.9**). Yet the differences were smaller when compared to yoga and chiropractic use (Clarke et al., 2018).

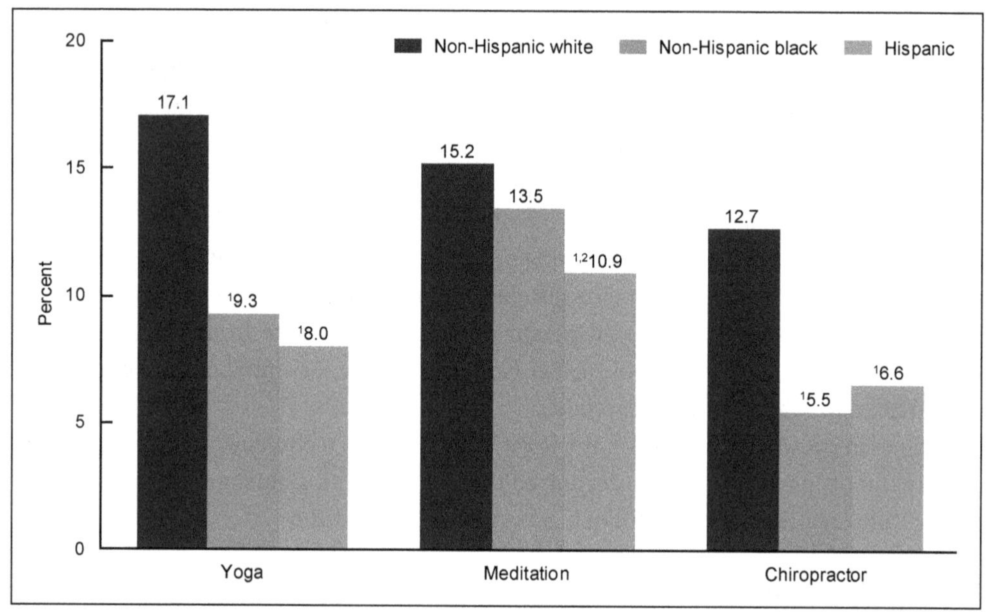

[1]Significantly different from non-Hispanic white adults ($p < 0.05$).
[2]Significantly different from non-Hispanic black adults ($p < 0.05$).
NOTES: Estimates are age adjusted using the projected 2000 U.S. population as the standard population and three age groups: 18–44, 45–64, and 65 and over. Estimates are based on household interviews of a sample of the civilian noninstitutionalized population. Access data table for Figure 4 at: https://www.cdc.gov/nchs/data/databriefs/db325_table-508.pdf#4.
SOURCE: NCHS, National Health Interview Survey, 2017.

Figure 4.9 Yoga, meditation, and chiropractic use by race/ethnicity, 2017.

Laws Affecting Cultural Practices and Health

Many cultures have traditions and practices that involve health and healing. The members of the cultural group are familiar with the healing practices and find them normative. However, those practices often conflict with state and federal laws intended to protect the welfare of the community.

Unlicensed Practices

Every state licenses those who engage in the provision of health care services. Physicians, nurses, pharmacists, dentists, and so on must meet certain state-mandated requirements for education and testing before receiving a license to practice their profession. Again, the state's concern is protecting its citizens from unsafe practitioners. Those who attempt to practice the healing arts without obtaining the requisite license and complying with the licensing laws are prosecuted for the unlicensed practice of the particular profession. Penalties for unlawful practice can be stiff and include both prison time and monetary penalties.

Practitioners of various cultural healing traditions must be aware of and cautious regarding these types of laws. An example of a common area where these laws come in conflict with cultural practices is midwifery. Many cultures have customs regarding childbirth. Those who assist the mother in the delivery must be aware of the state's laws regarding that practice. For many years the practice of midwifery was banned by the great majority of states on the premise propounded by the medical associations that modern medical care during childbirth was safer for the mother and infant. Although those ideas have changed, and many states now sanction the practice of midwifery, the midwife must comply with licensing laws or risk sanctions for the unlawful practice of medicine or nursing. Therefore, traditional practitioners must be informed about both the legal requirements and the liabilities that exist in their practice.

Another area of cultural practice that attracts scrutiny is the use of herbs and other natural products in the treatment of illness or disease. We are all familiar with herbal dietary supplements that are available in practically every store in the country. In ethnic areas of many cities in the United States, shops offer various products common to ethnic or cultural tradition. On the surface it appears that no difference exists between those herb shops and the over-the-counter dietary supplements at the local drug store. However, herbal treatments are often treated differently from dietary supplements.

Ethnic healers and herbalists risk running afoul of licensing laws in the manner in which they apply their healing practices. If the healer is merely making available various herbs or natural products to the public, then they are no different from over-the-counter preparations at the local drug store. However, when the healer begins to evaluate and diagnose symptoms and prescribe treatment, healers are considered to be invading the domain of medical practitioners and become subject to sanctions for unlicensed practice.

For example, Lee Wah was a healer in the ancient Chinese traditions. A patient came to Lee's herb shop, described her ailment to him, and he prescribed certain herbs for the problem. He then chose the herbs and prepared them for her use. Lee was convicted of the unlicensed practice of medicine and was imprisoned (*People v. Lee Wah*, 1886).

Mexican Americans are very familiar with *curanderas*, traditional Mexican healers. *Curanderas* have treated illness in rural areas of Mexico for hundreds of years. It is not unexpected, then, that they should continue those practices in Mexican communities in the United States. However, the licensing laws apply to their practices as well. When a *curandera* visited an ill person in his or her home and prescribed a mixture of rhubarb, soda, glycerin, and spirits of peppermint for the patient's ailment, he or she was found to be in violation of the licensing laws (*People v. Machado*, 1929).

Many states now have licensing or registration requirements for herbal practitioners, and anyone engaging in those activities should consult local and state regulations to determine the rules with which they must comply.

Ethnic Remedies

The remedies utilized by traditional healers are often prepared by the healer or herbalist or are brought to the United States from the native country. These remedies are subject to government oversight and regulation to ensure safety. The FDA is responsible for ensuring the safety of all foods, drugs, and medical devices marketed and distributed in the United States. How the FDA views a particular remedy, and therefore the amount of regulation applicable to it, depends on how that remedy is classified.

Pharmaceutical products are subject to stringent regulation and testing both before and after approval by the FDA for placement on the market. These drugs are researched for mass production and distribution. No traditional ethnic remedy has ever been taken through the rigorous process for FDA approval.

Because traditional folk remedies contain ingredients such as vitamins, minerals, herbs, or other botanicals and substances such as enzymes and glandular and organ tissues, they are more likely to be viewed as dietary supplements and subject to less stringent regulation. The Dietary Supplement Health and Education Act of 1994 (DSHEA) established the FDA's current authority to regulate dietary supplements. A dietary supplement is a product taken by mouth that contains a "dietary ingredient" intended to supplement the diet. Those ingredients often are the very things that were previously noted as the components of ethnic remedies.

According to the DSHEA, a producer is responsible for determining that the dietary supplements it manufactures or distributes are safe and that any representations or claims made about them are substantiated by adequate evidence to show that they are not false or misleading. Dietary supplements do not need approval from the FDA before they are marketed. After a dietary supplement is on the market, the FDA has the responsibility of monitoring its safety and, if found to be unsafe, to take action to remove it from the market. Further, a product may not be sold as a dietary supplement and promoted as a treatment, prevention, or cure for a specific disease or condition. Such an action would be considered the distribution of an illegal drug. Although most ethnic healers would not consider their practices to include marketing a dietary supplement, a traditional healer who provides any type of remedy is technically subject to these regulations and could be held responsible for their violation.

On a more local level, the state and county health departments are responsible for ensuring the health of the local community. It is not unusual for local health departments to investigate traditional healing practitioners for the unauthorized practice of medicine or the provision of remedies as treatments rather than as dietary supplements. For example, health investigators in Houston, Texas, investigated the lead poisoning of siblings where the children had been given a traditional Mexican remedy for stomach ailments that was found to be 90% lead (Rhor, 2008). Certain candy ingredients, such as chili powder and tamarind, may be a source of lead exposure. Lead can get into the candy when drying, storing, and grinding the ingredients are done improperly. Serious consequences for the health and welfare of an unwary population such as this demand government involvement to protect the general welfare.

Summary

This chapter includes descriptions of complementary and alternative health care modalities that are associated with a number of cultures. Many are ancient practices that continue to exist despite the emergence of modern Western medicine. Although research on the efficacy of many of these practices is scarce, their prevalence of use indicates a need for further investigation of the risks and benefits of these practices. People using these modalities and preparing ethnic remedies need to be aware of the laws in the United States to avoid violating them.

Review

1. Describe the advantages and disadvantages of three of the CAM modalities discussed in this chapter.
2. Discuss how meditation could be used in Western health care practice.
3. Describe how the laws in the United States affect CAM practitioners.

Activity

Select a CAM method that interests you. Conduct research on the topic and interview a practitioner in the field. Write a paper explaining what you learned from the research and the interview. Include a list of the questions that you asked the practitioner and his or her responses in the appendix of the paper.

Case Study 1

Some cultural practices used to treat illness produce marks on the body that can mimic abuse. Coining and cupping are two such examples. Coining is a form of dermabrasion commonly used in Southeast Asian cultures to rid the body of "bad winds" by bringing bad blood to the surface (Harris, 2010). The process of coining involves applying ointment to the skin and using a coin or spoon to firmly rub the skin until purple-colored spots and patches appear on the skin. The result is a distinct, symmetrical pattern of bruises typically on the back, shoulders, chest, temples, and forehead that resolve without residual effects (see **Figure 4.10**). Cupping is another cultural practice used to treat illness. Cupping has been practiced by Russian, Asian, and Mexican cultures (Harris, 2010). A heated cup is applied to the skin, which creates suction on the skin, causing bruises that have been mistaken for abuse (see **Figure 4.11**). Both of these practices leave burns or bruises on skin, but they are cultural norms.

1. Are coining and cupping child abuse? Why or why not?
2. When do cultural practices cross over to being abuse?

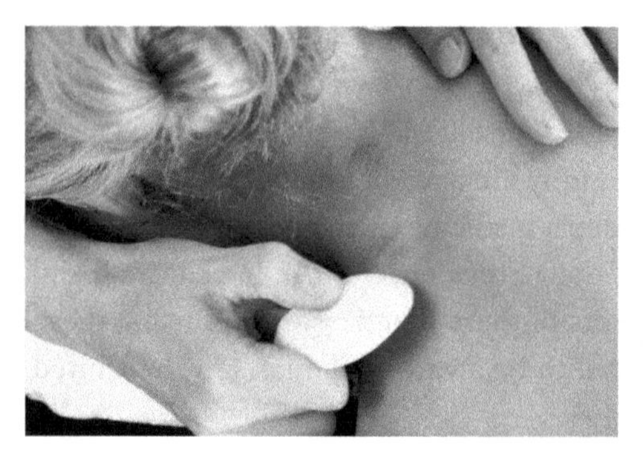

Figure 4.10 Coining.

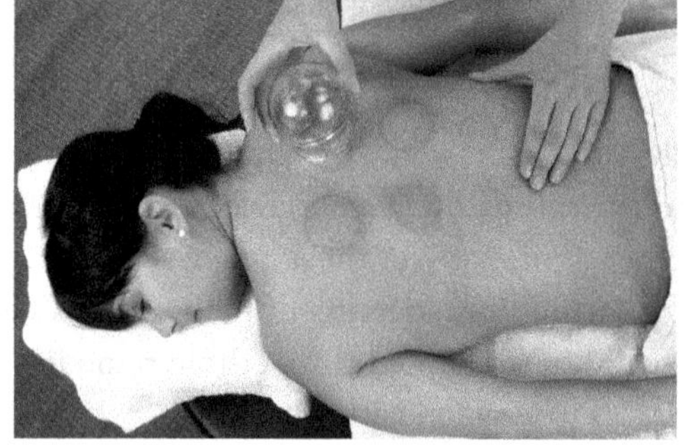

Figure 4.11 Cupping.

Case Study 2

Juan visits the doctor with his wife Luciana. They live in Arizona and return to Columbia a few times a year. Juan has very high cholesterol. The physician informs Juan that his high cholesterol can lead to heart problems. She asked Juan if he is taking his medication. He nods yes. The physician does not understand why the medication is not working. She reviews his medical record and sees that the medication prescription has not been refilled in 9 months. The physician asks Juan what medication he is taking. Juan states that he uses herbs and uses cat's claw in his tea. He smiles and looks at his wife. Cat's claw is used by men as an aphrodisiac.

The physician asks him if he is taking the medication she prescribed. Juan says no. He uses the herbs that his healer in Columbia recommends. The physician is aware that cat's claw is known to interact with the cholesterol medication she has prescribed. Therefore, if she encourages him to take the medication it may not be effective if he continues to consume cat's claw in his tea.

1. How can the physician show Juan the need to take the cholesterol medication that she prescribed?
2. She suspects that he will not want to stop drinking the cat's claw tea. How can she be culturally sensitive yet convey the possibility that the medication should not be used with cat's claw as it will inhibit its effectiveness?

References

American Cancer Society. (2012, March 8). *Reiki*.

Association of Accredited Naturopathic Medical Colleges. (2020). *The six principles of naturopathic medicine*. https://aanmc.org/6-principles/

Bansal, S. (2021, January 11). Study suggests use of medical marijuana might lead to multiple withdrawal symptoms. *Vice*. https://www.vice.com/en/article/4adqkp/medical-marijuana-cannabis-withdrawal-symptoms

Clarke, T. C., Barnes, P. M., Black, L. I., Stussman, B. J., & Nahin, R. L. (2018). *Use of yoga, meditation, and chiropractors among U.S. adults aged 18 and over*. National Center for Health Statistics. https://www.cdc.gov/nchs/data/databriefs/db325-h.pdf

Consumer Healthcare Products Association. (2021). *FAQs about dietary supplements regulations*. https://www.chpa.org/about-consumer-healthcare/faqs/faqs-about-dietary-supplements-regulations

Dahlhamer, J., Lucas, J., Zelaya, C., Nahin, R., Mackey, S., DeBar, L., Kerns, R., Von Korff, M., Porter, L., & Helmick, C. (2018). Prevalence of chronic pain and high-impact chronic pain among adults—United States, 2016. *Morbidity and Mortality Weekly Report, 67*(36), 1001–1006. http://dx.doi.org/10.15585/mmwr.mm6736a2

Freeman, L. (2004). *Complementary and alternative medicine: A research-based approach* (2nd ed.). Mosby.

Harris, T. S. (2010). Bruises in children: Normal or child abuse? *Journal of Pediatric Health Care, 24*(4), 216–221.

Hendel, C. (2015, November 25). *What you need to know about supplements and drug interactions.* Consumer Reports. https://www.consumerreports.org/vitamins-supplements/supplement-and-drug-interactions/

Johns Hopkins Medicine. (2020). *Types of complementary and alternative medicine.* https://www.hopkinsmedicine.org/health/wellness-and-prevention/types-of-complementary-and-alternative-medicine

Johns Hopkins Medicine (2021). *9 benefits of yoga.* https://www.hopkinsmedicine.org/health/wellness-and-prevention/9-benefits-of-yoga

Nahin, R. L., Barnes, P. M., Stussman, B. J., & Bloom, B. (2009). *Costs of complementary and alternative medicine (CAM) and frequency of visits to CAM practitioners: United States, 2007.* National Center for Health Statistics.

National Center for Complementary and Alternative Medicine. (2013). *Ephedra.* http://nccam.nih.gov/health/ephedra

National Center for Complementary and Alternative Medicine. (2021, January 3). *NCCIH 2016 strategic plan.* https://www.nccih.nih.gov/about/nccih-2016-strategic-plan

National Center for Complementary and Integrative Health. (2018, December). *Reiki.* https://www.nccih.nih.gov/health/atoz#linkH

National Center for Complementary and Integrative Health. (2019, October). *Cannabis (marijuana) and cannabinoids: What you need to know.* https://www.nccih.nih.gov/health/cannabis-marijuana-and-cannabinoids-what-you-need-to-know

National Center for Complementary and Integrative Health. (2021, January 10). *Introduction.* https://www.nccih.nih.gov/about/strategic-plans/introduction

People v. Lee Wah, 71 C. 80 (1886)

People v. Machado, 99 CA 702 (1929)

Rhor, M. (2008, January 23). Folk medicines pose poison risk. *San Francisco Chronicle,* p. A8.

Sanford, N. N., Sher, D. J., Ahn, C., Aizer, A. A., & Mahal, B. A. (2019). Prevalence and nondisclosure of complementary and alternative medicine use in patients with cancer and cancer survivors in the United States. *JAMA Oncology, 5*(5), 735–737. https://doi.org/10.1001/jamaoncol.2019.0349

Sharma H. (2015). Meditation: Process and effects. *Ayu, 36*(3), 233–237. https://doi.org/10.4103/0974-8520.182756

University of Maryland. (2011). *Naturopathy.*

White House Commission on Complementary and Alternative Medicine Policy. (2002). *Chapter 10: Recommendations and actions.*

CREDITS

Fig. 4.1: Source: https://www.nccih.nih.gov/about/use-of-complementary-and-integrative-health-approaches-in-the-united-states-2012.

Fig. 4.2: Source: https://www.nccih.nih.gov/about/use-of-complementary-and-integrative-health-approaches-in-the-united-states-2012.

Fig. 4.3: Source: https://www.nccih.nih.gov/about/use-of-complementary-and-integrative-health-approaches-in-the-united-states-2012.

Fig. 4.4: Source: https://www.nccih.nih.gov/about/use-of-complementary-and-integrative-health-approaches-in-the-united-states-2012.

Fig. 4.5: Source: https://www.nccih.nih.gov/research/expenditures-on-complementary-health-approaches-united-states-2012.

Fig. 4.6a: Copyright © 2011 Depositphotos/prezent.

Fig. 4.7: Copyright © 2018 Depositphotos/VectorMine.

IMG 4.1: Copyright © 2015 Depositphotos/Wavebreakmedia.

Fig. 4.8: Copyright © 2015 Depositphotos/DragonImages.

Fig. 4.9: Source: https://www.cdc.gov/nchs/data/databriefs/db325-h.pdf.

Fig. 4.10: Copyright © 2011 Depositphotos/SimpleFoto.

Fig. 4.11: Copyright © 2011 Depositphotos/SimpleFoto.

CHAPTER 5

Public Health

People who are Promotores(as) have a gift for service and a noble and kind heart. We think about things and take care of people. We identify with the people and the needs of the community.

—MIRIAN PEREZ, *PROMOTORA*

There is a push, sometimes—"what's the recipe" or "what are the ten things you have to do in every multicultural community." My experience says that there is a contextualization that needs to happen.

—ZOE CARDOZA CLAYSON

KEY CONCEPTS AND TERMS

Digital divide
Fotonovela
Multicultural evaluation
Promotores
Reciprocity

LEARNING OBJECTIVES

After reading this chapter, you should be able to do the following:

1. Explain at least three ways to deliver health information.
2. Identify at least four issues to consider when developing social media and printed materials.
3. Describe the health belief and PRECEDE–PROCEED models and how they can be utilized when working with diverse populations.
4. Describe at least three differences between traditional evaluation and multicultural evaluation.

In this chapter the focus is on public health and working with diverse communities. The chapter begins with a discussion about health communication, then addresses the delivery of the health message. It ends with a focus on models that can be used for developing a health promotion program and multicultural evaluation. Communication is the basis of any health promotion effort, but in this chapter special attention is paid to considerations that need to be taken into account when working with diverse populations.

Health Communication

Health communication encompasses the study and use of communication strategies to inform and influence individual and community decisions that enhance health. Its importance continues to escalate with the increasing amount of inaccurate information that is available to the public. Health communication can occur on a one-to-one basis or one-to-many. Communication is recognized as a necessary element of efforts to improve personal and public health. Health communication can contribute to all aspects of disease prevention and health promotion and is relevant in a number of contexts, including (a) health professional–patient relations; (b) individuals' exposure to, search for, and use and understanding of health information; (c) individuals' adherence to clinical recommendations and regimens; (d) the construction of public health messages and campaigns; (e) the dissemination of individual and population health risk information (i.e., risk communication); (f) images of health in the mass media and the culture at large; and (g) the education of consumers about how to gain access to the public health and health care systems.

Effective health communication can help raise awareness of health risks and solutions, provide the motivation and skills needed to reduce these risks, help individuals find support from other people in similar situations, and affect or reinforce attitudes. Health communication also can increase demand for appropriate health services and decrease demand for inappropriate health services. It can make information available to assist in making complex choices, such as selecting health plans, care providers, and treatments. For the community, health communication can be used to advocate for policies and programs, promote positive changes in the socioeconomic and physical environments, improve the delivery of public health and health care services, and encourage social norms that benefit health and quality of life. Health communication was contradictory, confusing, and murky during the COVID-19 pandemic. The messaging deepened the mistrust of public health authorities and created feelings of paternalism. Many researchers and experts noted the absence of timely and trustworthy guidelines from authorities and used social media to try and fill the void by communicating their findings directly to the public. Reporters tried to keep the public informed under time and knowledge constraints, which were made more severe by the worsening media landscape. Much of the public messaging focused on offering a series of clear rules to ordinary people, and it did not explain the mechanisms of viral transmission for this pathogen. Fallacies and pitfalls have affected public health messaging, as well as media coverage, and played an immense role in derailing an effective pandemic response (Tufekci, 2021).

Health messages can be shared through public education campaigns that seek to change the social climate to encourage healthy behaviors, create awareness, change attitudes and social norms, and motivate individuals to adopt recommended behaviors. Campaigns traditionally have relied on mass communication (e.g., public service announcements on billboards, radio, and television) and educational messages in printed materials (e.g., pamphlets) to deliver health messages. With advances in technology, newer methods of message delivery now exist, such as text messaging, social media, and podcasts. Many campaigns use social marketing techniques. Social marketing is the systematic application of marketing used to achieve specific behavioral goals for a social good. **Table 5.1** provides a list of attributes of effective health communication.

TABLE 5.1 Attributes of Effective Health Communication

Accuracy: The content is valid and without errors of fact, interpretation, or judgment.
Availability: The content is delivered or placed where the audience can access it. Placement varies according to audience, message complexity, and purpose, ranging from interpersonal and social networks to billboards and mass transit signs to television, radio, social media sites, and websites.
Balance: Where appropriate, the content presents the benefits and risks of potential actions or recognizes different and valid perspectives on the issue.
Consistency: The content remains internally consistent over time and is consistent with information from other sources (the latter is a problem when other widely available content is not accurate or reliable).
Cultural competence: The design, implementation, and evaluation process accounts for special issues for select population groups (e.g., ethnic, racial, and linguistic) and educational levels and disability.
Evidence based: Relevant scientific evidence that has undergone comprehensive review and rigorous analysis to formulate practice guidelines, performance measures, review criteria, and technology assessments for telehealth applications.
Reach: The content gets to or is available to the largest possible number of people in the target population.
Reliability: The source of the content is credible, and the content itself is kept up to date.
Repetition: The delivery of/access to the content is continued or repeated over time, both to reinforce the impact with a given audience and to reach new generations.
Timeliness: The content is provided or available when the audience is most receptive to, or in need of, the specific information.
Understandability: The reading or language level and format (including multimedia) are appropriate for the specific audience.

As stated previously, health improvement activities are taking advantage of digital technologies, such as social media sites, health games, mobile applications, blogs, podcasts, infographics, videos, Twitter, text messaging, and the internet, that can target audiences, tailor messages, and engage people in interactive, ongoing exchanges about health. As a result, a growing area is health communication to support community-centered prevention. Community-centered prevention shifts attention from the individual to group-level change and emphasizes the empowerment of individuals and communities to effect change on multiple levels.

On a community level, the promotion of topics such as regular physical activity, healthy weight, good nutrition, and responsible sexual behavior requires a range of information, education, and advocacy efforts. Public information campaigns are used to promote a variety of health messages such as Text-For-Baby and TRUTH ads.

Health communication alone, however, cannot change systemic problems related to health, such as poverty, environmental degradation, or lack of access to health care. However, comprehensive health communication programs should include a systematic exploration of all the factors that contribute to health and the strategies that could be used to influence these factors. Well-designed health communication activities help individuals better understand their own and their communities' needs so that they can take appropriate actions to maximize health.

The environment for communicating about health has changed significantly. These changes include dramatic increases in the number of communication channels and the number of health issues vying for public attention, as well as consumer demands for more and better quality health information and the increased sophistication of marketing and sales techniques, such as direct-to-consumer advertising of prescription drugs and sales of medical devices and medications over the internet.

The expansion of communication channels and health issues on the public agenda increases competition for people's time and attention; at the same time, people have more opportunities to select information based on their personal interests and preferences. The trend toward commercialization of the internet suggests that the marketing models of other mass media will be applied to emerging media, which has important consequences for the ability of noncommercial and public health–oriented communications to stand out in a cluttered information environment.

Communication occurs in a variety of contexts (e.g., school, home, and work); through a variety of channels (e.g., interpersonal, small group, organizational, community, text messages, and social media) with a variety of messages; and for a variety of reasons. In such an environment, people do not pay attention to all communications they receive but selectively attend to and purposefully seek information. One of the main challenges in the design of effective health communication programs is to identify the optimal contexts, channels, content, and reasons that will motivate people to pay attention to and use health information.

A one-dimensional approach to health promotion, such as reliance on mass media campaigns or other single-component communication activities, has been shown to be insufficient to achieve program goals. Successful health promotion efforts increasingly rely on multidimensional interventions to reach diverse audiences about complex health concerns, and communication is integrated from the beginning with other components, such as community-based programs, policy changes, and improvements in services and the health delivery system. Research shows that health communication best supports health promotion when multiple communication channels are used to reach specific audience segments with information that is appropriate and relevant to them. An important factor in the design of multidimensional programs is to allot sufficient time for planning, implementation, and evaluation and sufficient money to support the many elements of the program. Public–private partnerships and collaborations can leverage resources to strengthen the impact of multidimensional efforts. Collaboration can have the added benefit of reducing message clutter and targeting health concerns that cannot be fully addressed by public resources or market incentives alone.

Research indicates that effective health promotion and communication initiatives adopt an audience-centered perspective, which means that promotion and communication activities reflect audiences' preferred formats, channels, and contexts. These considerations are particularly relevant for racial and ethnic populations, who may have different languages and sources of information. In these cases, public education campaigns must be conceptualized and developed by individuals with specific knowledge of the cultural characteristics, media habits, and language preferences of intended audiences. While designing materials for your target audience, you also do not want to portray an issue as only relevant to part of that group. For example, providing a public message about HIV prevention in which all the photos show one ethnic or racial group could be of limited effectiveness or offensive as HIV affects everyone.

An audience-centered perspective also reflects the realities of people's everyday lives and their current practices, attitudes, beliefs, and lifestyles. Some specific audience characteristics that are relevant include gender, age, education and income levels, ethnicity, sexual orientation, cultural beliefs and values, primary language(s), and physical and mental functioning. Additional considerations include audience experience with the health care system, attitudes toward different types of health problems, and willingness to use certain types of health services. Particular attention should be paid to the needs of underserved audience members.

Targeting specific segments of a population and tailoring messages for individual use are two methods to make health promotion activities relevant to audiences. Examples include the targeted use of mass media messages for adolescent girls at increased risk of smoking, tailoring computer-generated nutritional information to help individuals reduce their fat intake and increase fruit and vegetable consumption, and a text campaign in Spanish to provide pregnant women with health information. In addition, there are new audiences to be aware of when creating public health messages. Examples include those who oppose vaccines, deny science, believe in conspiracy theories, and have political opposition to the government.

Compared to traditional mass media, interactive media may have several advantages for health communication efforts. These advantages include (a) improved access to personalized health information; (b) access to health information, support, and services on demand; (c) enhanced ability to distribute materials widely and update content or functions rapidly; (d) just-in-time expert decision support; and (e) more choices for consumers. The health impact of interactivity, customization, and enhanced multimedia is just beginning to be explored, and interactive health communication technologies are already being used to exchange information, facilitate informed decision-making, promote healthy behaviors, enhance peer and emotional support, promote self-care, manage demand for health services, and support clinical care.

Widespread availability and use of interactive health communication create at least two serious challenges. One is related to the risks associated with consumers' use of poor-quality health information to make decisions. Concerns are growing about the internet and social media making available large amounts of information that may be misleading, inaccurate, or inappropriate, which may put consumers at unnecessary risk. Although many health professionals agree that the technology is a boon for consumers, because they have easier access to much more information than before, professionals are also concerned that poor-quality information will undermine informed decision-making. These concerns are driving the development of a quality standards agenda to help health professionals and consumers find reliable health information.

The other challenge is related to the protection of privacy and confidentiality of personal health information, which are major issues for consumers, and these concerns are magnified when information is collected, stored, and made available online. As the availability and variety of interactive health applications grow, consumer confidence about developers' ability or intent to ensure privacy is concerning. The internet is awash with personal health information shared on social media and recorded on health and fitness apps.

With the rapidly growing volume of health information, advertising, products, and services available on web and social media sites, serious concerns arise regarding the accuracy, appropriateness, and potential health impact of these sites. People are using the internet to look up information, purchase medications, consult remotely with providers, and maintain their personal health records. The potential for harm from inaccurate information, inferior quality goods, and inappropriate services is significant. Many initiatives are under way to identify appropriate and feasible approaches to evaluate online health sites. Professional associations are issuing guidelines and recommendations. Federal agencies, such as the Federal Trade Commission, are actively monitoring and sanctioning owners of websites that are false or misleading, and developers and purchasers of online health resources are being urged to adopt standards for quality assurance.

To allow users to evaluate the quality and appropriateness of internet health resources, health-related sites should publicly disclose the following essential information: (a) the identity of the developers and sponsors of the site (and how to contact them) and information about any potential conflicts of interest or biases; (b) the explicit purpose of the site, including any commercial purposes and advertising; (c) the original sources of the content on the site; (d) how the privacy and confidentiality of any personal information collected from users is protected; (e) how the site is evaluated; and (f) how the content is updated. An additional mark of quality relates to the site's accessibility by all users.

Content should be presented in a way that it can be used by people with disabilities and low-end technology.

Culture affects how people perceive and respond to health messages and materials, and it is related to how health behaviors and materials convey culture. Although it is important to acknowledge and understand the cultures within an intended audience, developing separate messages and materials for each cultural group is not necessary or even advisable. For example, when print materials for a state program for low-income people depicted people of only one race, some intended audience members felt singled out and said the materials suggested that only members of their racial group were poor. Careful audience research can help your program identify messages and images that resonate across groups or identify situations in which different messages or images are likely to work best.

That being said, it does not mean that culture should be ignored. Culturally sensitive communications:

1. Acknowledge culture as a predominant force in shaping behaviors, values, and institutions.
2. Understand and reflect the diversity within cultures. In designing messages that are culturally appropriate, the following dimensions are important:
    - *Primary cultural factors* linked to race, ethnicity, language, nationality, and religion
    - *Secondary cultural factors* linked to age, gender, sexual orientation, educational level, occupation, income level, and acculturation to mainstream society
3. Reflect and respect the attitudes and values of the intended audience; some examples of attitudes and values that are interrelated to culture include:
    - Whether the individual or the community is of primary importance
    - Accepted roles of men, women, and children
    - Preferred family structure (nuclear or extended)
    - Relative importance of folk wisdom, life experience, and value of common sense compared to formal-education-specific situations and advanced degrees
    - Ways that wealth is measured (material goods, personal relationships)
    - Relative value put on different age groups (youth versus elders)
    - Whether people are more comfortable with traditions or open to new ways
    - Favorite and forbidden foods
    - Body language, particularly whether touching or proximity is permitted in specific situations
    - Manner of dress and adornment

4. Refer to cultural groups using terms that members of the group prefer (e.g., many people resent the term "minority" or "nonwhite." Preferred terms are often based on nationality, such as Japanese or Lakota).
5. Substituting culturally specific images, spokespeople, language, or other executional detail is not sufficient unless the messages have been tested and found to resonate with the intended audience.
6. Use the language of the intended audience, carefully developed and tested with the involvement of the audience. (Nursing Paper Slayers, n.d.)

You may have a message that you want to target to a particular cultural group in which you need to take specific cultural factors into consideration. For example, if you have developed a suicide prevention hotline for Asian Americans that provides services in a variety of Asian languages, you would not want the hotline number to contain a number that means death in any of the Asian cultures. Colors also have a wide variety of meanings in different cultures, so do your research. Also, some cultures do not respond well to health messages that try to induce change through fear, so be cautious of the images that you use. Some cultures, such as African Americans, tend to distrust the government, so you need to think about who is delivering the message and how. Of course, be sure to deliver your message at the appropriate language(s) and literacy levels.

Health Literacy

The definition of health literacy includes personal and organizational health literacy:

- **Personal health literacy** is the degree to which individuals have the ability to find, understand, and use information and services to inform health-related decisions and actions for themselves and others.
- **Organizational health literacy** is the degree to which organizations equitably enable individuals to find, understand, and use information and services to inform health-related decisions and actions for themselves and others (CDC, 2021).

Even with access to information and services, disparities still exist because many people lack health literacy, which is increasingly vital to help people navigate a complex health care system and better manage their own health. Health literacy is a key issue in the Health Care Access and Quality domain in *Healthy People 2030*. The Office of Disease Prevention and Health Promotion (2020) defines health literacy as "the degree to which individuals have the capacity to obtain, process, and understand basic health information needed to make appropriate health decisions." The capacity to obtain and process information is important to individual health literacy. For instance, the spotty and sometimes absence of COVID-19 vaccine appointment information led many people to complain and become confused and frustrated with the inability of many health care providers to provide accurate and timely appointment information. The resulting perceived futility of trying individually to follow through on the public health messaging that everyone should be vaccinated led to new access programs being included in the $1.9 trillion 2021 American Rescue Plan Act. A new single website and a single 800 number were approved to facilitate access to decentralized information and access by people without internet.

Low health literacy is more prevalent among

- older adults,
- minority populations,
- those who have low socioeconomic status, and
- medically underserved people (Health Resources and Service Administration [HRSA], 2019).

Differences in the ability to read and understand materials related to personal health and knowing how to navigate the health system contribute to health disparities. People with low health literacy are more likely to report poor health, have an incomplete understanding of their health problems and treatment, and be at greater risk of hospitalization. People with chronic conditions, such as asthma, hypertension, and diabetes, and with low reading skills, have been found to have less knowledge of their conditions than people with higher reading skills.

To complicate the issue is the fact that health care has a language of its own. There is certainly no shortage of acronyms and complex medical terms. In addition, how words are used can be a cause of communication errors. For example, to say that someone has tested positive for cancer may be interpreted as good news to even someone whose first language is English. After all, positive means good, right?

Adequate health literacy may include being able to read and comprehend essential health-related materials (e.g., prescription bottles, appointment slips, etc.). It may increase a person's capacity to take responsibility for their health and their family's health and to navigate the complex health care system.

Approximately 80 million or greater than 30% of adults in the United States are thought to have limited health literacy (Hersh et al., 2015). Even people with strong literacy skills may have trouble obtaining, understanding, and using complex health information.

Some of the greatest disparities in health literacy occur among racial and ethnic minority groups from different cultural backgrounds and those who do not speak English as a first language. Recent health literacy data is sparse. Results from the National Assessment of Adult Literacy demonstrated that Hispanic adults have the lowest average health literacy scores of all racial/ethnic groups, followed by Black and then American Indian/ Alaska Native adults (Kutner et al., 2006). People with low health literacy and limited English proficiency are twice as likely as individuals without these barriers to report poor health status (Sentell & Braun, 2012). According to the Agency for Healthcare Research and Quality (AHRQ), low health literacy is linked to higher risk of death and more emergency room visits and hospitalizations. Health literacy may not be related to years of education or general reading ability. A person who functions adequately at home or work may have marginal or inadequate literacy in a health care environment (National Network of Libraries of Medicine, 2014).

The National Assessment of Adult Literacy (NAAL) measures the health literacy of adults living in the United States. Health literacy was reported using four performance levels: below basic, basic, intermediate, and proficient. According to the NAAL, approximately 36% of adults in the United States have limited health literacy: 22% have basic and 14% have below basic. An additional 5% of the population is not literate in English. Only 12% of the population has a proficient health literacy level (National Network of Libraries of Medicine, 2014).

Here are some tips for working with people with low literacy:

- Speak slowly and clearly, not loudly.
- Repeat if necessary. Make it clear at the outset that you are happy to repeat anything you say in conversation.
- Avoid acronyms, idioms, and abbreviations. The medical culture has a language of its own that includes many acronyms such as ED, HMO, and NPO. Take the time to say words the long way and avoid terms that will create confusion for nonnative speakers. It is best when setting appointments to say "eight o'clock in the morning" instead of "8 a.m." Common expressions and idioms also can block communication. If you say "I'll run that past the doctor," a patient with limited English proficiency may literally picture you running to the doctor, which sounds urgent when you intended a casual tone.
- Write it down and demonstrate while speaking. Providing simple notes about the key points of an office visit and expectations for patient follow-up can be very useful to patients and families with limited English proficiency. Written material with more detailed information about medications and treatments also can be very helpful. Checking for understanding via open-ended questions, gesturing while speaking, and demonstrating actions is recommended. Instead of explaining how a topical medication is applied, the health professional can demonstrate how it is done (Carteret, 2012).

For health communication to contribute to the improvement of personal and community health stakeholders, health professionals, researchers, public officials, and the lay public must collaborate on a range of activities. These activities include (a) initiatives to build a robust health information system that provides equitable access; (b) development of high-quality, audience-appropriate information and support services for specific health problems and health-related decisions for all segments of the population, especially for underserved segments; (c) training health professionals in the science of communication and the use of communication technologies; (d) evaluation of interventions; and (e) promotion of a critical understanding and practice of effective health communication.

Closing the gap in health literacy is an issue of fundamental fairness and equity and is essential to reduce health disparities. Public and private efforts need to occur in two areas: the development of appropriate written materials and improvement in skills of those persons with limited literacy. Effective, culturally and linguistically appropriate, plain language health communications can be created. Professional publications and federal documents provide the criteria to integrate and apply the principles of organization, writing style, layout, and design for effective communication. These criteria should be widely distributed and used. Many organizations, such as public and medical libraries; voluntary, professional, and community groups; and schools could offer health literacy programs that target skill improvement for low-literacy and limited-English proficient individuals. If appropriate materials exist and people receive the training to use them, measurable improvements in health literacy for the least literate can occur.

Delivering Your Health Message

There are many ways to deliver your health message. Some methods have been shown to work better with specific cultures. For example, *promotores(as)* programs often are successful with the Hispanic population, and ethnic newspapers work well with older Asian Americans. It is important to look for model programs (also known as promising practices) when designing your implementation strategy. Two interventions you may not be familiar with that have been shown to be popular among certain groups are presented in the following sections, but first we discuss social media communication and printed materials.

Social Media

You will want to select the correct social media platforms for your target audience. For younger target groups you may want to use Instagram and Facebook and for older groups use Facebook only. It is important to review data about technology use among your target audience to assist with using the proper channel. As shown in **Figure 5.1**, social media use varies by geography, age, race and ethnicity, as well as gender. The channel you select may require different messaging, and multiple platforms may be needed to reach your target population.

In addition, you want to design your social media messages to be inclusive. Inclusive design is a "design that considers the full range of human diversity with respect to ability, language, culture, gender, age and other forms of human difference" (Inclusive Design Research Centre, n.d.). Without inclusive design you miss the opportunity to reach out to everyone and to provide interventions ethically.

While we will not go into this topic extensively here, a few items to think about are highlighted:

1. Think about color. Some people are color-blind, so you want to avoid some colors and color combinations.

% of U.S. adults in each demographic group who say they ever use ...

	Facebook	**Instagram**	**Linkedin**
Total	69%	40%	28%
Men	61%	36%	31%
Women	77%	44%	26%
Ages 18–29	70%	71%	30%
30–49	77%	48%	36%
50–64	73%	29%	33%
65+	50%	13%	11%
White	67%	35%	29%
Black	74%	49%	27%
Hispanic	72%	52%	19%
Less than $30K	70%	35%	12%
$30K–$49,999	76%	45%	21%
$50K–$74,999	61%	39%	21%
More than $75K	70%	47%	50%
High school or less	64%	30%	10%
Some college	71%	44%	28%
College graduate	73%	49%	51%
Urban	70%	45%	30%
Suburban	70%	41%	33%
Rural	67%	25%	15%

Note: Respondents who did not give an answer are not shown. White and Black adults include those who report being only one race and are not Hispanic. Hispanics are of any race.
Source: Survey of U.S. adults conducted Jan. 25-Feb. 8, 2021.
PEW RESEARCH CENTER

Figure 5.1 Social media use.

2. Video. Several social platforms have made accessibility updates to include video captioning. Automatic captioning is available on Facebook Live and Instagram IGTV. You will want to check if your communication channel preference has captioning available. Transcribing videos and posting the transcriptions also in encouraged.

3. Text. Items to consider include font type, size, literacy, and language, among other issues. Alt-image description fields are now available on some social media sites. Alt-image description fields, "alt tags," are the written text that appears in place of an image on a webpage if the image fails to load on a user's screen. This text helps screen-reading tools describe images to visually impaired readers. Lastly, you will want to consider the font type, as some work better than others for people with dyslexia.

Printed Materials

Printed materials can be created in numerous forms, including newsletters, booklets, pamphlets, flyers, and newspapers. They can be placed on billboards, bathroom walls, and buses, or they can be inserted in envelopes with paychecks. Regardless of where they are, be sure your message is appropriate for your target audience.

You need to consider literacy levels. You can check the literacy level by using the Fry readability graph (see **Figure 5.2**) or the Flesch-Kincaid grade level score, which is built into Microsoft Word.

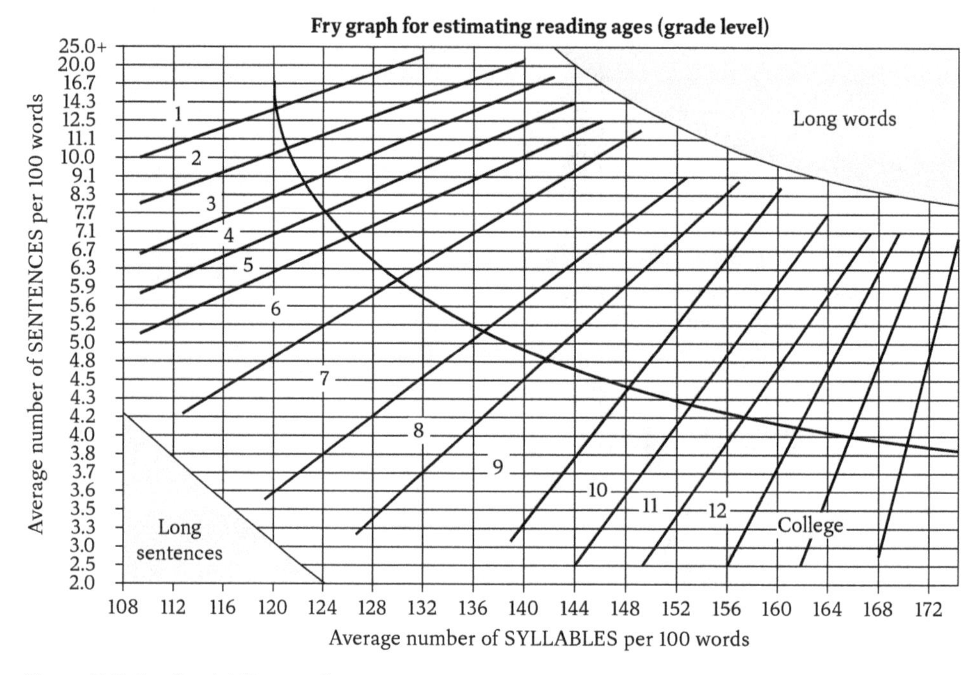

Figure 5.2 Fry Readability graph.

Pizcando Sueños
Un Camino Poblado de Sueños
La Otra Cara del Amor
La Otra Cara del Amor
¡Ay!, ya despierta mujer. Amása los tamales.
¡Cuánto le gustaban los tamales!...Pedro Luis...
¡Ay, mami! ¿no estás pensando en mi padre otra vez? ¡Mejor piensa en otra cosa!
Las cosas son diferentes ahora tía. Hablemos de otra cosa por favor.

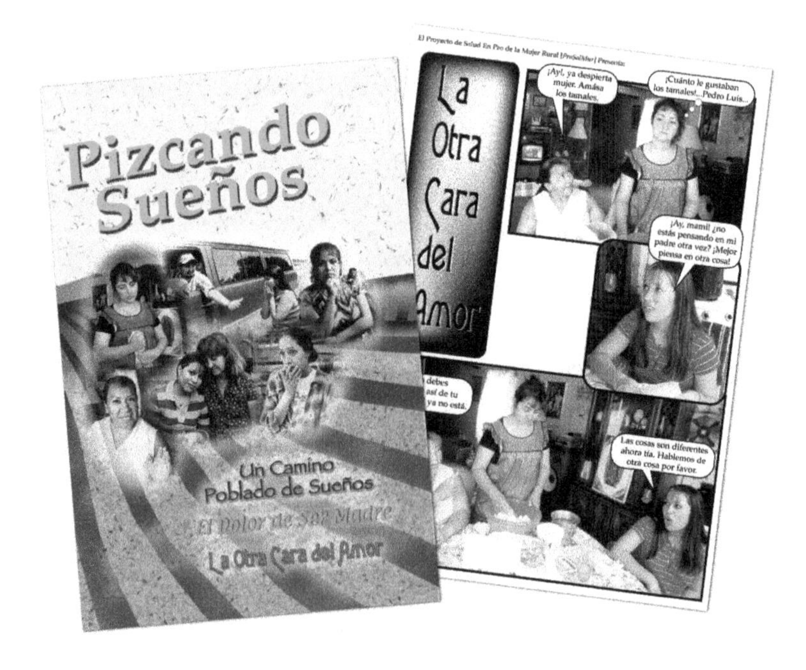

Image 5.1

Fry Readability Graph

Follow these directions for using the Fry readability graph:

- Randomly select three 100-word passages from a book or an article.
- Plot the average number of syllables and the average number of sentences per 100 words on the graph to determine the grade level of the material.
- Choose more passages per book if great variability is observed and conclude that the book has uneven readability.
- Few books will fall into the solid black area, but when they do, grade-level scores are invalid.

Promotores

Promotores and *promotoras* are community members who promote health in their own communities. They provide leadership, peer education, and resources to support community empowerment. As members of minority and underserved populations, they are in a unique position to build on strengths and to address unmet health needs in their communities. *Promotores(as)* integrate information about health and the health care system into the community's culture, language, and value system, thus reducing many of the barriers to health services. They provide peer education, support, and links to services. They also help make health care systems more responsive. With the appropriate resources, training, and support, *promotores(as)* improve the health of their communities by linking their neighbors to health care and social services, by educating their peers about disease and injury prevention, by working to make available services more accessible, and by mobilizing their communities to create positive change.

Organizations may refer to *promotores(as)* as *promotores(as) de salud*, which literally means "health promoters." In English, most *promotores(as)* call themselves community health workers.

Promotores(as) conduct outreach in clients' homes and at community centers, clinics, hospitals, schools, work sites, shelters, and farmworker labor camps. Many *promotor* programs focus on serving the needs of specific ethnic or racial groups, and others focus on vulnerable segments of the population or prominent health problems. *Promotores(as)* engage in a broad range of activities, but they share a number of common roles by providing the following:

- A link between communities and health and human service agencies
- Informal counseling and support
- Culturally competent health education
- Advocacy
- First aid and emergency assistance translation services

Promotores(as) effectively address many barriers to better health for underserved populations. Some of their accomplishments include the following:

- Helping people understand and access the health and social service system
- Enhancing client and health provider communication
- Encouraging people to make and keep doctor's appointments
- Decreasing costs for organizations and government programs
- Improving adherence to health recommendations
- Reducing the need for emergency and specialty services
- Improving overall community health status
- Building community capacity

Promotores programs have partnered with community members to address issues related to affordable housing, improving health services, equal education opportunities, neighborhood safety, access to healthy foods, and combatting discrimination. ***Fotonovelas*** are imaged-based interventions that are popular among Mexicans and Latin Americans. *Fotonovelas* are illustrated with photos, and these comic books with complex perspectives and dark imagery have had a long history and a far-reaching impact within the Latino communities in the United States as well as Mexico and Latin America, where they continue to thrive in the popular culture (Independent Television Service, 2020).

In the United States, the *fotonovela/historieta* has a distinct manifestation in the Latino community, providing a unique idiom through which the community addresses social concerns using a highly innovative visual language (Independent Television Service, 2020). Because of its popularity and flexibility, the *fotonovela* has been used in increasingly fresh ways by visual artists and writers to address important social issues within the Latino community (Independent Television Service, 2020). Activists and religious groups also have turned to the form as an organizational tool for outreach and education, and to induce someone to convert to their own religious faith or political party. *Fotonovelas* are becoming more commonly used in public health as a way of delivering health information in a more creative manner. A representative from the Rural Women's Health Project (RWHP, n.d.) stated,

> RWHP fotonovelas reflect the struggles of communities in a positive light, incorporating role models who balance socio-cultural obstacles and disease prevention. The visual aspects of the novela are enticing and the style allows the reader to explore the health topics, increase self-identification and risk, and strengthen cultural identity.

According to RWHP, the organization utilizes community actors and messages specific to the target community, and the *fotonovelas* successfully present health messages, document the work of communities, and unify them to both improve individual and community well-being. "The minimal text, popular language, and visuals of the fotonovelas allow them to be easily read by any community. These elements make fotonovelas an excellent educational tool for outreach workers, youth, and discussion groups" (RWHP, n.d.).

Después de la misa...
¡Hola, prima!
¿Qué pasó Marta? No fuiste a la fiesta de Noelito.
¡Ay Socorro!, tuve un susto la semana pasada y he estado un poco distraída por eso.
El Susto de Marta
Vamos a mi casa y platicamos, prima.
¡Está bien!
Mi madre es mi ejemplo. Ella me enseñó desde la pubertad cómo hacerme el auto-examen del seno.
Amiga, tienes que hacer tu parte...
Lo Que Dicen Mis Amigas Sobre El Cáncer Del Seno

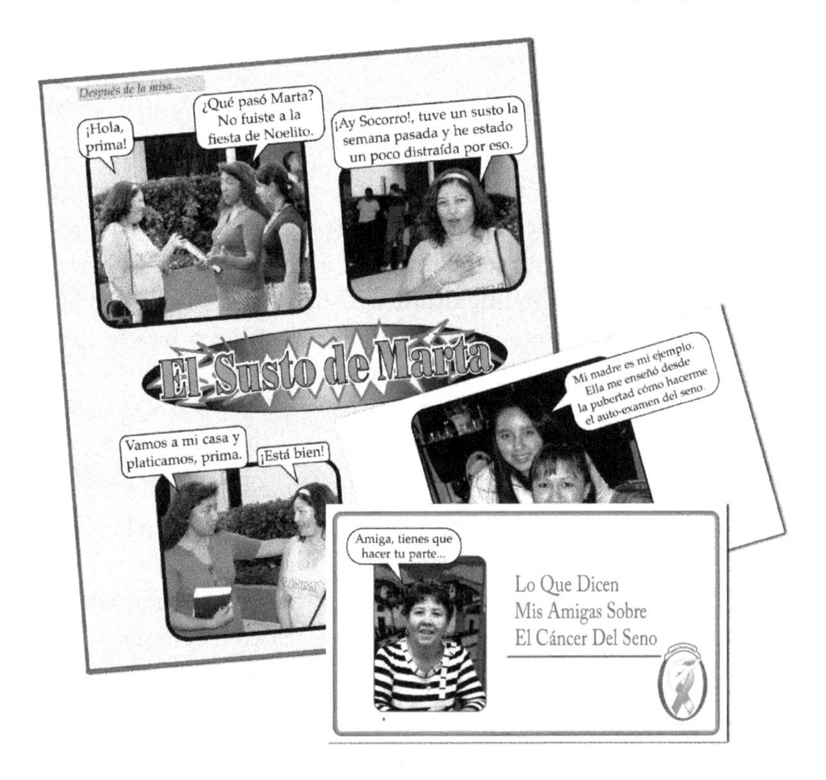

Image 5.2

WHAT DO YOU THINK?

What are some communication methods that would work well with your culture? What images or phrases do you suggest? What communication channels would work well? Why would you recommend these? What methods, images, phrases, or channels would not work well and why?

Public Health Programs

Public health efforts focus on health promotion and disease and injury prevention through research, community intervention, and education. To accomplish these goals, health promotion activities need to be delivered within a cultural context. One-size-fits-all health promotion programs fail to take into consideration that there are unique ideals and goals regarding health and various ways to initiate health behavior change. Health education and promotion programs for diverse populations are challenging, but to be successful, the cultural dimensions of the target audience must be considered.

Interventions for promoting health and disease prevention in any population require systematic planning. This organized effort requires an understanding of the culture of the target audience, because culture is a strong force in the determinants of health and behavior change. Although the overall steps to program development are the same, distinct factors need to be taken into consideration when your audience is diverse. Planning models can be useful in this process.

Planning Models

Models and theories are planning tools that assist with understanding the causes of behaviors, predicting behaviors, and evaluating programs. Models are the starting place on which to build, and they can serve different purposes, which is why so many models exist. Promoting health in a multicultural setting requires using models that take the cultural context into consideration. Two planning models are briefly described here: the health belief model and the PRECEDE–PROCEED model.

Health Belief Model

The health belief model (HBM) is a psychological model that attempts to explain and predict health behaviors by focusing on the attitudes and beliefs of individuals. The HBM was developed in the 1950s as part of an effort by social psychologists in the U.S. Public Health Service to explain the lack of public participation in health screening and prevention programs (e.g., a free and conveniently located tuberculosis screening project). Their focus was on increasing the use of preventive services, such as chest X-rays for tuberculosis screening and immunizations.

The developers assumed that people feared diseases and that health actions were motivated in relation to the degree of fear (perceived threat). If the potential benefits outweighed practical and psychological obstacles to taking action (net benefits), they expected that action would occur. The HBM was one of the first models that adapted theory from the behavioral sciences to health problems, and it remains one of the most widely recognized conceptual frameworks of health behavior. The HBM has been adapted to explore a variety of long- and short-term health behaviors, including sexual risk behaviors and the transmission of HIV. The key variables of the HBM are given in **Figure 5.3**.

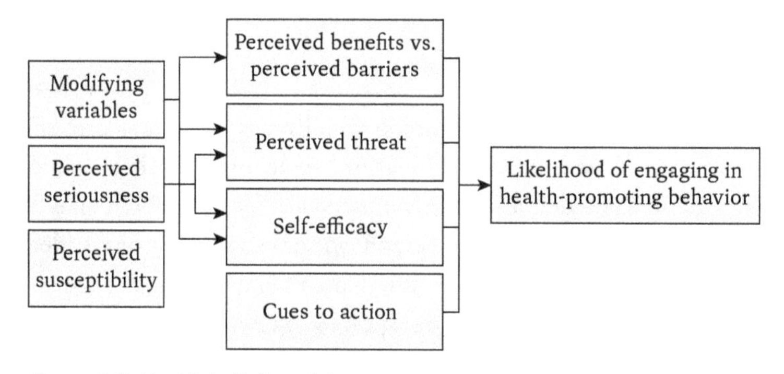

Figure 5.3 Health belief model.

It is important to note that a wide variety of demographic (i.e., age, gender, ethnicity, race), social and psychological (i.e., personality, social status, group pressure), and structural (i.e., prior experience with the disease, knowledge about the health condition) variables may also influence people's perceptions and have an impact on their health behaviors. Ways that these constructs can be applied are described in **Table 5.2**.

TABLE 5.2 Applications of the Health Belief Model

Concept	Definition	Application
Perceived threat	Consists of two parts: perceived susceptibility and perceived severity of a health condition	Explain how anyone can contract the disease and how easily it is spread.
Perceived susceptibility	One's opinion of chances of getting a condition	Define population(s) at risk and the degree of risk. Personalize risk based on a person's features or behavior. Heighten perceived susceptibility if it is too low.
Perceived severity	One's opinion of how serious a condition and the condition that follows as a result of the disease	Explain the consequences of the risk and the condition.
Perceived benefits	One's opinion of the benefits of the action to reduce risk or seriousness of impact	Clarify the positive effects to be expected from the behavior change.
Perceived barriers	One's opinion of the tangible and psychological costs of the advised action	Identify and reduce barriers through reassurance, incentives, education, and assistance.
Cues to action	Strategies to activate change	Provide how-to information, promote awareness, initiate media campaigns, write a newspaper or magazine article, provide reminders such as a postcard from a dentist or physician, obtain a friend's or family member's recommendation.
Self-efficacy	Confidence in one's ability to take action	Provide training, guidance in performing action, and role modeling.

Source: Adapted from National Cancer Institute, "Theory at a Glance: A Guide for Health Promotion Practice," 2003.

The HBM can be applied to multicultural health in several ways. For example, if a person has a fatalistic perception of how disease develops, the program planner should work with that ideology because that person's idea about perceived susceptibility would be very different from that of a person with a Western perspective.

PRECEDE–PROCEED Framework

The PRECEDE-PROCEED framework, illustrated in **Figure 5.4**, is an approach to planning that examines the factors that contribute to behavior change. PRECEDE is an acronym for **pre**disposing, **r**einforcing, and **e**nabling **c**onstructs in **e**ducational/**e**cological **d**iagnosis and **e**valuation, and PROCEED is an acronym for **po**licy, **r**egulatory, and **o**rganizational **c**onstructs in **e**ducational and **e**nvironmental **d**evelopment (McKenzie et al., 2009).

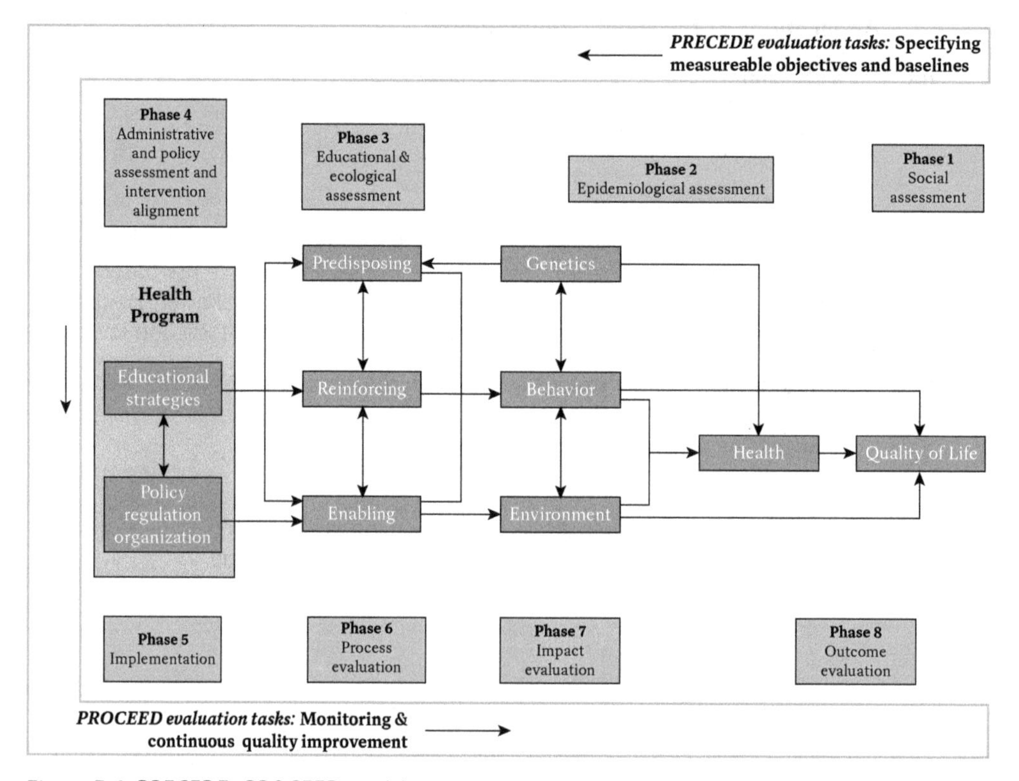

Figure 5.4 PRECEDE–PROCEED model.

The factors that contribute to behavior change are described as follows:

- *Predisposing factors.* The individual's knowledge, attitudes, behavior, beliefs, and values before the intervention that affect their willingness to change
- *Enabling factors.* Factors in the environment or community of an individual that facilitate change
- *Reinforcing factors.* The positive or negative effects of adopting the behavior that influence continuing the behavior

The PRECEDE part of the model entails the planning steps that should occur prior to the intervention, and the PROCEED component includes the phases that should occur during and after the intervention.

Evaluating Your Multicultural Health Program

Effective program evaluation is a systematic way to improve and account for public health actions by involving procedures that are useful, feasible, ethical, and accurate. The CDC (2017) developed a framework to guide public health professionals in using program evaluations. It is a practical, nonprescriptive tool designed to summarize and organize the essential elements of effective program evaluation (see **Figure 5.5**).

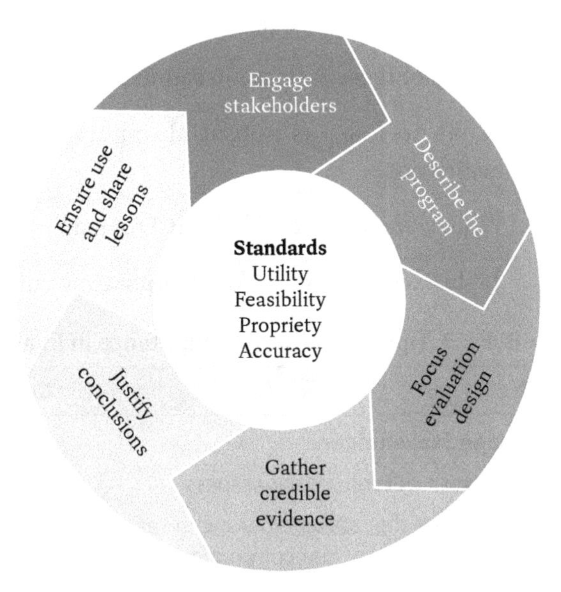

Figure 5.5 Recommended framework for program evaluation.

The framework is composed of six steps that must be taken in any evaluation. They are starting points for tailoring an evaluation to a particular public health effort at a particular time. Because the steps are all interdependent, they might be encountered in a nonlinear sequence; however, an order exists for fulfilling each—earlier steps provide the foundation for subsequent progress (see **Figure 5.5**).

Evaluation is a large subject and will not be covered in detail here because there are many other resources on the topic. The focus of this section is on illuminating the differences between traditional evaluation and **multicultural evaluation** and presenting strategies for making your program evaluation sensitive to diverse populations.

Multicultural evaluation integrates cultural considerations into its theory, measures, analysis, and practice. It requires a conceptual framework that incorporates different worldviews and value systems, engages in data collection strategies that take into account potential cultural and linguistic barriers, includes a reexamination of established evaluation measures for cultural appropriateness, and incorporates creative strategies for ensuring culturally competent analysis and creative dissemination of findings to diverse audiences. Multicultural evaluation, like traditional evaluation, prioritizes impartial inquiry designed to provide information to decision-makers and other parties interested in a particular program, policy, or intervention.

The CDC developed tips and guiding questions aligned with the six steps of CDC's framework for program evaluation in public health. The self-reflection questions for evaluators were developed to help explore your own identity:

1. Where am I from (nationality, region, and heritage)?
2. What are my beliefs, values, and religious and political orientation?
3. What is my biological sex and gender identity?

4. What is my age group?
5. What is my social class?
6. Which of these factors are significant to me?
7. What do I see as potential opportunities, challenges, or conflicts for this evaluation?
8. What stereotypes do I hold? (CDC, n.d.).

Table 5.3 contains tips for incorporating culture into evaluation.

TABLE 5.3 Tips for Cultural Competence in Evaluation

Tips	Guiding Questions
Engage Stakeholders • Assess cultural self-awareness. • Request that stakeholders who reflect the diversity of the community be included throughout the evaluation. • Lay clear ground rules for participation to establish equality. • Build trust by talking openly with the community about the evaluation.	• Does the stakeholder group fully represent the diversity of the program's participants and others affected by the program? • Are meaningful roles planned for stakeholders throughout the evaluation? • Is there a distribution of power among stakeholders? To other distinctions related to status and social class? • Are there multiple voices in planning, implementing, interpreting, and decision-making?
Describe the Program • Conduct key informant interviews to clarify stakeholders' perspectives of the program. • Hold an information-gathering session for stakeholders about the social and historical context of the program. • Use models that resonate with the community.	• Are stakeholders' perspectives appropriately reflected? • What is known about the strengths, assets, challenges, and barriers of the community, including the talents and expertise that individual community members or organizations bring? • Are there "gatekeepers of knowledge" within the community that can help describe the social and political context of the program/community?
Focus the Evaluation Design • Engage an experienced facilitator familiar with the community who can guide the development of evaluation questions that reflect stakeholders' values. • Develop a visual chart that describes evaluation design options in such a way that all stakeholders understand the choices and the implications.	• What/whose values and perspectives are represented in the evaluation questions? • Is the design appropriate to the evaluation questions as well as the cultural context and values of the community? • Is the evidence considered credible by the community and stakeholders?

(continued)

TABLE 5.3 Tips for Cultural Competence in Evaluation (*Continued*)

Tips	Guiding Questions
Gather Credible Evidence • Select culturally appropriate data collection instruments. • Develop data collection methods that factor in cultural and linguistic distinctions. • Adapt data collection processes to the stakeholder context.	• Whose perspectives are accepted as credible evidence? Credible to whom? • Are the language, content, and design of the instruments culturally sensitive? Have the instruments been validated with their intended audiences? • Have verbal and nonverbal communication been addressed?
Justify Conclusions • Prior to developing final conclusions, discuss cultural implications during data analysis. • Involve diverse stakeholders in interpreting data. • Ensure that many stakeholders' voices are heard when making judgments.	• How are different stakeholders' perspectives and values addressed in the analysis and interpretation of the evaluation findings? Are conclusions validated by participants? • Are conclusions balanced with culturally appropriate recommendations and community capacity? • Are findings meaningful to the group or community of interest?
Ensure Use and Share Lessons Learned • Generate recommendations through an inclusive process by providing a role for various stakeholders to implement the evaluation findings. • Tailor dissemination of evaluation results to stakeholder needs. • Encourage the use of evaluation information by holding an inclusive meeting about developing an action plan for evaluation use.	• Are communication mechanisms culturally appropriate? • Does the reporting method meet stakeholder needs (both the message and the messenger)? • Are the data presented in context, with efforts made to clarify issues and prevent misuse? • Has the community benefited as anticipated? How?

Source: Centers for Disease Control and Prevention, Excerpt from "Program Evaluation Tip Sheet: Integrating Cultural Competence into Evaluation."

Multicultural evaluation is built from core elements of sound evaluation practices, such as data-based inquiry, valid and reliable measures, and impartial assessment. When the principles of multicultural evaluation are applied to all aspects of evaluation—from the evaluator to design and planning, to data collection, analysis, reporting, and application of findings—the result is a significant shift in how evaluation is implemented. The characteristics of a multicultural evaluation are shown in **Table 5.4**.

Traditional evaluation is based on a long history in which formally trained evaluators implement needs or impact assessments based on established measures of what is good practice. Multicultural evaluation is characterized by **reciprocity**. Evaluators

TABLE 5.4 Characteristics of a Multicultural Evaluation

	Traditional Evaluation	→	Multicultural Evaluation
Evaluator			
Where knowledge resides	Formally trained evaluators are the experts	→	Grantees, community members, and formally trained evaluators each have expertise. Each knows best their issues and strengths.
Evaluator role	Leader, judge, expert	→	Facilitator, translator, convener.
Design and planning	Evaluator presents design to commissioning entity for approval	→	Prioritizes developing rapport and trust with stakeholders to engage them in an inclusive planning process that infuses multiple worldviews.
Data collection	Conducted by evaluation professional	→	Conducted by all players. Facilitated by the evaluator; stakeholders are often trained in some collection methods and then implement them.
Data analysis	Results and their meaning are analyzed by evaluation professionals	→	Results and their meaning are derived with a focus on culture and system analysis.
Reporting	Written report, usually accompanied by brief presentation to commissioning entity	→	Jointly disseminated and presented in nontraditional formats. Results have relevance and utility to diverse communities.
Application of findings	Findings used as monitoring, judging device	→	Findings used to build capacity of community and community organizations.

Source: Traci Endo Inouye, Hanh Cao Yu and Jo-Ann Adefuin, "Exhibit I-2: Characteristics of a Multicultural Evaluation," *Commissioning Multicultural Evaluation: A Foundation Resource Guide*, p. 10.

integrate their own expertise throughout the evaluation, but the evaluator does not presume to understand the cultural context of diverse communities that are being studied. As a result, multicultural evaluation is characterized by a fundamental shift in how the evaluation is conceptualized and designed, how communities are engaged in data collection and analysis, and how the findings from the evaluation are ultimately communicated and used.

Closely related to understanding the principles and characteristics of multicultural evaluation is defining the characteristics of evaluators that make them culturally competent. Attributes of multicultural evaluators' competence do not lend themselves to a checklist or a formula. Rather, the multicultural knowledge, attitudes, and skill sets that evaluators bring to their work can best be viewed as evolving human skills that are developed over time. Some of the most often described characteristics are as follows:

- *Experience in diverse communities.* Although evaluators may not necessarily be from the same cultural background as the people in the communities they are evaluating, cultural competence involves a broader world perspective, often gained from experience living or working with different cultural groups.
- *Openness to learning about cultural complexities.* Culturally competent evaluators exhibit humility about what they think they already know and are open to in-depth understanding of the nuances and complexities of inter- and intracultural influences and variations.
- *Flexibility in evaluation design and practice.* Rather than coming in with prescriptive evaluation strategies, culturally competent evaluators realize limitations to established approaches and are willing to adapt to honor different cultural contexts.
- *Rapport and trust with diverse communities.* Culturally competent evaluators prioritize relationship building with diverse communities rather than viewing them solely as data sources. Relationships are viewed as mutually beneficial.
- *Acknowledgment of power differentials.* Culturally competent evaluators acknowledge the various power differentials possible in an evaluation, including those between the evaluator and those being evaluated, or between the commissioning entity (often a foundation) and those being evaluated.
- *Self-reflection for recognizing cultural biases.* Culturally competent evaluators take the time to become mindful of potential biases and prejudices and how they might be incorporated into their research.
- *Translation and mediation across diverse groups.* Culturally competent evaluators are skilled in translating jargon-laden evaluation findings to those who may not be trained in evaluation or have high levels of education, literacy, or English-language fluency. Likewise, evaluators must be adept in communicating cultural paradigms and community voice back to funders.
- *Comprehension of historic and institutional oppression.* An understanding of oppression is critical for designing evaluations that integrate how historic and current social systems, institutions, and societal norms contribute to disparities among different communities.

The power imbalances that are inherent within both funder-grantee relationships and evaluator-community relationships require specific and explicit attention throughout the evaluation process. Understanding and implementing multicultural evaluation approaches is an ongoing process. A meaningful shift toward multicultural evaluation will be determined greatly by the individual and collective beliefs, experiences, and will of the people within the organization. Therefore, as with many personal or institutional journeys toward change, the path toward multicultural evaluation can be considered a progression along a continuum.

Table 5.5 maps the implementation of multicultural evaluation principles (outlined earlier) along a stepwise continuum. This continuum is adapted from the stages of cultural competency that were developed for the service delivery field. It assumes that the implementation of evaluation principles unfolds in four stages:

- *Cultural incompetence.* Diverse cultures are not acknowledged in evaluation.
- *Cultural blindness.* Awareness of diversity may exist but is not presumed to be a critical factor within evaluation design or implementation.
- *Cultural sensitivity.* Acknowledgment of cultural differences exists, and steps are taken to incorporate cultural considerations within existing evaluation models.
- *Cultural proficiency.* The way that evaluations are designed and implemented are fundamentally shifted to honor and capitalize on the diverse cultural contexts in which target populations exist.

TABLE 5.5 Continuum of Multicultural Evaluation

Principle	Cultural Incompetence	Cultural Blindness	Cultural Sensitivity	Cultural Proficiency
Inclusive design and implementation	Evaluation designed to be accountable to the board; community largely unaware evaluation is happening and is uninvolved in any aspect of the evaluation.	Communities may be involved in evaluation, but no consideration for representation of multiple and diverse community voices.	Recognizing different cultural contexts, evaluation gathers input from diverse communities, typically through one-time requests for feedback. Community members may feel that their input is tokenized.	Diverse communities are involved in meaningful ways from start to finish. Evaluation is accountable to multiple stakeholders, including grantees and community beneficiaries.
Acknowledgment and infusion of multiple worldviews.	Funder assumptions and beliefs drive the evaluation; different perspectives and worldviews not acknowledged.	Mainstream values, beliefs, and perspectives drive evaluation; these are presumed to apply to diverse communities being studied.	Culturally competent evaluation strategies in place (e.g., translation of survey instruments; evaluators that reflect the diversity of community being studied; co-interpretation of findings). Evaluator still holds primary expertise.	Culturally competent evaluation strategies in place; evaluator approaches study with an intentional sense of humility; and expert knowledge is equally shared by evaluator and community being studied.

(continued)

TABLE 5.5 Continuum of Multicultural Evaluation (*Continued*)

Principle	Cultural Incompetence	Cultural Blindness	Cultural Sensitivity	Cultural Proficiency
Cultural and systems analysis.	Cultural and systemic power differences are not recognized.	Cultural and systemic power differences are ignored.	Cultural and systemic power differences are acknowledged, but not analyzed.	In-depth analysis of cultural and systemic power influences on a community is incorporated into findings.
Appropriate measures of success.	Evaluation does not consider the diversity of data sources or the relevance of methodology or measures.	Diversity may be acknowledged, but grantees and/or community success still judged using traditional methods and measures (often for the sake of "technical rigor").	Although traditional evaluation measures may still be used, additional strategies are in place to strengthen multicultural validity of findings (e.g., multimethod data collection, diversity considerations incorporated in analysis).	Validity of frameworks, tools, measures tested across multiple cultural groups, languages, and contexts; they are accordingly modified and/or new measures are developed.
Relevance and utility to diverse community.	Funder and/or evaluator priorities drive evaluation; results kept from communities because there is no recognition of their value to community or because it is assumed that they won't understand.	Results might be shared back but with no consideration of how they might be interpreted or used. Results are not useful because they are not rooted in multicultural analysis.	Results consider cultural context and are shared with community, but community may not feel ownership of results and dissemination because of their limited role in the evaluation.	Because of joint development, results are culturally relevant and used constructively for program improvement for diverse communities. There is consideration of how to share findings in culturally appropriate ways.

Source: Traci Endo Inouye, Hanh Cao Yu and Jo-Ann Adefuin, "Exhibit I-5: Continuum of Multicultural Evaluation (MCE)," *Commissioning Multicultural Evaluation: A Foundation Resource Guide,* pp. 15-16. Copyright © 2005 by The California Endowment. Reprinted with permission.

A true shift to a multicultural paradigm takes time. The extent to which some or all of the multicultural evaluation steps are incorporated into evaluation practice will determine whether researchers and foundations are harbingers of the shifts that can revolutionize the evaluation world.

Summary

Communication, program planning, and program evaluation are central to public health and must take cultural, literacy, and language barriers into consideration. When developing and delivering a health promotion program, there are additional considerations when the audience is a cultural group other than your own or composed of a diverse group. It is important that planners are sensitive and considerate of these differences to avoid wasting resources and possibly offending people.

In this chapter models for program planning and ways to deliver and evaluate your program were provided. The delivery method includes considering the content of your message as well as how it is disseminated. Some methods of delivery, such as *promotores(as)*, work better with some cultural and ethnic groups than others. After the program is complete, evaluation is essential. You will want to be sure that your message is received as you intended and see what impact it has had on your target audience. We outlined some differences between traditional and multicultural evaluation, which should be considered.

Review

1. What is health communication?
2. What are some issues to consider when using written communication?
3. What is health literacy and why is it important?
4. How can you check the reading level of a document? Social media?
5. What are *promotores(as)* and *fotonovelas*?
6. What are the concepts of the health belief model and the PRECEDE-PROCEED model?
7. How are traditional and multicultural evaluations different?

Activity

Locate six to eight written health communication documents that are targeted to the same population. In a paper, describe the similarities and differences in the outreach documents and discuss why you expect they would be successful or unsuccessful. Support your statements by referring to published literature. For example, if you state that the images include staple foods in that culture, cite literature indicating that the foods in the written materials are staple foods in that culture.

Case Study 1

In a city in Northern California, the director in the Department of Public Health, Alice, noticed that the county has a very high rate of hepatitis B among the Asian American population. Hepatitis B is a disease caused by the hepatitis B virus. The most common ways people get hepatitis B are sexual contact with a person infected with hepatitis B, exposure to needles, medical or dental procedures where instruments are contaminated with the hepatitis B virus, or when a mother passes hepatitis B to an infant at birth. The virus can live outside of the body for up to 7 days. The disease can be prevented by a vaccine, and blood tests are used to determine if someone is infected. Alice knows that most Asian Americans become infected while in the womb and not by sexual contact or exposure to needles from drug use. She is concerned that a major public information campaign must be designed to engage the Asian American population but not imply to the general community that Asian Americans have a major drug addiction problem. She has organized a meeting with her staff to discuss how to address the disparity.

1. What information should Alice ask her staff to collect about the Asian American population in the county?
2. How should Alice and her team decide what communication campaign is best to use?
3. How should the materials be developed and tested?

Case Study 2

Eudora is interested in reducing substance addiction among the American Indian community. She specifically wants to focus on reducing underage drinking and opioid use among teens and adults. She is writing a proposal to obtain funding.

1. How can Eudora utilize either the health belief model or the PRECEDE-PROCEED framework in her approach to making the programs effective for her target population?
2. What are some ways that she can make her social media campaigns more effective for the American Indian community?
3. What evaluation strategies might she use to make the process take culture into consideration?

References

Carteret, M. (2012, October 21). *8 tips for communicating with limited English proficiency patients.* http://www.dimensionsofculture.com/2010/10/8-tips-for-communicating-with-limited-english-proficiency-patients/

Centers for Disease Control and Prevention. (n.d.). *Program evaluation tip sheet: Integrating cultural competence into evaluation.* https://www.cdc.gov/dhdsp/docs/cultural_competence_tip_sheet.pdf

Centers for Disease Control and Prevention. (2017, September 17). Framework for public health and evaluation. *Morbidity and Mortality Weekly Report, 48.*

Centers for Disease Control and Prevention. (2021, January 28). *Health literacy.* https://www.cdc.gov/healthliteracy/learn/index.html

Communication Initiative Network. (2003). *Health belief model.*

Community Toolbox. (2007). *PRECEDE–PROCEED.*

Discovery Education. (1995). *Kathy Schrock's guide for educators. Fry's readability graph.*

Health Resources and Service Administration. (2019, August). *Health literacy.* https://www.hrsa.gov/about/organization/bureaus/ohe/health-literacy/index.html

Hersh, L., Salzman, B., & Snyderman, D. (2015). Health literacy in primary care practice. American Family Physician, *92*(2), 118–124.

Inclusive Design Research Centre. (n.d.). *What is inclusive design.* https://legacy.idrc.ocadu.ca/about-the-idrc/49-resources/online-resources/articles-and-papers/443-whatisinclusivedesign

Independent Television Service. (2020). *What is a foto-novela?*

Inouye, T. E., Yu, H. C., & Adefuin, J. (2005). *Commissioning multicultural evaluation: A foundation resource guide.*

Kutner, M., Greenburg, E., Jin, Y., & Paulsen, C. (2006). *The health literacy of America's adults: Results from the 2003 national assessment of adult literacy.* National Center for Education Statistics.

McKenzie, J. F., Neiger, B. L., & Thackeray, R. (2009). *Planning, implementing, and evaluating health promotion programs: A primer.* Pearson

National Network of Libraries of Medicine. (2014). *An introduction to health literacy.* http://nnlm.gov/outreach/consumer/hlthlit.html#A4

Nursing Paper Slayers. (n.d.). *Manner of dress and adornment.* https://nursingpaperslayers.com/manner-of-dress-and-adornment/

Office of Disease Prevention and Health Promotion. (2020, October 8). *Health literacy.* https://www.healthypeople.gov/2020/topics-objectives/topic/social-determinants-health/interventions-resources/health-literacy

Pew Research Center. (2019, June 12). *Social media fact sheet.* https://www.pewresearch.org/internet/fact-sheet/social-media/

Rural Women's Health Project. (n.d.). *What is a fotonovela?* http://www.rwhp.org/catalog_info/whatis.html

Sentell, T., & Braun, K. L. (2012). Low health literacy, limited English proficiency, and health status in Asians, Latinos, and other racial/ethnic groups in California. *Journal of Health Communication*, *17*(3), 82–99. https://doi.org/10.1080/10810730.2012.712621

Tufekci, Z. (2021, February 26). 5 pandemic mistakes we keep repeating. *The Atlantic.* https://www.theatlantic.com/ideas/archive/2021/02/how-public-health-messaging-backfired/618147/

CREDITS

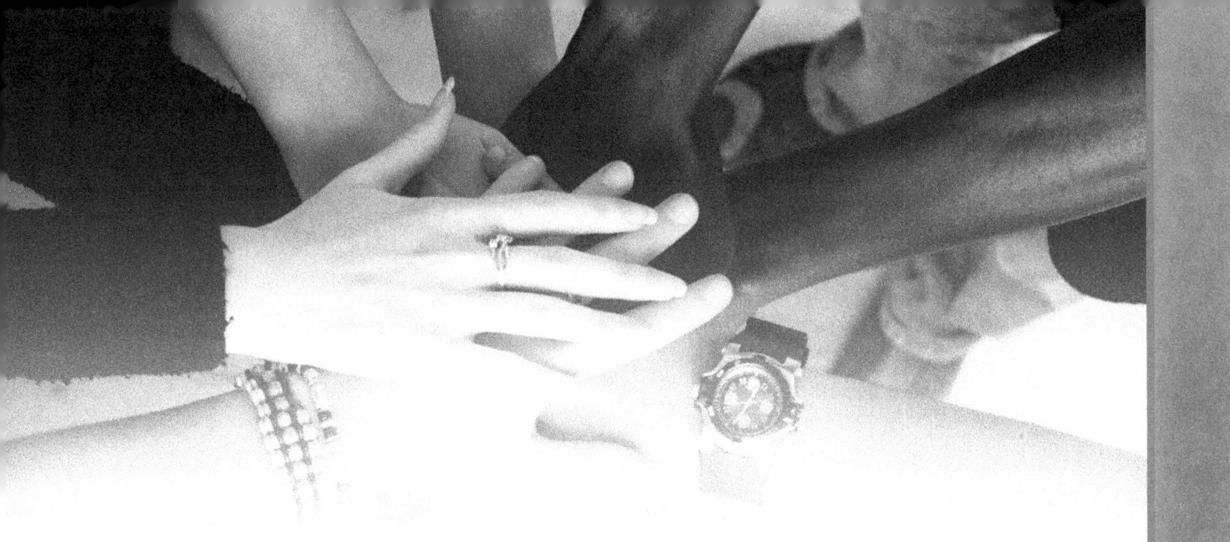

UNIT II

Specific Cultural Groups

CHAPTER 6

Hispanic and Latino American Populations

Preservation of one's own culture does not require contempt or disrespect for other cultures.

—CESAR CHAVEZ

KEY CONCEPTS AND TERMS

Curandero(a)
Empacho
Espiritismo
Evil eye
Familismo
Hispanic paradox
Mal de ojo
Orishas
Respeto
Santeria
Susto

LEARNING OBJECTIVES

After reading this chapter, you should be able to do the following:

1. Provide an overview of the social and economic circumstances of Hispanics in the United States.
2. Provide an overview of Hispanic beliefs about the causes of illness.
3. Describe at least three culture-bound illnesses among Hispanics.
4. Describe Hispanics' health risk behaviors and common illnesses.
5. List at least six tips for working with Hispanic populations.

Introduction

Predating the establishment of the United States, Hispanic people founded many of their own communities in land now part of the United States. These communities were based on the tradition of strong family relationships. Building on a general framework of respect, some Indigenous religions, and Catholic beliefs, there is a sense of class and hierarchy within Hispanic families. There is also a tradition of integrating others into their community through understanding and the development of rapport between friends and business associates. These factors contribute to a community that looks to both modern medicine and traditional practices within a context of cohesive families and mutual support.

In this chapter, we begin by clarifying terminology and provide a brief discussion about the history and current information about Hispanics in the United States. We then provide information about general Hispanic beliefs related to health and illness and discuss in more detail beliefs about specific health issues and events, such as pregnancy. We end the chapter with information about culture-bound illnesses, healing traditions and healers, risk factors and disease prevalence, and tips for working with this population.

Terminology

The Hispanic American population is composed of people who come from as many as 20 different countries. The well-known terms *Latin American, Hispanic, Latino,* and *Chicano* derive from various geopolitical and linguistic categorizations of this diverse group of people.

Latin America includes all the countries in the Americas that speak languages derived from Latin, which include Spanish, Portuguese, and French. The term *Latino* refers to everyone from Latin America and therefore includes people from Brazil (who speak Portuguese). The term *Hispanic* (derived from the Spanish word *Hispano*) refers to an ethnic group that shares a culture derived from the Spanish. In the United States, this term gained acceptance when it was picked up by the government and used in forms and on the Census to identify people with a Spanish heritage. A recent trend by some to use the term *Latinx,* which is intended to include lesbian, gay, bisexual, transgender, questioning, intersex, and asexual/aromantic/agender (LGBTQIA+) people is thought not to be as gender biased as "Latino." The term became publicly used after the Pulse Massacre in 2016, a mass shooting that occurred at a gay nightclub in Orlando, Florida (Roth, 2021). However, according to the Merriam-Webster (n.d.) dictionary "Latinx purposefully breaks with Spanish's gendered grammatical tradition" and "has been especially embraced by members of Latin LGBTQIA communities ... and it is unclear whether it will catch on in mainstream use." According to a study by Pew Research, about 3% of Spanish-speaking Americans use the term, and only about 25% have even heard the term (Bustamonte, 2020). Therefore, in this text we will us the traditional terms *Latino* and *Latinos* that are inclusive of multiple genders and generally recognized in the Hispanic and Latino cultures.

Hispanic is not a race but an ethnic distinction; Hispanics come from a variety of geographic regions and are not all genetically related. The ethnic label *Hispanic* was the result of the desire to quantify the Spanish-speaking population for the U.S. Census Bureau. For years, the U.S. Census Bureau considered Hispanic a race. They changed that definition before the 1970 Census, and in 1977 the U.S. racial classifications became American Indian, Alaskan Native, Asian or Pacific Islander, Black, and White, with the added ethnic classifications of "Hispanic origin" and "not of Hispanic origin."

Chicano, which is an abbreviation of the word *Mexicano,* is a more exclusive term and is used solely to refer to people of Mexican descent who are Americans with Mexican heritage (Mexican American). Originally, this label was used by non-Hispanics as a racial slur. Around the 1950s, however, Mexican Americans adopted this word, and it changed from a derogative term to an expression of confidence for Mexican Americans. Although *Chicano* is an old word, many elderly Hispanics of Mexican descent do not like it because of its history as a derogatory reference to Mexican people.

If you are trying to figure out how to refer to a group of people, the one concept on which most Hispanics and Latinos agree is that they prefer to be referred to based on their immediate ethnic group, for example, Mexican Americans. The U.S. government continues to use "Hispanic," and we will use that label throughout this chapter unless the data source identifies the ethnic group differently.

History of Hispanics in the United States

People often hold the misconception that Hispanics recently migrated to the United States. This erroneous perception is mostly due to the media attention given to Hispanic groups in the 1980s, when the Census revealed that Hispanics were the fastest growing population group in the southwestern United States. The reality is that Hispanics have a long history in the land now encompassed by the United States.

On the other side of the continent, Puerto Rico is a territory of the United States. The United States acquired Puerto Rico at the end of the Spanish-American War in 1898 and has retained sovereignty over it. By enacting the Jones–Shafroth Act in 1917, the U.S. Congress provided that all Puerto Ricans are U.S. citizens, enabling free migration between the island and the mainland.

Hispanics in the United States

According to the 2019 U.S. Census Bureau, there are roughly 60.5 million Hispanics living in the United States, which represents 18.5% of the total U.S. population (U.S. Census Bureau, 2020). The Hispanic population is projected to grow to about 111 million by 2060 (Vespa et al., 2018). In 2019, among Hispanic subgroups, Mexicans represented 61.4%. Puerto Ricans totaled 9.6%, followed by Central Americans (9.8%), South Americans (6.4%), and Cubans (3.9%) (HHS, OMH, 2021a).

The greatest number of Hispanics live in California, Texas, and Florida. In 2017, 31.5% of Hispanics were under the age 18 in comparison to 18.8% of non-Hispanic Whites (HHS, OMH, 2021a). U.S. Hispanics age 5 and older speak either English only or speak English very well (U.S. Census Bureau, 2014).

Hispanics tend to highly value the family. Families are very close, broadly defined, and emotionally and financially supportive. This characteristic is referred to as ***familismo***. The eldest male is typically the authority figure, and gender roles are traditional. Important decisions are made by the whole family, not the individual, because they tend to have a collectivist type of social structure. Respect (**respeto**) is fundamental to communication and relationships. The value of respeto places social worth and ultimate decision-making power on authority figures such as parents, teachers, leaders, elders, and government officials. All members of the family are expected to be respected and give it in return. Traditionally, Hispanic elderly were highly valued for their role and function as well as their ability to contribute their knowledge and experience to their family. They serve as a source of history, tradition and values. Children are socially and morally obligated to support their elderly parents, which may result in parents moving in with their children's family once they become too old to care for themselves (UKEssays, 2018).

Hispanics place higher value on individuals as opposed to institutions. The American culture values independence and individualism while the Hispanic culture values interdependence and collectivism. Hispanics tend to trust and cooperate with individuals they know personally, and many dislike impersonal and formal structures. Hispanic customers may identify a health care worker by name rather than by job title or institution. In a professional situation, many Hispanics expect to be addressed formally (e.g., Mrs. Martinez), but also personally (e.g., How are your children?). The length of the social interaction is often viewed to be less important than the quality.

Hispanics tend to avoid conflict and criticism and prefer smooth social relations based on politeness and respect. Overt disagreement is not considered appropriate behavior. Many Hispanics are characterized by warm, friendly, and affectionate relationships. Personal space is close and frequently shared with family members or close friends. Many Hispanics, particularly if they were not raised in the United States, may avoid direct eye contact with authority figures or in awkward situations. Many will nod affirmatively but not necessarily mean agreement. Silence may mean failure to understand and embarrassment about asking or disagreeing.

The family is considered a reliable source of health information. The family also is influential in health-seeking behaviors. They generally have a fatalistic worldview and an external locus of control, and this influences their help-seeking behaviors as well. There also is a belief that poor health is the fault of the individual and hence illness is a punishment from God. Expressing negative feelings is impolite, and people from this cultural group may not complain when health problems occur. Consistent with the importance of respect, modesty and privacy are important; therefore, health issues that are stigmatized should be discussed through an interpreter and not family members. Sexual issues are difficult to discuss. Often the word for sex (*sexo*) is not even used: *tener relaciones* (to have relations) is used instead.

It is believed that the close family structure is a contributing factor to what is called the **Hispanic paradox**. In 1986, Kyriakos Markides coined the expression "Hispanic epidemiological paradox" to refer to what appears to be surprisingly good health outcomes for Hispanics for mortality relative to non-Hispanic Whites and other minorities (Markides & Coreil, 1986). For example, between 2000 and 2017, the age-adjusted death rates for Hispanic adults aged 25 and over ranged from 39% through 42% lower compared with non-Hispanic Black adults, whereas the difference between rates for Hispanic and non-Hispanic White adults widened, from 23% lower for Hispanic adults in 2000 to 31% lower in 2017 (National Center for Health Statistics, 2019). Several efforts to explain this as errors in reporting, self-selection of healthy people entering the United States, or that Hispanics who are ill return to their prior country have not been sustained. It has likewise been suggested and conceded by Kyriako Markides that the support and "love" associated with strong family ties may contribute to the apparent positive outcomes (Yasmin, 2014).

Despite the history of the Hispanic paradox, the COVID-19 pandemic of 2020 proved to have a great impact on the Hispanic population. Generally, the elderly and minority groups, particularly African Americans, Native Americans, and Hispanics, have been highly susceptible. According to the CDC (2022), Hispanics had 1.5 times the number of cases of COVID-19, 2.3 times the number of hospitalizations, and 1.7 times the number of deaths than White Americans as of February 2022.

General Philosophy About Disease Prevention and Health Maintenance

Hispanics generally view health as being and looking clean, being able to rest and sleep well, feeling good and happy, and having the ability to perform in one's expected role as mother, father, worker, and so forth. In Puerto Rico, the phrase *llenitos y limpios* (clean and not too thin) is used. A person's well-being depends on a balance of emotional, physical, and social factors, and when they are not in balance, illness occurs. Some attribute physical illness to *los nervios*, believing that illness results from having experienced a strong emotional state (Nogueira et al., 2015).

Thus, they try to prevent illness by avoiding intense rage, sadness, and other emotions. Depression is not talked about openly.

DID YOU KNOW?

Even though you might think low income is always associated with health risks, the CDC estimates the infant mortality rate in the United States at 5.79 per 1,000 live births (Ely & Driscoll, 2019). The Hispanic infant mortality rate in 2017 was 5.1 per 1,000 live births (Ely & Driscoll, 2019). Infants born to Hispanic women, especially foreign-born mothers, have lower rates of low birth weight and mortality than the national average, a phenomenon known as the Latina birth outcomes paradox (Velasco Mondragon et al., 2016).

Worldview

Hispanics tend to value closeness, so touching and embracing are common. Sustained eye contact with an older person is considered rude; direct eye contact with superiors is viewed as being disrespectful. This may not be relevant to second- and third-generation Hispanics. Using formal names and greeting with a handshake are signs of respect, and health care providers should address and greet Hispanics in this way. Inquiring about family before discussing the health issues is a way of gaining trust. Health care providers should engage in "small talk" before addressing the patient's health concerns (Purnell, 2021 p. 448). Hispanics are reluctant to speak about some topics with health care providers, such as sexuality, but otherwise they are open to discussing their physical problems with providers. This group uses both complementary and alternative medicine (CAM) and allopathic medical care. It is important for health care providers to inquire about the CAM used.

Hispanics tend to be present oriented, so disease prevention may not be a priority. They may arrive late for appointments due to their relaxed sense of time. The social structure is a collectivistic one that values interdependence and cooperation. In the family, traditional gender roles are followed, with women making decisions related to the health of the family. Families are close, and decisions are made jointly. This closeness is why Hispanics tend to refrain from putting family members in long-term care, caring for them at home instead.

Catholicism is the predominant religion among Hispanics, and the spirit is important in terms of health. Most people in this culture discuss spirituality, especially in times of illness. This may make some health care practitioners uncomfortable. Families may occasionally pray as a group, and rosaries may be present. Hispanics have a fatalistic worldview and believe that their health is in God's hands. Illness may be viewed as a punishment from God. Many Hispanics view pain as a test of faith, and this view may affect a health care provider's pain management interventions. Hispanic patients are more likely to have their pain underestimated by physicians, to receive less medication, and to be prescribed lower analgesic dosages (Torres et al., 2017). The Hispanic community holds beliefs about pain and pain medications that contribute to such disparities, including a fear of addiction, stoicism, preference for folk remedies, and religious beliefs that pain is "God's will." Blood transfusions are acceptable to Hispanics, but organ donations are infrequent, especially with regard to donating organs while the person is still living. Some frown upon organ transplants. Over 60% of organs donated from Hispanic patients in 2019 were from deceased donors and only comprised 14.6% of all organ donors in 2019 (HHS, OMH, 2021b). Hispanic individuals, compared to White counterparts, are unlikely to discuss their end-of-life care before death, are unlikely to have any legal arrangements regarding their care, and are unlikely to choose withholding any treatment (Orlovic et al., 2019).

Pregnancy, Birth, and Child Rearing

Family, marriage, and child rearing are highly valued in Hispanic culture. In 2017, Hispanic females aged 15 to 19 had a birthrate more than twice as high as Non-Hispanic Whites: 25.3 per 1,000 versus 11.2 per 1,000 (Ely & Driscoll, 2019). While teen births have declined across all groups by around 4%, Hispanic teen birth rates have dropped by 5.3% between 2018 and 2019 (HHS, CDC 2021c).

Birth control, no matter how practiced, is against Catholic doctrine but is utilized by many (Purnell, 2021 p. 626). While the Catholic Church continues to instruct against the use of contraception, a 2016 study by the Pew Research Center found that only 13% of weekly Mass-going Catholics in the United States thought contraception was morally wrong (Rocca, 2018). At the prenatal state, avoiding foods that are considered "hot" (spicy or physically hot) is thought to be beneficial because eating hot foods can cause the baby to be born with spots and be susceptible to rashes. Eating foods with iron, avoiding greasy foods, eating soup and dairy products, keeping active, and seeking advice from older family members is customary. Not wearing tight clothing and wearing a rosary or talisman to ward off malformation are also traditions. It is believed that pregnant women should not walk in the moonlight because it might cause a birth deformity. Other ways to prevent birth deformities include wearing a metal key, safety pin, or some other metal object on the abdomen (Purnell, 2021 p. 626).

During labor and delivery, medication is thought to be detrimental to the baby, as is screaming during labor. Makeup is not worn during labor and delivery. Some Hispanic traditions hold that the mother and child should be in the *cuarentena* for about 40 days after the birth, remaining home with limited visitors to enable the mother–child bond to develop and to avoid exposure to infections. During this period family members prepare *purgantes* (laxatives) for the mother to eliminate impurities from the birth. The belief is that postpartum depression will not occur if these *purgantes* are taken. Women are cared for by other women but are expected to care for their newborn child on their own. New mothers are discouraged from taking showers for several days, and also discouraged from getting out of bed for the first few hours after birth. Light foods are provided, including *caldo de pollo* (chicken bouillon), herbal teas, and tortillas; beans are avoided. The reasoning behind the length of the 40-day period is that it's believed to take 40 days for the mother's reproductive organs to heal and regain their ordinary shape after giving birth. During the *cuarentena*, carrots and chicken soup (of any kind) are often the approved foods of choice. Chicken soup is chosen because it is known to not be too spicy or heavy for someone who is trying to heal (Benton, 2018).

Child rearing is consistent with the concepts of formality, distinctly defined parental roles, and extended family. The child is raised by a family not only to reach adulthood but also to be part of a family throughout life. Child-rearing goals for social, educational, and financial development are important not only for the child but also so that the child becomes a sustaining member of the extended family.

Older children often have significant responsibility for younger siblings or relatives and are generally actively engaged in the care of older family members. Grandparents are also involvement in child rearing as it not only helps the parent but also helps engender a deep sense of family loyalty in the child and a sense of responsibility for providing extended social support to other family members, including the elderly.

Nutrition and Exercise

Many Hispanics retain core elements of the traditional Hispanic diet, including grains, beans, and fresh fruits and vegetables. The typical diet is high in fiber, with beans and grains (rice) as staple foods, and they generally rely on beans as a source of protein rather than meat. Leafy green vegetables are not as large a part of the diet as non-Hispanic Whites. Generally, Hispanics eat a good deal of tropical fruits, fruit juices, and starchy root vegetables (e.g., potatoes, cassava, and plantains). The food pyramid for the traditional Latino diet is shown in **Figure 6.1**.

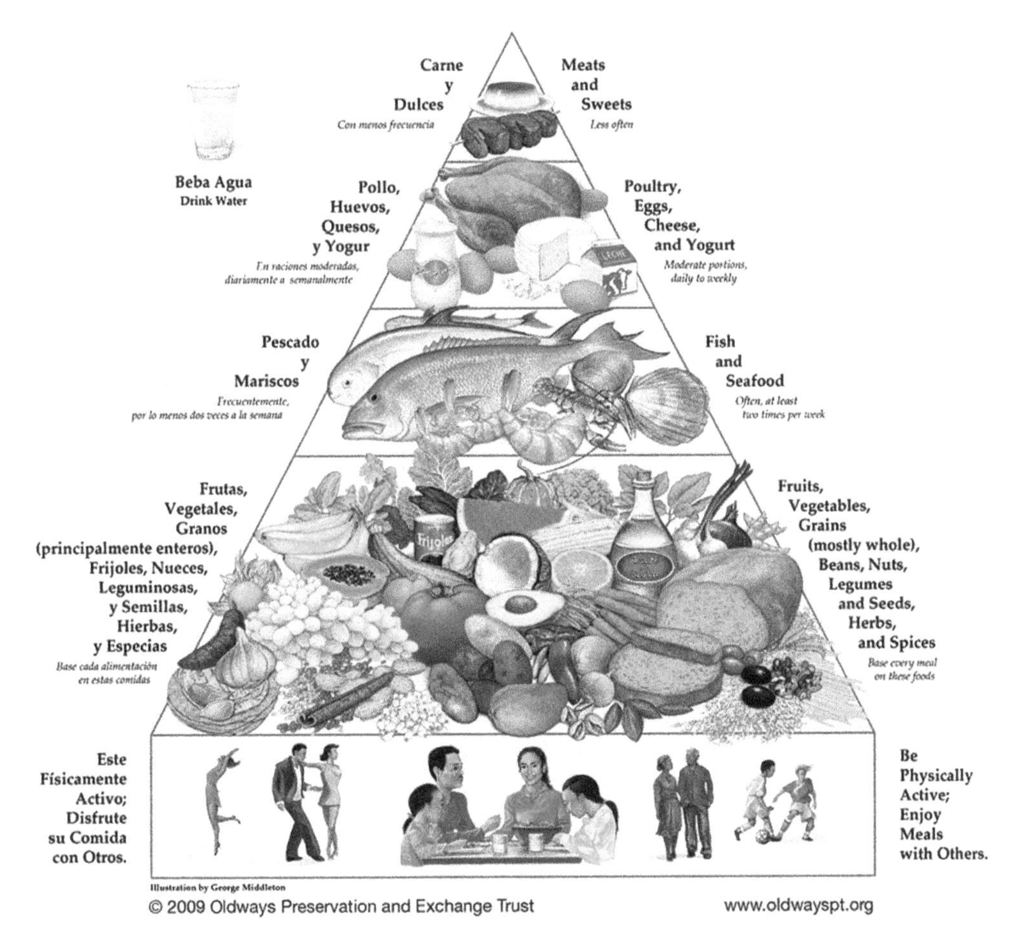

Figure 6.1 Food pyramid for traditional Latino diet.

Family life has traditionally occupied a central place in Hispanic culture and contributed to dietary behaviors supporting home preparation of meals and families eating together. Ironically, the lifestyle of Hispanic Americans is undergoing a transition as they begin to adopt the values and behaviors of the United States. Acculturation typically results in a more sedentary lifestyle and a change in dietary patterns even as economic status increases. A large study measuring physical activity among middle-aged and older adults found that Hispanic adults were less likely to report walking (leisure time) and vigorous physical activity than non-Hispanic adults (Meir, 2017).

Mental Health

Religion can be a protective factor for mental health in Hispanic communities (faith, prayer) but can also project stigma against mental illness and treatment (demons, lack of faith, sinful behavior) (Caplan, 2019).

Hispanics living in poverty are over twice as likely to report psychological distress when compared to Hispanics living over the poverty level (HHS, OMH, 2021c). In 2017,

- the death rate from suicide for Hispanic men was four times the rate for Hispanic women;
- The suicide rate for Hispanics was less than half that of the non-Hispanic White population, yet suicide was the second leading cause of death for Hispanics, ages 15 to 34;
- suicide attempts for Hispanic girls, grades 9–12, were 40% higher than for non-Hispanic White girls in the same age group (HHS, OMH, 2021c).

Despite these problems, non-Hispanic Whites received mental health treatment twice as often as Hispanics in 2018 (HHS, OMH, 2021c).

Contemporary empirical studies tend to support the assertion that acculturation is an important correlate of mental health among immigrants. Foreign-born Asians and Latinos have significant mental health advantages, such as lower rates of depression and anxiety, compared to their U.S.-born counterparts. This phenomenon has been referred to as the "immigrant paradox," where foreign nativity serves as a protective factor against psychiatric disorders, despite the stresses often associated with immigrating and settling into a new country. Acculturation into U.S. society may also have a negative impact on mental health for Hispanics. U.S.-born and long-term residents have significantly greater rates of mental disorders and substance dependency than recent Hispanic immigrants (Salas-Wright et al., 2018). The prevalence of current prescription opioid misuse was significantly lower among White students (5.5%) compared with Black (8.7%) or Hispanic students (9.8%). Conversely, the prevalence of current alcohol use was lower among Black students (16.8%) compared with White (34.2%) or Hispanic students (28.4%) (Jones et al., 2020).

Suicide risk increases across generations of Hispanics, the risk greatest amongst U.S.-born Hispanics. Acculturative stress has been linked to increased risk for suicide ideation, attempts, and fatalities among Hispanics. Acculturative stress may increase suicide risk via disintegration of cultural values (e.g., familism and religiosity) and social bonds (Silva & Van Orden, 2018).

Thousands in this population often go without professional mental health treatment. Many do not look for treatment due to stigma or fear of being perceived as crazy as well as often not having the means to access services to manage their mental health needs (Naso, 2016).

Death and Dying

Women tend to care for the seriously ill and dying. Men may stay close but usually do not provide hands-on care. While some Indigenous and other customs still have some influence, death rites are generally derived from Catholic Church customs and generally include confession and last rites. Based on both family respect and religious custom, funerals usually involve burial and often include a wake or social gathering where food is served and the life of the deceased is remembered positively and without grim mourning (Hidalgo, 2020).

Cultural-Bound Illnesses

Hispanics are diagnosed with many unique illnesses that are not part of the Western medical system. Some common illnesses and their causes are listed in **Table 6.1.**

TABLE 6.1 Culture-Bound Illnesses in the Hispanic Culture and Their Characteristics and Causes

Diagnosis	Characteristics	Traditional Treatment
Ataque de nervios ("nervous attack")	Intense but brief release of emotion thought to be caused by family conflict or anger	No immediate treatment other than calming the patient
Bilis (anger)	Outburst of anger	Herbs, including wormwood
Caida de la mollera ("fallen fontanel")	Childhood condition characterized by irritability and diarrhea thought to be caused by abrupt withdrawal from the mother's breast	Holding the child upside down or applying gentle pressure to the hard palate
Empacho (indigestion)	Constipation, cramps, or vomiting thought to be caused by overeating	Abdominal massage and herbal purgative teas; an egg passed over the abdomen supposedly "sticks" to the affected area
Fatiga (shortness of breath, fatigue)	Asthma symptoms and fatigue	Steam inhalation and herbal treatments, including eucalyptus and mullein (*gordolobo*)
Frio de la matriz (decreased libido)	Pelvic congestion and decreased libido thought to be caused by insufficient rest after childbirth	Damiana tea, rest

(continued)

TABLE 6.1 Culture-Bound Illnesses in the Hispanic Culture and Their Characteristics and Causes (*Continued*)

Diagnosis	Characteristics	Traditional Treatment
Mal aire ("bad air")	Cold air that is thought to cause respiratory infections and earaches	Steam baths, hot compresses, stimulating herbal teas
Mal de ojo ("evil eye")	A hex cast on children, sometimes unconsciously, that is thought to be caused by the admiring gaze of someone more powerful	The hex can be broken if the person responsible for the hex touches the child, or if a healer passes an egg over the child's body; the egg is then broken into a bowl of water and placed under the child's bed; child may wear charms for protection
Mal puesto (sorcery)	Unnatural illness that is not easily explained	Magic
Pasmo ("frozen face")	Temporary paralysis of the face or limbs, often thought to be caused by a sudden hot-cold imbalance	Massage
Susto ("soul loss")	Posttraumatic illness (e.g., shock, insomnia, depression, anxiety)	*Barrida* ritual purification ceremony (herbs used to sweep patient's body) repeated until the patient improves

Source: Gregory Juckett, "Caring Latino Parents," *American Family Physician*, vol. 87, no. 1, p. 50.

Susto (literally "fright" in Spanish) is illness that occurs from a frightful experience, and it is similar to anxiety in modern medicine. Symptoms include withdrawal from social interactions, listlessness, not sleeping well, and loss of appetite. Most people who believe in susto say that anyone can get it; both adults and children can be affected. The soul leaves the body due to a frightening experience, and the body becomes susceptible to illness and disharmony. It can be caused by events such as the sudden, unexpected barking of a dog, tripping over an unnoticed object, having a nighttime encounter with a ghost that keeps your spirit from finding its way back into your body before you wake, or being in a social situation that causes you to have fear or anger.

Mal de ojo, sometimes called "**evil eye**," is an illness that is a result of an envious glance from another individual. It mostly affects children. It has been defined as a hex caused by a gaze from a more powerful or stronger person looking at a weaker person (usually an infant or child but sometimes a woman). It may be someone from outside the family looking at the child with envy, or a stare from a powerful person who is admiring the child. It is usually caused inadvertently. Those affected may suffer from headaches, high fever, diarrhea, sleeplessness, increased fussiness, and weeping. It is not fully known what diseases in modern medicine correlate with *mal de ojo*; however, in severe cases, the symptoms are similar to those of sepsis (the presence of pathogenic organisms or their toxins in the blood or tissues) and should warrant a medical evaluation. Cases of *mal de ojo* with frequent crying and no other symptoms are thought to be similar to colic.

Empacho (blocked intestines) describes stomach pains and cramps that are believed to be caused by a ball of food clinging to the stomach due to a change in eating habits, eating spoiled food, overeating, or swallowing chewing gum. The disease state of empacho has often been defined as a perceived stomach or intestinal blockage. In most cases, it is not an actual obstruction but rather indigestion or gastroenteritis. Abdominal pain and bloating are symptoms of *empacho*. Some Hispanic populations also add nausea, vomiting, diarrhea, and lethargy as symptoms that may occur in some cases. Empacho tends to occur more in young children, but people of all ages are susceptible. *Empacho* is considered a cold illness. Folk medicines used to treat *empacho* include *greta* (lead monoxide) and *azarcón* (lead tetroxide), which are dangerous and can cause lead poisoning. There have been case reports of deaths from these substances.

The ideology of illness and health is rooted in the fabric of the culture, and it is the fundamental element of traditional values. Even though the Mexican American culture utilizes modern medicine, they rely primarily on folk practitioners to treat traditional illnesses.

Healing Traditions, Healers, and Healing Aids

Even though Hispanics generally look to standard primary care doctors and facilities for care, some treatments for illness are provided by family or nonfamily members. On a secondary basis, Hispanics may rely on traditional healing traditions.

In Hispanic cultures, illnesses, treatments, and foods are viewed as having hot or cold properties, although how these are ascribed may vary by country. Some Hispanics consider health to be the product of balance among four body humors (blood and yellow bile are hot; phlegm and black bile are cold). One would balance a hot illness with cold medications and foods and vice versa. This might result in not following a doctor's advice to drink lots of fluids for a common cold, if one believes such drinks add more coldness to the body. Instead, hot liquids (tea, soup, broth) could be recommended (Rhode Island Department of Health, n.d.). **Table 6.2** lists some hot and cold illnesses.

TABLE 6.2 Hot Versus Cold Latino Diagnoses

Cold Conditions	Hot Conditions
• Cancer	• *Bilis* (bile, rage)
• Colic	• Diabetes mellitus
• *Empacho* (indigestion)	• Gastroesophageal reflux or peptic ulcer
• *Frio de la matriz* (frozen womb)	• Hypertension
• Headache	• *Mal de ojo* (evil eye)
• Menstrual cramps	• Pregnancy
• Pneumonia	• Sore throat or infection
• Upper respiratory infections	• *Susto* (soul loss)

Source: Juckett (2013).

Healers

Healer names are specific to cultural groups and may include *curanderos* in Mexico and much of Latin America, Santeria in Brazil and Cuba, and *espiritismo* in Puerto Rico. Most of these traditions distinguish natural illnesses from supernatural illnesses. The healing traditions include a variety of methods, as shown in **Table 6.1**.

Curanderos

A *curandero* (*curandera* for a female) is a traditional folk healer or shaman who is dedicated to curing physical and/or spiritual illnesses. *Curanderos* (plural term including both males and females) are often respected members of the community and seen as highly religious and spiritual. In Spanish the word *curanderos* means healers. These healers often use herbs and other natural remedies to cure illnesses, but their primary method of healing is the supernatural. They believe that the causes of many illnesses are lost malevolent spirits, a lesson from God, or a curse. There are different types of *curanderos*. *Curanderos* use herbs and verbal charms or spells to produce a magic effect, *sobadores* practice manipulation, *parteras* are midwives, and *abuelas* (literally "grandmothers," although they are not necessarily related to the patient) provide initial care. *Yerberos* are primarily herbalists, and *hueseros* and *sabaderos* are bone/muscle therapists who specialize in physical ailments.

Curanderos treat ailments such as *espanto* (Spanish for shock), *empacho* (Spanish for surfeit, which means to feed in excess), *susto*, *mal aire* (literally "bad air"), and *mal de ojo* with religious rituals, ceremonial cleansing, and prayers. Often *curanderos* contact certain spirits to aid them in their healing work. The remedies of the *curanderos* are often helpful but sometimes have a negative effect on the health of their patients. For example, a common method of healing *mollera caída*, a condition in which an infant's fontanelle has sunken, is to hold the infant's feet with its head down and perform a ceremonial ritual. Some other traditional treatments, such as *azarcón* and *greta* (lead salts) and *azogue* (mercury), are also harmful because of their lead and mercury content. Other remedies are harmless. For example, a common method of treating *mal de ojo* is to rub an egg over the body of the sick to draw out the evil spirit that is causing the disease.

These methods of treating health problems often lead to conflict with modern medicine because doctors reject the *curandero*'s healing as superstitious and worthless. As a result, *curanderos* have often experienced discrimination and been likened to witches by the medical profession and non-Hispanic communities. However, these remedies are important to the Hispanic culture, and disbelief may lead to insult, conflict, or the rejection of modern medicine. Other medical doctors, recognizing the benefits of the spiritual and emotional healing offered by *curanderos*, have begun to work in conjunction with them, supporting their use of rituals and ceremonies in the healing of the sick while insisting that patients receive modern medical attention as well.

Santeria

Santeria, also known as the "Way of the Saints," is an Afro-Caribbean religion based on beliefs of the Yoruba people in Nigeria, Africa. The traditions have been influenced by

Roman Catholic beliefs. Santeria incorporates elements of several faiths and is therefore called a syncretic religion. It has grown beyond its Yoruba and Catholic origins to become a religion in its own right and a powerful symbol of the religious creativity of Afro-Cuban culture. For a long time, Santeria was a secretive underground religion, but it is becoming increasingly visible in the Americas.

Because of the history of secrecy, it is not known how many people follow Santeria. There is no central organization for this religion, and it is practiced in private, which makes it more difficult to determine the number of followers. There are no scriptures for this religion, and it is taught through word of mouth. The Santeria tradition consists of a hierarchical structure according to priesthood level and authority.

Santeria practices include animal offerings, dance, and appeals for assistance sung to the **orishas**, which resemble the Catholic saints and are spirits that reflect one of the manifestations of *Olodumare* (God). Animal sacrifice also is a part of Santeria and is very controversial. Followers of Santeria point out that ritual slaughter is conducted in a safe and humane manner by the priests who are charged with the task. Furthermore, the animal is cooked and eaten afterward by the community. Chickens, a staple food of many African-descended and Creole cultures, are the most common sacrifice; the chicken's blood is offered to the orisha, and the meat is consumed by all.

Followers believe that orishas will help them in life if they carry out the appropriate rituals and will enable them to achieve the destiny God planned for them before they were born. This is very much a mutual relationship because the orishas need to be worshipped by human beings if they are to continue to exist. In a 1993 Supreme Court case, Justice Kennedy said in his decision:

> The Santeria faith teaches that every individual has a destiny from God, a destiny fulfilled with the aid and energy of the orishas. The basis of the Santeria religion is the nurture of a personal relation with the orishas, and one of the principal forms of devotion is an animal sacrifice. According to Santeria teaching, the orishas are powerful but not immortal. They depend for survival on the sacrifice. (*Church of Likumi Babalu Aye v. City of Hialeah*, 1993)

Drum music and dancing are forms of prayer and will sometimes induce a trance state in an initiated priest, who becomes possessed and then channels the orisha.

Espiritismo

Espiritismo is the Spanish word for "spiritism." It is the belief in Latin America and the Caribbean that good and evil spirits can affect human life, such as one's health and luck. An opinion, doctrine, or principle (tenet) of *espiritismo* is the belief in a supreme God who is the omnipotent creator of the universe. There also is a belief in a spirit world inhabited by discarnate spiritual beings who gradually evolve intellectually and morally.

Espiritismo has never had a single leader or epicenter of practice, so practice varies greatly among individuals and groups. *Espiritismo* has absorbed various practices from other religious and spiritual practices endemic to Latin America and the Caribbean, such as Roman Catholicism, *curanderismo*, Santeria, and voodoo.

Behavioral Risk Factors and Common Health Problems

The behaviors described here are linked to the common health problems that Hispanics face, but it is important to note that some of illnesses are not related to behaviors. Many health problems are related to other social factors as well, such as poverty or lack of access to care.

The 10 leading causes of death among Hispanics/Latinos in 2017 were as follows (Heron, 2019):

1. Cancer
2. Heart disease
3. Unintentional injuries
4. Stroke
5. Diabetes mellitus
6. Alzheimer's disease
7. Chronic liver disease and cirrhosis
8. Chronic lower respiratory disease
9. Intentional self-harm (suicide)
10. Nephritis, nephrotic syndrome, and nephrosis

Hispanics have higher rates of obesity than non-Hispanic Whites. Approximately 34.36% of Hispanic men and 35.4 of women 20 years old and older are obese (body mass index of 30 or greater), compared to 31.2% for non-Hispanic White men and 28.7% for women (Jones et al., 2020). Diabetes and hypertension are closely linked to obesity; 14.3% of Latinos more than 20 years old have type 2 diabetes, making it the foremost health issue in this population (CDC, 2021b).

Hispanics have lower rates of smoking than most racial and ethnic groups. In 2015, 10.1% of Hispanics smoked while 16.6% of non-Hispanic Whites and 21.9% of Native Americans smoked (American Lung Association, 2020). There are significant variations in smoking rates among Hispanic subgroups: 19.8% of Cuban Americans, 28.5% of Puerto Ricans, 19.1% of Mexican Americans, and 15.6% of Central and South Americans were smokers in 2016 (CDC, 2021a).

Overall, Hispanics are less likely to drink at all than are non-Hispanic Whites. Hispanics have high rates of abstinence from alcohol, but Hispanics who choose to drink are more likely to consume higher volumes of alcohol than non-Hispanic Whites (National Institute on Alcohol Abuse and Alcoholism, 2019).

Although the Hispanic paradox shows that Hispanics have health issues similar to non-Hispanic Whites or even less in several categories such as cancer, Hispanics do have a particular risk of diabetes with adults having more than a 50% chance to contract the disease (CDC, 2021b).

WHAT DO YOU THINK?

Life expectancy among Hispanics is 3 years longer than for Whites (Arias & Xu, 2020). Hispanics also have lower mortality rates than Whites (Ely & Driscoll, 2019). even though they are two times more likely to be economically under the poverty line and three times more likely to be without health insurance. Hispanics have markedly reduced mortality from cancer (−14%) and heart disease (−22%), two leading causes of death in the United States (National Center for Health Statistics, 2019). Hispanics also have lower smoking rates, better diet, and better general health during the first few years after immigrating. However, CDC statistics show that Hispanics are more prone to die of diabetes, as well as cirrhosis and other chronic liver diseases. What do you think accounts for the paradox related to mortality? Could it be better genetics? Could it be due to lower smoking rates? What about the problems of diabetes and cirrhosis? Could this be due to efforts to try to adapt to the majority culture?

QUICK FACTS

Examples of some important health disparities include the following (Carratala & Maxwell, 2020):

Chronic health conditions

- Ten percent of Hispanics reported having fair or poor health compared with 8.3% of non-Hispanic Whites.
- Almost 22 percent of Hispanic adults over age 20 have been diagnosed with diabetes compared with 13% of White adults over age 20.
- Approximately 25% of Hispanics have high blood pressure.
- Hispanic women are 40% more likely to have cervical cancer and 20% more likely to die from cervical cancer than non-Hispanic White women.

Mental health

- In 2018, 8.8% of Hispanic adults received mental health services compared with 18.6% of non-Hispanic White adults.
- Almost 7% of Hispanic adults received prescription medication for mental health services compared with 15.4% of non-Hispanic White adults.
- In 2018, 4.6% of Hispanic adults reported serious psychological distress.

(continued)

QUICK FACTS (*CONTINUED*)

- In 2017, the number of suicide attempts by adolescent Hispanic females was 40% higher than that of adolescent non-Hispanic White females.

Leading causes of death

- The leading causes of death among Hispanics are cancer, heart disease, and accidents.
- The life expectancy for Hispanics, 81.9 years, is longer than that of non-Hispanic Whites.
- In 2017, the infant mortality rate for Puerto Ricans was 40% higher than for non-Hispanic Whites.
- There are 5.1 infant deaths per 1,000 live births among Hispanic and Latinx Americans.

Source: Sofia Carratala and Connor Maxwell, "Health Disparities by Race and Ethnicity," https://www.americanprogress.org/issues/race/reports/2020/05/07/484742/health-disparities-race-ethnicity/.

Considerations for Health Promotion and Program Planning

Consider the following concepts when planning and implementing a health promotion program for this target audience:

- Preventive medicine is not a norm for most Hispanics. This behavior may be related to the Hispanic here-and-now orientation, as opposed to a future-planning orientation. It also is related to their fatalistic belief system.
- Some common Hispanic sayings suggest that events in one's life result from luck, fate, or other powers beyond an individual's control. See the following examples:
  - *Que sea lo que Dios quiera.* (It's in God's hands.)
  - *Esta enfermedad es una prueba de Dios.* (This illness is a test of God.)
  - *De algo se tiene que morir uno.* (You have to die of something.)
- People with acute or chronic illness may regard themselves as innocent victims of malevolent forces. Severe illness may be attributed to God's design, bad behavior, or punishment. Genetic defects in a child may be attributed to the parents' actions.
- Consider sitting closer to Hispanic patients and clients than you would with people from other cultures.

- Be particularly aware of your nonverbal communication messages. Sustained eye contact when speaking to an older person may be considered rude, and avoiding eye contact with a superior is a sign of respect (Purnell, 2021 p. 641).
- Be aware that Hispanics often have higher exposure rates to environmental hazards due to living in urban environments, and males have high exposure due to their jobs.
- Family and friends may indulge patients, allowing them to be passive, which is an approach that may conflict with the Western view that active participation is required to prevent or heal much disease.
- Some Hispanic sayings support health promotion and illustrate the considerable status given to health and prevention:
    - *La salud es todo o casi todo.* (Health is everything, or almost everything.)
    - *Es mejor prevenir que curar.* (An ounce of prevention is worth a pound of cure.)
    - *Ayúdate que Dios te ayudará.* (Help yourself and God will help you.)
- Vaccination is very important and adhered to for children.
- Western medicine is expected and preferred in case of severe illness, but some Hispanics may also use native healers. The educator and health provider should inquire about the utilization of other healers.
- Use appropriate titles to show respect, such as *señor* and *señorita.*
- To show respect, greet the person with a handshake.
- A botanica is a resource store for herbs and other traditional remedies. Some Hispanics may go there before going to a physician or clinic. In many Latin American countries, pharmacists prescribe medications, and a wider range of medications is available over the counter. People may share medicines or write home for relatives to send them medications. Individuals may discontinue medication if it does not immediately alleviate symptoms or after their symptoms abate.
- When providing nutritional advice or education, use positive examples from Hispanic cultural foods.
- Consider suggesting family-based methods for increasing physical activity, such as dancing or walking with family members.
- If you have the patient's permission, involve the family members in the consultation because it may assist with increasing the listener's adherence to the recommendation(s).
- Consider using peer educators (*promotoras*) as community outreach workers for community-based efforts; they have been shown to be successful with this community.

- Check for understanding and agreement because Hispanics tend to avoid conflict and are hesitant to ask questions.
- Inquire about complementary and alternative treatments being used as they are frequently utilized by Hispanics.
- Because of historic events, some Hispanics may distrust the health care system (e.g., many Puerto Rican women experienced involuntary sterilization and were adversely affected by birth control pill trials), view the health care system as an extension of a repressive government (Central Americans), or fear deportation, especially if they are in the country illegally. Some Hispanics confuse public health programs with welfare and avoid them due to stigma.
- They have a relaxed perspective related to time and may be "late" for appointments.
- When using interpreters the following tips may be helpful:
  - Speak clearly and use short simple sentences.
  - Look at and speak directly to your employee rather than the interpreter.
  - Listen carefully to the employee and watch them for nonverbal cues.
  - Use clarification questions such as "Did I understand you correctly?" and "Tell me more about ..." to avoid misinterpretation (Holliday, n.d.).

Tips for Working with the Hispanic Population

When working with a Hispanic patient or family, it is important to convey respect, some formality combined with a demonstration of personal interest. Traditional family values, diet, reliance on modern medicine, and respect for authority should be encouraged and reinforced. It may be useful to mention the importance of retaining traditional values and practices rather than abandoning them to be more like the U.S. majority, which could be detrimental to their health both physically and mentally.

Caring for Hispanic Patients

Make sure to greet and acknowledge everyone in the room, even the children. Do not act rushed during the appointment. It is better to ask "How can I serve (help) you today?" than "How are you?" which may be taken as a greeting and be answered "Fine and you?"

Avoid instant familiarity, especially when meeting a new person such as during an initial office visit. Formality is a sign of respect when you do not know someone well. The Spanish language differentiates between the formal and the familiar forms of salutations and should be literally translated and communicated by your conduct. After you have explained something to your patient, use inquiring comprehension checks such as "Tell me what I am proposing to do" because "Do you understand?" may be misunderstood as an insult.

Remember that Latinos embrace alternative therapies and healers. Herbal remedies are second nature to Latinos, and these alternative medicines are typically found in neighborhood stores (botanicas).

Also remember that decisions may need to be made in consultation with family members who may not be present. The Latino family unit has well-defined gender roles. The husband is the provider, protector, and the authority figure. The wife is the homemaker, child raiser, and adviser. Even an educated and competent Latino wife may not consent to any significant treatment without the specific permission of the husband (Jimenez, 2002).

Summary

Hispanics total approximately 60.5 million people in the United States today and are a rapidly growing population (U.S. Census Bureau, 2020). Hispanics have strong family ties and have held on to their cultural belief systems and practices. Hispanics incorporate unique features in their health belief systems and healing practices. They have types of healers that are not seen in other cultures. Consider these major differences when providing health care services to this population. One particular challenge is that Hispanic health outcomes deteriorate with the loss of traditional lifestyle patterns. Hispanics have equal or better health outcomes, even when in lower economic status, but with increasing economic status and acculturation into the majority U.S. culture these advantages are soon lost.

In this chapter, an overview of the history of Hispanics was described, including that part of the United States previously belonged to Mexico. Several culture-bound illnesses have been discussed, such as *empacho* and *susto,* along with treatment modalities that include the treatment of hot and cold illnesses. Various types of healing systems have been discussed, such as *curanderismo* and *Espiritismo.* Common health behaviors and illnesses among this group have been explained, along with issues for consideration when developing health promotion and education efforts for this target population.

Review

1. Define the terms *Hispanic* and *Latino* and explain why this population is not considered a race.
2. Provide an overview of the history of Hispanics in North America and the United States.
3. Explain the socioeconomic conditions of Hispanics in the United States.
4. What are *susto, empacho,* and *mal de ojo*?
5. What are *curanderismo,* Santeria, and *espiritismo*?

6. What are some of the common health risk behaviors and diseases among Hispanics in the United States?

7. What are some tips for working with the Hispanic population?

Activities

1. Conduct research on health programs that have been implemented for members of the Hispanic culture. Summarize the literature and identify some best practices.

2. Develop a *fotonovela* on a specific health topic. Be sure that the text, images, and other content are appropriate for this target audience.

Case Study 1

Jerome is a 30-year-old Hispanic man who has presented at his dentist's office with a complaint of a sore on the roof of his mouth. Dr. Perez has been Jerome's dentist for the past 4 years. On initial examination, she sees a lesion on the hard palate that looks like a bruise the size of a pea. Without any further investigation or examination she explains her finding to Jerome by saying, "What you have on the roof of your mouth is a sore that could indicate that you have a kind of cancer called Kaposi's sarcoma. Have you ever heard of Kaposi's sarcoma?"

Jerome looks stunned and says, "Isn't that the kind of cancer gay guys get when they have HIV?" Dr. Perez answers, "It is often associated with HIV infection. It sounds like you know something about HIV. Do you know anyone with HIV or this kind of cancer? Do you think you are HIV positive?"

1. How was health literacy taken into account in the way that Dr. Perez described the lesion?

2. What do you think Dr. Perez is trying to achieve with this line of questioning? Would you approach Jerome in a different manner? If so, how? How would you approach health literacy issues?

3. What do you know about the Hispanic concept of machismo? If Jerome is influenced by machismo, how do you think it would affect his health literacy and his ability to understand a diagnosis of HIV? Do you think Dr. Perez is taking this—and other cultural factors—into consideration as she progresses in the discussion?

4. What do you think would be the best way to continue this conversation with Jerome? Would you consider offering him a chance to talk to a male provider? What kind of materials or referrals would be appropriate?

5. Based on the case study discussion, what strategies to address health literacy might you include in an action plan for Jerome's care?

6. What ethical responsibility does Dr. Perez have to the patient?

7. Should Dr. Perez have made an effort to exclude other possible lesions that could be present first that are not associated with HIV, before explaining her findings to the patient? Why or why not?
8. Discuss other cultural competence issues that may impact retention into care and treatment.

Source: AETC-NMC, "Case Study 22: Addressing HIV Care and Health Literacy," https://www.aetcnmc.org/documents/case-study-22.pdf. Copyright © by AIDS Education and Training Center-National Multicultural Center (AETC-NMC) at Howard University. Reprinted with permission.

Case Study 2

Maria is a 54-year-old Mexican immigrant with type 2 diabetes mellitus, hypertension, and obesity. Her visits to your clinic have been challenging because of her limited English proficiency, late arrivals, and nonadherence to several medications. She agrees to start taking medications but does not refill her prescriptions or lose weight.

During Maria's next visit, you arrange for a telephone interpreter, which enables you to take a brief social history. She has three grown children: two still live in Mexico, and the third lives in a distant U.S. city. Her husband died in an industrial accident 4 years ago, and she is still grieving. She asks about your family, and hesitantly, through the interpreter, you share a bit about your own children. Her face lights up when you share this.

Using the LEARN model,[1] you listen to her story about her poor control of diabetes and frustration with her diet. She says that she does not feel better when taking the medicine and says the diet you prescribed does not include tortillas or any of the foods she likes. She says that since her husband died, she has lost interest in what might happen to her in the future. You explain why these interventions are necessary but acknowledge her frustration and agree to revise her diet. You recommend a compromised treatment plan for her diabetes and grief. After some negotiation, she agrees to see a dietitian and a bilingual counselor and agrees to take just two medications, metformin (Glucophage) and lisinopril (Zestril), although she understands that they will not make her feel better right away. You use "teach back" to ensure that Maria understands your directions, and you provide her with Spanish-language handouts about the benefits of controlling her diabetes and hypertension. You then schedule a return visit, during which an interpreter will be available.

You call the dietitian to alert him to this patient's cultural concerns. Maria needs to eat fruit; she should also consume more fiber to counteract her high-carbohydrate diet. One suggestion she readily agrees to is to include *nopales* (prickly pear cactus pads), a

1 *Editor's note:* The LEARN model described here involves listening to the patient's perception, explaining your perception of the problem, acknowledging differences in the perceptions, recommending treatment, and negotiating agreement (Juckett, 2013).

favorite from her childhood in Mexico. This traditional food is high in fiber and pectin and lowers lipid levels by binding bile acids; when eaten with other foods, it reduces the glycemic index of the meal by 50 percent. Because *nopales* may inhibit the absorption of drugs as well as glucose, Maria was told not to take her medications within a few hours of eating it. Other vegetables and fruits she likes are added to replace some other carbohydrates. The counselor helps her with her grief and gets her involved in an exercise and weight loss group at her church.

Your efforts pay off at the next visit, when Maria expresses much more interest in controlling her diabetes and shows personal warmth that was missing from earlier encounters. She has lost 10 pounds (4.5 kg), and for the first time has acceptable blood pressure and fasting glucose levels. It took extra time in relationship building (*personalismo*), a team approach, an interpreter, negotiation, and a bit of research to make it all happen.

Source: Gregory Juckett, "Caring for Latino Parents," *American Family Physician*, vol. 87, no. 1, p. 51. Copyright © 2013 by American Academy of Family Physicians. Reprinted with permission.

1. Do you think it can be appropriate to share your personal family information with patients?
2. Do you think providing Spanish language handouts to this patient was effective given you modified your oral communication style, engaged an interpreter, and provided personalized counseling?
3. What could be dangers of adapting food recommendations to accommodate patients' food traditions? What are the possible consequences of not adapting to patients' food customs?

References

American Lung Association. (2020). *Tobacco use in racial and ethnic populations.* https://www.lung.org/quit-smoking/smoking-facts/impact-of-tobacco-use/tobacco-use-racial-and-ethnic

Arias, E., & Xu, J. (2020, November 17). United States life tables, 2018. *National Vital Statistics Report, 69*(12). https://www.cdc.gov/nchs/data/nvsr/nvsr69/nvsr69-12-508.pdf

Benton, E. (2018, September 21). *5 rejuvenating soups women around the world drink for postpartum recovery.* Healthline. https://www.healthline.com/health/pregnancy/nourishing-soups-postpartum

Bustamonte, L., Mora L., & Lopez, M. (2020, August 11). *About one-in-four about U.S. Hispanics have not heard of Latinx, but just 3% use it.* Pew Research Center. https://www.pewresearch.org/hispanic/2020/08/11/about-One-in-four-u-s-hispanics-have-heard-of-latinx-but-just-3-use-it/

Caplan, S. (2019). Intersection of cultural and religious beliefs about mental health: Latinos in the faith-based setting. *Hispanic Health Care International: The Official Journal of the National Association of Hispanic Nurses, 17*(1), 4–10. https://doi.org/10.1177/1540415319828265

Carratala, S., & Maxwell, C. (2020, May 7). *Health disparities by race and ethnicity.* Center For American Progress. https://www.americanprogress.org/issues/race/reports/2020/05/07/484742/health-disparities-race-ethnicity/

Centers for Disease Control and Prevention. (2021a). *Hispanics/Latinos and tobacco use.* https://www.cdc.gov/tobacco/disparities/hispanics-latinos/index.htm

Center for Disease Control and Prevention. (2021b). *Hispanic/Latino Americans and type 2 diabetes.* https://www.cdc.gov/diabetes/library/features/hispanic-diabetes.html

Centers for Disease Control and Prevention. (2021c). About teen pregnancy. https://www.cdc.gov/teenppregnancy/about/index.htm

Centers for Disease Control and Prevention. (2022). *Risk for Covid-19 infection, hospitalization and death by race/ethnicity.* https://www.cdc.gov/coronavirus/2019-ncov/covid-data/investigations-discovery/hospitalization-death-by-race-ethnicity.html

Church of Likumi Babalu Aye v. City of Hialeah, 508 U.S. 520 (1993).

Cross Cultural Health Care Case Studies. (n.d.). *The case of Alejandro Flores.* http://support.mchtraining.net/national_ccce/case3/case.html

Curtin, S. C., & Arias, E. (2019, July). *Health, United States, 2018.* National Center for Health Statistics. https://www.cdc.gov/nchs/hus/contents2018.htm?search=,Hispanic_or_Latino

Ely, D. M., & Driscoll, A. K. (2019, August 1). Infant mortality in the United States, 2017: Data from period linked birth/infant death data set. *National Vital Statistics Report, 68*(10). https://www.cdc.gov/nchs/data/nvsr/nvsr68/nvsr68_10-508.pdf

Heron, M. (2019, June 24). Deaths: Leading causes for 2017. *National Vital Statistics Report, 68*(6), 12. https://www.cdc.gov/nchs/data/nvsr/nvsr68/nvsr68_06-508.pdf

Hidalgo, I., Brooten, B., Youngblut, J. M., Roche, R., Li, J., & Hinds, A. M. (2020). Practices following the death of a loved one reported by adults from 14 countries or cultural/ethnic group. *Nursing Open.* https://onlinelibrary.wiley.com/doi/epdf/10.1002/nop2.646

Holliday, N. (n.d.). *Working with Hispanics.* https://www.nrcs.usda.gov/Internet/FSE_DOCUMENTS/nrcs142p2_007143.pdf

Howard University College of Medicine, AIDS Education and Training Center, National Multicultural Center. (n.d.). *Case study 22.* https://www.aetcnmc.org/documents/case-study-22.pdf

Jimenez, R. (2002). *Culturally competent patient encounter tips. American Academy of Orthopaedic Surgeons: Bulletin: October 2002.* http://www2.aaos.org/bulletin/oct02/comm.htm

Jones, C. M., Clayton, H. B., Deputy, N. P., Roehler, D. L., Yo, J. K., Esser, M. B., Brookmeyer, K. A., & Hertz, M. F. (2020, August 21). Prescription opioid misuse and use of alcohol and other substances among high school students—Youth risk behavior survey, United States, 2019. *Morbidity and Mortality Weekly, 69*(1), 38. http://dx.doi.org/10.15585/mmwr.su6901a5

Juckett, G. (2005). Cross-cultural medicine. *American Family Physician.* 72(11), pp. 6722–2274. http://www.aafp.org/afp/20051201/2267.html

Juckett, G. (2013). Caring for Latino patients. *American Family Physician, 87*(1), 48–54. https://www.aafp.org/afp/2013/0101/p48.html

Markides, K. S., & Coreil, J. (1986). The health of Hispanics in the southwestern United States: An epidemiological paradox. *Public Health Reports, 101,* 253–265.

Meir, N., Smith, M. L., Wang, X., Towne, S., Carillo, N., Garza, N., & Ory, M. (2017). Factors associated with diet and exercise among overweight and obese older Hispanics with diabetes. SAGE Open, 7(2). https://doi.org/10.1177/2158244017710840

Merriam-Webster. (n.d.). *"Latinix" and gender inclusivity.* https://www.merriam-webster.com/words-at-play/word-history-latinx}.

Naso, A. (2016, September 12). *Mental illness and stigma in the Latino community.* Center For Health Journalism, USC Annenberg. https://centerforhealthjournalism.org/fellowships/projects/mental-illnesses-stigma-among-latino-community

National Center for Health Statistics. (2019). *Mortality trends by race and ethnicity among adults aged 25 and over: United States, 2000–2017.* https://www.cdc.gov/nchs/products/databriefs/db342.htm

National Institute on Alcohol Abuse and Alcoholism. (2019). *Factsheet alcohol and the Hispanic community.* https://www.niaaa.nih.gov/publications/brochures-and-fact-sheets/alcohol-and-hispanic-community

National Kidney Foundation. (2021). *Social determinants of kidney disease.* https://www.kidney.org/atoz/content/hispanics-kd

Nogueira, B., Mari, J., & Rassouk, D. (2015). Culture-bound syndromes in Spanish speaking Latin America: The case of *nervios, susto* and *ataques de nervios*. *Archives of Clinical Psychiatry, 42*(6). https://doi.org/10.1590/0101-60830000000070

Orlovic, M., Smith, K., & Elias, M. (2019). Racial and ethnic differences in end-of-life care in the United States: Evidence from the Health and Retirement Study (HRS). *SSM - Population Health,* 7(100331). https://www.sciencedirect.com/science/article/pii/S2352827318302714

Purnell, L. & Fenkl E., Eds. (2021). Textbook for transcultural health care: A population approach (5th ed., pp. 426–626). F. A. Davis.

Rhode Island Department of Health, n.d. *Latino/Hispanic culture & health.* http://www.health.ri.gov/chic/minority/lat_cul.php

Rocca, F. X. (2018, May 10). After 50 years, birth control still divides Catholics. *Wall Street Journal.* https://www.wsj.com/articles/after-50-years-a-popes-birth-control-message-still-divides-catholics-1525962322

Roth, M. S. (2021, August 2). What does Latinix mean. *Good Housekeeping.* https://www.goodhousekeeping.com/life/a33806428/what-latinx-means/

Salas-Wright, C., Vaughn, M., Clark, T., Miller, D., & Schwartz, S. (2018). Immigrants and mental disorders in the United States: New evidence on the healthy migrant hypothesis. *Psychiatry Research, 267,* 438–445. https://doi.org/10.1016/j.psychres.2018.06.039

Silva, C., & Van Orden, K. (2018). Suicide among Hispanics in the United States. *Current Opinion in Psychology,* 22, 44–49. http://www.sciencedirect.com/science/article/pii/S2352250X17301938

Torres, C. A., Thorn, B. E., Kapoor, S., & DeMonte, C. (2017, February 2). An examination of cultural values and pain management in foreign-born Spanish-speaking Hispanics seeking care at a federally qualified health center. *Pain Medicine, 18*(11), 2058–2069. https://academic.oup.com/painmedicine/article/18/11/2058/2967135

UKEssays. (2018, November). Hispanic cultural views and traditional values. https://www.ukessays.com/essays/sociology/hispanic-cultural-views-and-traditional-values-sociology-essay.php

U.S. Census Bureau. (2014, September 8). *Facts for features: Hispanic heritage month 2017: Sept. 15–Oct. 15.* http://www.census.gov/newsroom/facts-for-features/2014/cb14-ff22.html

U.S. Census Bureau. (2020). *American community survey table. 1* https://www.census.gov/data/tables/2019/demo/hispanic-origin/2019-cps.html

U.S. Department of Health and Human Services, Office of Minority Health. (2020). Obesity and Hispanic Americans. https://minorityhealth.hhs.gov/omh/browse.aspx?lvl=4&lvlid=70

U.S. Department of Health and Human Services, Office of Minority Health. (2021a). *Profile: Hispanic/Latino profile.* https://www.minorityhealth.hhs.gov/omh/browse.aspx?lvl=3&lvlid=64

U.S. Department of Health and Human Services, Office of Minority Health. (2021b). Organ donation and Hispanic Americans. https://www.minorityhealth.hhs.gov/omh/browse.aspx?lvl=4&lvlid=72

U.S. Department of Health and Human Services, Office of Minority Health. (2021c). *Mental and behavioral health—Hispanics.* https://www.minorityhealth.hhs.gov/omh/browse.aspx?lvl=4&lvlid=69

Velasco-Mondragon, E., Jimenez, A., Palladino-Davis, A. G., Davis, D., & Escamilla-Cejudo, J. A. (2016). Hispanic health in the USA: A scoping review of the literature. *Public Health Reviews, 37*(31). https://doi.org/10.1186/s40985-016-0043-2

Vespa, J., Medina, L., & Armstrong, D. M. (2018). *Demographic turning points for the United States: Population projections for 2020 to 2060.* https://www.census.gov/content/dam/Census/library/publications/2020/demo/p25-1144.pdf

Yasmin, S. (2014, January 17). Decoding the Hispanic paradox. *The Dallas Morning News.* https://www.dallasnews.com/opinion/commentary/2014/01/17/decoding-the-hispanic-paradox/

CREDIT

CHAPTER 7

American Indian and Alaskan Native Populations

What we see as science, Indians see as magic. What we see as magic, they see as science. I don't find a hopeless contradiction. If we can appreciate each other's views, we can see the whole picture more clearly.

—HAMMERSCHLAG (1988, p. 14)

Everything on the earth has a purpose, every disease an herb to cure it, and every person a mission. This is the Indian theory of existence.

—MOURNING DOVE SALISH, 1888-1936

KEY CONCEPTS AND TERMS

Medicine bundle
Medicine wheel
Peyote
Sand painting
Sweat lodges

LEARNING OBJECTIVES

After reading this chapter, you should be able to do the following:

1. Provide an overview of the social and economic circumstances of American Indian and Alaskan Native populations in the United States.
2. Provide an overview of American Indian and Alaskan Native beliefs about the causes of illness.
3. Describe at least three American Indian and Alaskan Native healing practices.
4. Describe American Indian and Alaskan Native health risk behaviors and common illnesses.
5. List at least six tips for working with American Indian and Alaskan Native populations.

Introduction

The American Indian and Alaskan Native populations include a broad range of people and cultures that existed in North America at the time of the arrival of Christopher Columbus. The U.S. Census Bureau (2020) identifies this population as a race that includes anyone having origins in any of the original peoples of North and South America (including Central America) who maintains a tribal affiliation or community attachment. A wide range of other terms have been used to describe "American Indian and Alaska Native," such as Native Indians, American Indians, Native American Indians, Indians, Aborigines, Native Alaskans, and Original Americans. Other American Indian and Alaskan Native populations include the Hawaiian and Pacific Islanders, but they are now counted separately by the U.S. Census Bureau. Race is not the same as culture, but Census Bureau information provides a general profile of the combined populations.

Health conditions among the original tribes were directly associated with living off the land and holding a holistic philosophy regarding promoting health. American Indian and Alaskan Native populations lived a pre-industrial lifestyle much like hunter-gathers and small-scale farmers on other continents. Each tribe or nation had its own practices based on its own culture and geographic region. The Seminoles in Florida, Quinault in Washington, Chumash in California, Inuit in Alaska, and Iroquois in the Northeast were all very different, living on different foods, facing different weather conditions, and developing their own cultural practices and languages. Yet all eventually suffered conquest, and many endured forced dislocation and generally became economically disadvantaged. In 2018, the approximately 6.9 million American Indian and Alaskan Native people (alone or in combination with other races) are culturally diverse and geographically dispersed (U.S. Census Bureau, 2019).

Current disease patterns among American Indians and Alaska Natives are associated with negative consequences of poverty, limited access to health services, and cultural dislocation generally imposed by colonization practices of Europeans. Inadequate education, high rates of unemployment, discrimination, and cultural differences all contribute to unhealthy lifestyles and disparities in access to health care for many American Indian and Alaska Native people and the disparities in money, power, and resources have existed since colonization (Jernigan, 2015).

In a special message on Indian affairs delivered to Congress July 8, 1970, President Richard Nixon (1970) declared,

> But the story of the Indian in America is something more than the record of the white man's frequent aggression, broken agreements, intermittent remorse and prolonged failure. It is a record of enormous contributions to this country—to its art and culture, to its strength and spirit, to its sense of history and its sense of purpose.

This chapter provides a brief history of American Indian and Alaskan Native populations and information about their current status in the United States, their beliefs about the causes of illness and healing practices, behavioral risk factors, and the common health problems they face.

Terminology

The various words used to describe American Indian and Alaskan Native populations have varied in popularity and use. None of these terms is accurate, because they are derived from mistaken identity of peoples by Columbus and from naming the country after a post-Columbian Italian explorer and map maker, Amerigo Vespucci. Each is based on labels created by Europeans who generally saw the great variety of cultures as one large group of native people. Certainly, the Europeans learned to recognize and deal with individual tribes, but a tribe was seen as a subset of a group of generally less worthy people.

Like most people, American Indian and Alaskan Native people prefer to be referred to by the society with whom they themselves identify. So, for example, Navajo and Blackfeet prefer being identified by their specific tribe or nation. When we refer to American Indian and Alaskan Native people, we are referring to a broad group of cultures similar in scope to the group of cultures included in the label "Europeans." It is intended as a neutral and all-encompassing term for pre-Columbian cultures located in North America. Certainly, Germans still prefer to be called German as much as the English prefer to be called English or British. Some broad generalizations can be made about such classifications of peoples, but cultural practices and differences can lead to great partnerships as well as great conflicts and wars. In this chapter, we refer to American Indian and Alaskan Native populations generally, but we also describe some groups more specifically, such as American Indians located within what is now the contiguous 48 United States, Alaska Natives, and specific tribes or nations depending on the context and available data.

History of American Indians and Alaska Natives in the United States

The American Indian and Alaskan Native populations are descendants of the first humans who migrated from Asia and Europe to North America about 30,000 years ago. Christopher Columbus reached North America in 1492 during a voyage in search of the East Indies. The explorer used the name "Indians" to describe the people of the land, because of the mistaken idea the European sailors were in the Far East.

The European migration initiated what is sometimes called the Columbian Exchange and began in the 15th century. It changed the lives of American Indian and Alaskan Native populations as well as Europeans even before there was physical contact. In the Columbian Exchange, foods, wealth, and customs were transferred back and forth between America, Europe, and Africa. For instance, the modern horse was introduced to North America by the Spanish. When a thousand captured horses were released by American Indians in 1580 after a skirmish with the Spanish, the horses spread into the American Great

Plains and changed the way of life for tens of thousands of people who began to use the horse for the first time. This transformed many cultural and economic practices among Plains Indians. It changed their culture into one based on horses that allowed mobility and effective hunting of the vast quantities of bison on the Great Plains. Likewise, corn, potatoes, and tomatoes were transferred to Europe from the Americas.

As transportation and trade increased, new diseases were transmitted by the Europeans, such as smallpox and measles, which spread between American Indian and Alaskan Native tribes before many even heard of the Europeans. American Indian and Alaskan Native Americans had no immunities to these diseases. While actual population counts for the United States area are based only on estimates, about 18 million Native Americans lived north of Mexico at the beginning of the 16th century (Thornton, 2019). The data-driven best estimate of the death toll throughout the Americas is 56 million by the beginning of the 1600s, which was about 90% of the pre-Columbian Indigenous population and around 10% of the global population at the time. This makes the "Great Dying," due to illness and European colonialization policies and practices, the largest human mortality event in proportion to the global population, putting it second in absolute terms only to World War II, which led to approximately 80 million deaths. However, disease transfer was not all in one direction. In a similar way, it is believed that syphilis was first transported to Europe from the Americas.

Vast differences in culture caused misunderstanding and conflict. The American Indian and Alaskan Native populations were viewed by the Europeans as a problem. The solution was to control them through wars and to push any survivors to low-valued lands. The Europeans viewed land as something to be held by an owner with various groups managing their own parcels of land. The American Indian and Alaskan Native populations generally viewed land as unbounded except for physical barriers; land was something to be used but not owned. This does not mean life was easy or peaceful. Intertribal wars and preindustrial living off the land presented ongoing dangers and challenges to health and survival. Once it became evident that the Europeans intended to stay and seize land in any way necessary, American Indian and Alaskan Native populations began to initiate their own acts of violence against the Europeans.

In the 19th century, the westward expansion of the United States caused large numbers of American Indians to be moved farther west, often by force, almost always reluctantly. The U.S. Congress, under President Andrew Jackson, passed the Indian Removal Act of 1830, which authorized the president to conduct treaties to exchange American Indian land east of the Mississippi River for lands west of the river. As many as 100,000 Native Americans eventually were compelled to relocate in the West as a result of the Indian Removal Act. In theory, relocation was supposed to be voluntary, but in practice great pressure was put on American Indian leaders to sign removal treaties.

The United States purchased Alaska from Russia in 1867. In 1906, the Homestead Act granted land to the following individuals:

> Indian or Eskimo of full or mixed blood who resides in and is a native of said district, and who is the head of a family, or is 21 years of age; and the land so

allotted shall be deemed the homestead of the allotted and his heirs in perpetuity and shall be inalienable and nontaxable until otherwise provided by Congress.

This act was the first to establish land for Alaska Natives, but it left out many tribes. Discrimination and segregation were prevalent in Alaska, especially between Alaska Natives and Whites (Russians and European Americans). In 1945, Alaska passed a law that ended legal segregation, and this marked the start of a new beginning. According to the Alaska Native Claims Settlement Act of 1971, 40 million acres of land and nearly a billion dollars was awarded to Alaska Natives.

Many steps were taken to subjugate the American Indian and Alaskan Native populations and to change their cultural practices, such as not permitting them to speak their native language and creating Indian boarding schools to keep children away from their tribal setting. The Indian Citizenship Act of 1924 gave U.S. citizenship to American Indians, in part because of an interest by many existing American citizens to see them merged with the American mainstream and also because of the service of many American Indian and Alaskan Native Americans in World War I.

American Indian and Alaskan Native Populations in the United States

There are 574 federally recognized tribes and more than 100 state-recognized tribes. As a result of early treaties, the federal government provides health care services to federally recognized tribes through the Indian Health Service (IHS), part of the U.S. Department of Health and Human Services. Comprehensive health services are available to approximately 2 million American Indians and Alaska Natives (Federal Register, 2020). Some groups of people identify themselves with "tribes" but are not recognized by the states or the federal government.

The majority of those who receive IHS services live on reservations and in rural communities in 37 states, generally in the western United States and Alaska. Thirty-six percent of the IHS service area population resides in non-Indian areas, with 2.56 million served in 2020. The urban clientele has less access to hospitals, health clinics, and contract health services provided by the IHS or to health programs in tribal areas. Studies on the urban American Indian and Alaskan Native populations have frequently documented issues that prevent them from receiving quality medical care. These issues include cultural barriers, geographic isolation, inadequate sewage disposal, and low income (HHS, OMH, 2018).

Since 1972, IHS has embarked on a series of initiatives to fund health-related activities in off-reservation settings to make health care services accessible to urban American Indians and Alaska Natives. In 2020, the IHS funded 41 urban Indian health organizations, which operated at sites located in cities throughout the United States. Approximately 2.56 million American Indians and Alaska Natives are eligible for this program (Indian Health Service, 2021). The 41 programs administer medical services, dental services, community services, alcohol and drug dependency prevention, education and treatment, AIDS and sexually transmitted disease education and prevention services, mental health services, nutrition education and counseling services, pharmacy services, health education, optometry services, social services, and home health care.

In 2017, 26.9% of American Indians and Alaskan Natives spoke a language other than English at home (HHS, OMH, 2018). American Indian and Alaskan Native populations use many different languages. The Census Bureau recognizes 169 American Indian and Alaskan Native languages, but these languages are spoken by only 364,331 people at home (U.S. Census Bureau, 2015).

In 2017, the median family income for American Indian and Alaska Natives was $45,448, compared to $65,845 for non-Hispanic Whites. Thirty-five percent of American Indians and Alaskan Natives aged 16 and over worked in management and professional occupations, compared to 42.9% of Whites. Also, 21.9% of this racial group lived at the poverty level, compared to 9.6% of non-Hispanic Whites (HHS, OMH, 2018).

Like many other peoples, American Indian and Alaskan Native populations generally believe in a Supreme Creator; most tribes also have lesser deities and mediators between the spirit world and the earth, while others hold pan- or atheistic beliefs. Most believe that people should try to maintain constant, daily harmony and contact with the Creator or natures, follow all sacred teachings, and treat all life (people, animals, plants, rocks, rivers, rainbows, etc.) with respect.

American Indian and Alaskan Native populations are family based and are taught to respect and obey their elders. The elders are seen as people with much knowledge, and they are considered the head of the household. After the elders, men are considered the leaders of the house. Men also are viewed as the leaders of the tribe, protectors, and fighters. Traditionally, the men would hunt to bring food for the whole community; as a result, they are still seen as the providers for the family.

Women are often viewed as being responsible for housework and for teaching the children the ways of the people. The children have to learn the traditions of the tribe and the community and have to respect the elders. The older family members keep an eye on the new generation to make sure that they are following traditions.

In addition to believing in close family relations, American Indian and Alaskan Native populations also believe in living as a community. A person does not need to be from the same tribe or even have blood relations with anyone from the community to be a member of the community. As many as 80 different tribes can live together in one community. The elders are in charge of teaching and guiding the community in the ways of the tribes. They have the responsibility to pass on their history orally and to teach the community the traditional ways of the tribe. They show the new generation how to make traditional arts and crafts and show them the traditional rituals.

One of the rituals is storytelling, or experiencing stories through songs or other performances. Songs play an important part in the lives of American Indian and Alaskan Native populations. These songs are usually ancestral songs that tell the story of the ancestors and of hardships they had to face. Many of the songs are related to nature and hunting. The songs are considered the property of the person who created or dreamt them or of the community after that person passes away. If someone wants to reenact the song, they must obtain special permission from the community.

Alaskan Native populations include people from villages or tribes such as Aleut, Inupiat, Yupik, Eskimo, and Athabaskan peoples. Villages consist of mostly related families; however, if residents are not related, they are still treated as one big family. Alaska Natives typically develop close-knit relationships with one another. Village members watch out for one another, and food is always shared when an animal is caught. Alaska Natives believe that if people share their food, they will catch more animals in the future. When a young hunter experiences a first kill, it is tradition to give the entire kill to the elders, as a sign of respect and as a way to indicate passing on tradition from generation to generation. The tradition of sharing and giving is a major part of Alaskan Native culture.

General Philosophy About Disease Prevention and Health Maintenance

Traditionally, health was a continual process of staying strong spiritually, mentally, and physically. This strength keeps away or overcomes the forces that cause illness. People must stay in harmony with themselves, other people, their natural environment, and their Creator. Adhering to traditional and tribal beliefs and obeying tribal religious codes is another part of staying healthy; violating tribal tenets or laws may have consequences such as physical or mental illness, disability, ongoing bad luck, or trauma. The violation must be set right before harmony and health can be restored. Some American Indians believe illness is the price to be paid either for something that happened in the past or for something that will happen in the future; therefore, everyone is responsible for their own health. Illness is not looked upon as abnormal. However, this group does not believe in biomedicine or germ theory; they believe illness is caused by personal responsibility, qualities, and spirits (Spector, 2017).

Even though some Alaska Natives are nonreligious, traditional Natives believe that the cause of illness is derived from spirits (Alexandria, 1994). To get rid of an illness, a shaman is needed to remove the ill spirit and restore health. Healing ceremonies can take place in public, and the shaman encourages village members to participate to get rid of the bad spirit that is causing the illness. In addition, some shamans have medical skills that include treating burns with fat, cleaning wounds with urine, amputating frozen gangrenous limbs, and setting broken bones. Traditional Natives believe that shamans have the ability to fly and reach the heavens.

Currently, beliefs about the causes of illness are beginning to shift. Alaska Natives noticed that they were less likely to get sick when they traveled in small nomadic bands. However, when Alaska Natives began to settle, they noticed that people were more likely to become ill and die. As a result, they have begun to lean toward germ theory. Shamans are still used today because it is often difficult to reach health care clinics. In some instances, both a shaman and Western medicine are used in combination to treat illness.

Worldview

Being in harmony is important to the people in these collectivist cultures. Group success is more important than the success of the individual. American Indian and Alaskan Native populations tend to see property as communal. A strong sense of connectedness and an understanding of the world comes from the cycles and natural rhythms of life. Health is achieved through balance. Autonomy is important, but illness is viewed as a family matter. Participation in religious ceremonies and prayer is believed to promote health.

Generally having a fatalistic view, Native peoples may not take preventative actions, such as participating in health screenings or treating health issues. American Indian and Alaskan Native peoples also do not recognize silent disease—in other words, if there are no symptoms, then one is not ill. This provides another barrier to participating in health screenings and to treating illnesses that are "invisible" such as cancer.

American Indian and Alaskan Native populations have no precise beliefs regarding what might occur after death. Some believe that humans return as ghosts or that people go to another world. Others believe that nothing definite can be known about one's fate after this life. Combinations of belief are common. Organ donations and autopsies are generally not desired. Do not resuscitate orders are not acceptable in many tribes, because they are believed to bring about negative thoughts and, hence, inevitable loss.

There is high respect for elders, and elders play an important role is passing down cultural traditions to children and grandchildren. In general, respect is a core value and central to all interactions. Respect is viewed as not talking about oneself, bragging, or talking back.

American Indian and Alaskan Native populations select their words carefully and may take long pauses during conversations. Do not interrupt when a person is speaking. Avoiding eye contact and keeping a respectful distance is encouraged. "A primary social premise is that no person has the right to speak for another" (Purnell, 2021, p. 164). Their perspective on time is that it cannot be controlled, and planning for the future may be seen as being foolish (Purnell, 2021).

Amulets, sacred objects, and medicine bags are valued. Do not remove them without asking permission. If you are given permission to remove them, do it carefully and replace them as soon as possible.

American Indian and Alaskan Native populations tend to complain of pain in general terms. For example, the patient may report discomfort. Pain is often undertreated in this population. This is, in part, because it is viewed as a violation of proscriptive behaviors. When sick, they are often stoic and quiet.

DID YOU KNOW?

For some American Indian and Alaskan Native populations, having long hair is not an issue of style; it is related to culture. Cutting one's hair can be related to health or mourning the death of a close relative or loved one. If a health procedure requires that hair be cut or shaved, ask if the hair should be returned to the patient or to a family member. This includes needing to shave an area of the body for a surgical procedure. Some members of this culture will wash the hair of the ill person as a custom or ceremony. Touching the hair of a pregnant woman should be avoided.

Pregnancy, Birth, and Child Rearing

Although each American Indian and Alaskan Native culture has its own beliefs and rituals, there are many descriptions of American Indian and Alaskan Native childbirth practices involving the pregnant woman secluding herself, with perhaps a woman helper, and having a private birth experience out of the sight of men. Early accounts of the childbirth practices of the American Indian and Alaskan Native population indicate that pregnant women were to limit their activities and watch their diet and behavior to protect the baby. Certain foods might affect the fetus and cause unwanted physical characteristics. For example, the Cherokee believed that eating raccoon meat would cause illness or death of the baby. They believed that speckled trout could cause birthmarks. Mothers- and fathers-to-be performed rituals to guarantee a safe delivery, such as washing hands and feet daily.

As the birth grew closer, women and their families observed other rituals to ensure an easy and healthy birth. Some newborns were ceremonially plunged into water on a daily basis for up to 2 years to gain strength. European descriptions of Native American women's quick recovery from childbirth may have been exaggerated. But generally, the excellent physical conditioning of women would have facilitated their recovery from childbirth, allowing most women to return to their regular duties quickly.

Children are considered specially linked to the spiritual world and in general are indulged rather than punished. Europeans were surprised at the absence of physical punishment as a means to discipline children. Sometimes the children were chastised by having a little water thrown in their faces, and there were reports of Creek parents occasionally scratching disobedient children and, along with the Chickasaws, allowing young ones to be beaten by someone outside the household. Corporal punishment was clearly the exception rather than the rule, although ridicule or fear of the supernatural might be used to produce obedience.

The transition from childhood to adulthood is well defined. For girls there are sometimes rituals surrounding the onset of menstruation. For boys, whose passage through puberty is less biologically evident, there are more elaborate ceremonies such as the *huskinaw*, a rigorous physical trial, and the vision quest, a spiritual journey. Both involved isolation as well as sensory deprivation and stimulation; their purpose was to begin a new path without forfeiting their upbringing.

Marriage partners might be tentatively chosen by parents, and a prospective groom could be expected to consult the parents of the intended spouse. Yet there was no coercion: both partners had a choice when it came to marrying and deciding whether to remain wed.

Nutrition and Exercise

With regard to their dietary practices, American Indian and Alaskan Native populations believe that certain foods are sacred. For example, some believe the Great Spirit Hashtali gave the people corn as a present, so it is considered sacred. Corn is used quite frequently for meals because it can be easily grown and does not require much work. Another sacred food is blood soup, which is made from a mixture of animal blood and corn flour cooked in broth. Blood soup may be used as a sacred meal during the nighttime Holy Smoke ceremony of the Sioux, which is a celebration of Mother Earth that involves the use of the peace pipe (Garces, n.d.). Wolves and coyotes are the only animals that are not hunted for food, because they are regarded as teachers or pathfinders and held sacred by all tribes (Garces, n.d.). At marriage ceremonies, the bride and groom exchange food instead of rings. The groom brings venison or some other meat to indicate intention to provide for the household, and the bride provides corn or bean bread to symbolize willingness to care for and provide nourishment for the household (Garces, n.d.).

American Indian and Alaskan Native populations have changed their diet and food practices probably more than any other group in the United States. The current diet of American Indian and Alaskan Native closely resembles that of the U.S. White population (Garces, n.d.).

A food guide for American Indians is illustrated in **Figure 7.1**. Although current nutritional practices are similar to those of the general U.S. population, American Indian and Alaskan Native populations originally relied largely on meat, fish, plants, berries, and

A Guide to Daily Food Choices
KEY
These symbols show fats, oils, and added sugars in foods.
Fat (Naturally occuring and added)
Sugars (added)
Fat's, Oils & Sweets
use sparingly
Low or Non-fat Dairy Products
Milk, Yogurt & Cheese Group
2-3 Servings
Meat, Poultry, Fish, Dry Beans
Eggs & Nuts Group
2-3 Servings
MILK
NUTS
beans
YOGURT
PEANUT BUTTER
Vegetable Group
3-5 Servings
Fruit Group
2-4 Servings
WILD RICE
OATS
Bread, Cereal Group
6-11Servings
Rice, Pasta Group
6-11Servings

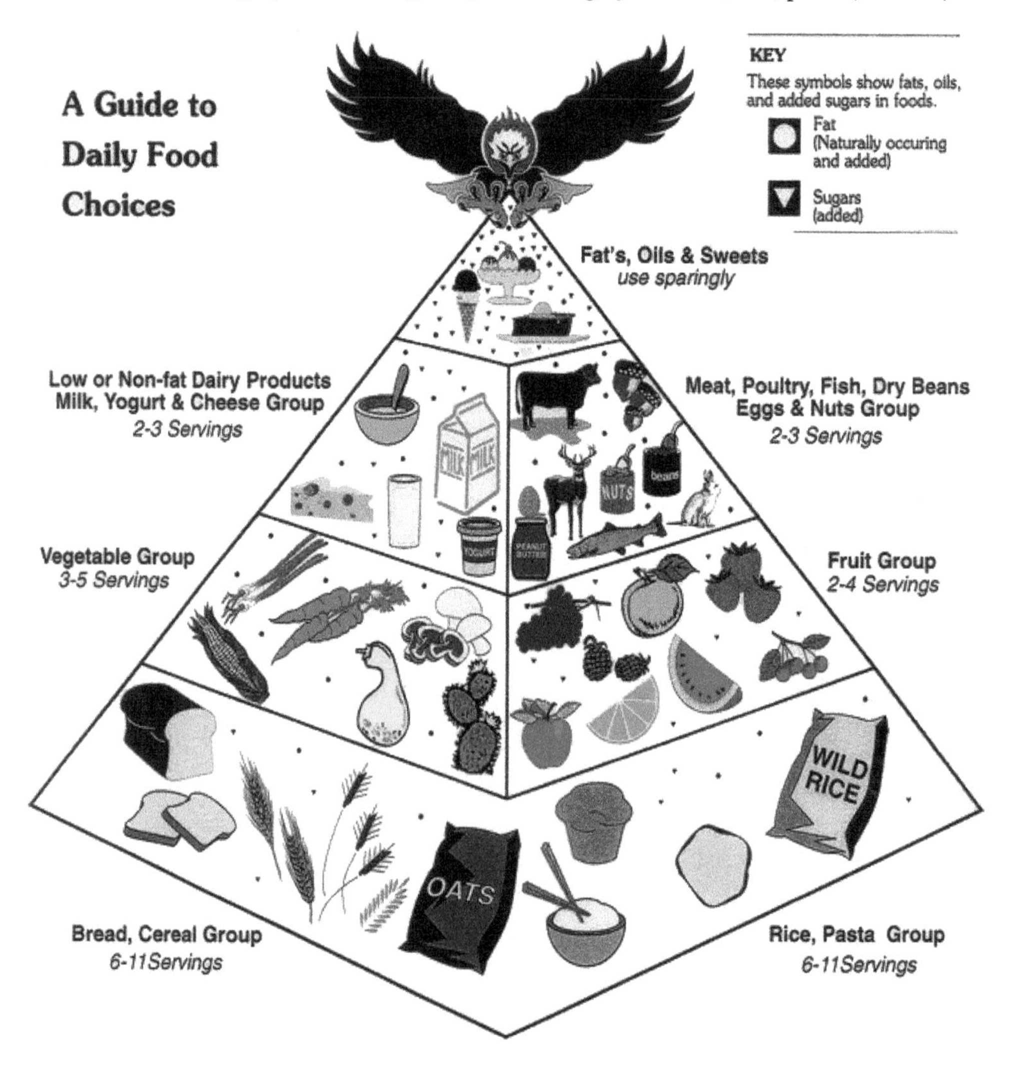

Figure 7.1 Native American food guide.

nuts. The most widely grown foods were maize (corn) and wild rice. Many tribes grew beans and enjoyed them as *succotash,* a dish made of beans, corn, dog meat, and bear fat. Tubers (roots) were also a common food and were cooked slowly in underground pits until the hard tough root became a highly digestible gelatin-like soup.

The American Indian and Alaskan Native populations were shunned and marginalized, but their foods have been integrated into the modern American menu. These include succotash in the South, wild rice dishes in the northern Plains, pumpkin soup in New England, chili in the Southwest, broiled salmon in the Pacific Northwest, and corn on the cob in most areas of the country. Traditionally, American Indian and Alaskan Native peoples lived an active farming and hunting lifestyle that was conducive to better health than the sedentary lifestyle now customary for all population groups in the United States.

Alaska Natives continue to rely substantially on subsistence foods such as fish, terrestrial mammals, marine mammals, and wild plants. Subsistence uses are central to the customs and traditions of many cultural groups in Alaska, including Aleut, Athabascan, Alutiiq, Haida, Inupiat, Tlingit, Tsimshian, and Yupik. Fish and wildlife harvests for food provide a major part of the nutritional requirements of Alaska's rural population, and lesser, but notable, percentages in urban areas. The annual rural harvest of 276 pounds per person contains 176% of the protein requirements of the rural population (i.e., it contains about 81 grams of protein per person per day; about 46 grams is the mean daily requirement. The subsistence harvest contains 25% of the caloric requirements of the rural population (i.e., it contains about 518 kcal daily, assuming a 2,100 kcal/day requirement). The urban wild food harvests contain 12% of the protein requirements and 2% of the caloric requirements of the urban population (Alaska Department of Fish and Game, n.d.).

When obtaining traditional foods, the men usually do the strenuous hunting, and the women gather berries and plants that will aid in nutrition. Women also prepare and store the food after it is gathered.

Mental Health

American Indian and Alaskan Native populations experience serious psychological distress at rates similar to those of the overall population. The most significant mental health issues are depression, substance abuse, and anxiety, including posttraumatic stress disorder (PTSD). In 2019, suicide was the second leading cause of death for American Indian/Alaska Natives between the ages of 10 and 34, and the overall death rate from suicide for American Indian/Alaska Native adults is about 20% higher compared to the non-Hispanic White population. Adolescent American Indian/Alaska Native females, age 15–19, have a death rate that is five times higher than for non-Hispanic White females in the same age groups, but older women have a lower suicide rate (HHS, OMH, 2021a). In some, but not all, American Indian and Alaskan Native groups, alcoholism and illicit drug use disorder rates are much higher than U.S. averages.

Cultural factors can influence how people feel or describe mental health and their acceptance of mental health issues and treatment. Among Indians/Native people, the concept of mental health has different meanings and interpretations. Often physical concerns and psychological concerns are not separated, and emotional distress may be expressed in different ways. In fact, words for "depressed" and "anxious" were not part of the American Indian and

Alaskan Native languages, and culturally different expressions of illness, such as ghost sickness, do not correspond to modern medicine diagnoses (National Alliance on Mental Illness, n.d.).

Death and Dying

There is a great variety of beliefs about death and dying across the various American Indian and Alaskan Native populations. Some American Indian and Alaskan Native cultures do not speak of death, dying, or negative outcomes to medical procedures because any mention might cause a negative outcome. Other tribal communities have no difficulty speaking directly about death or dying situations and wish to have all the information available (e.g., some Pueblo, Lakota, northern Plains, Midwestern, and northeastern tribes). These tribes tend to look at death as a natural part of the circle of life, not to be feared, as it may include a reunion with the ancestors who went before.

Cultural-Bound Illnesses

There are no particular illnesses associated with American Indian and Alaskan Native peoples, but many illnesses are associated with a cultural response to acculturation with Europeans. For instance, alcohol, now a major problem for a significant percentage of American Indian and Alaskan Native people, was plied to the tribes for trade and subjugation. The loss of traditional economic and cultural ways to mark life transitions, such as reduction or elimination of rite of passage into adulthood ceremonies, may contribute to the onset of early smoking. Blatant prejudice has contributed to conditions symptomatic of poor, undereducated, and purposely marginalized peoples of any minority group.

A couple of illnesses attributed to American Indian and Alaskan Native peoples may not have a defined cultural base. Ghost sickness is a psychological condition in which a person has an obsessive fear and preoccupation with the death of a person who meant a great deal to them. This can be associated with a person's concern that proper burial rites were not followed and that the deceased may not be able to move forward in the afterlife. Some attribute this illness to a severe case of grief and mourning. Concern about burial practices may be just one of many fears that might trigger the condition in any population.

Similarly, a condition called heartbreak syndrome has been attributed to American Indian and Alaskan Native populations, but it is more probably a general human condition. The American Heart Association (n.d.) has described this condition as involving a sudden onset of heart pain, and even damage, shortly after an intense event such as the death of a loved one or a divorce.

Healing Traditions, Healers, and Healing Aids

Most American Indian and Native American tribes have healing traditions related to their beliefs about the causation of illness and disease, which are not based on Western science. Therefore, many healing traditions and rituals focus on harmony, and the overall purpose is to bring participants into harmony with themselves, their tribe, and all of life. Healing occurs when someone is restored to harmony and connected to universal powers.

Traditional healing is holistic. It focuses on the person, not the illness, so the process does not focus on symptoms or diseases but addresses the total individual.

Alaska Native traditional healing practices are rooted in a 10,000-year history and are reemerging today as a holistic healing approach for individuals and communities. These methods are often used in combination with Western-based medical therapies for the purpose of health promotion, disease prevention, pain reduction, and enhancement of psychological wellness (Stanford Medicine, 2020). Many ancient traditions for healing are still used by Alaskan Natives today.

Despite the emergence of a complementary relationship between Alaskan traditional healing and Western medicine, traditional healing practices are quite distinguishable when compared to the Western medicine mode of treatment. Allopathic medicine focuses on identifying and treating a specific diagnosis, whereas traditional healing strives to restore the patient's sense of natural balance and harmony with self, community, and culture. Traditional healing attempts to nurture the mind-body-spirit connection and to actively involve the patient in finding renewed commitment to lifelong health and wellness. Complementary or integrative approaches, which bring traditional and nontraditional practices together, are becoming more common and provide some support by the National Center for Complimentary and Integrative Health at the U.S. National Institutes of Health.

Medicinal plants, such as roots, berries, leaves, and flowers, have historically been used as healing agents by American Indians and Alaska Natives. These medicinal plants are used in numerous ways to heal everything from the common cold, flesh wounds, and mouth sores to promoting healthy pregnancy and for many other applications. North American Indians have medicinal purposes for more than 2,500 plant species. For example, willow bark (the bark of the tree) is widely known to have been ingested as an anti-inflammatory and pain reliever. In fact, it contains a chemical called *salicin*, which is a confirmed anti-inflammatory that when consumed generates salicylic acid—the active ingredient in modern-day aspirin tablets (Roberts, 2020). The medicinal plants are aimed more at healing bodily ailments, but other traditional healing modalities focus on the spirit and the mind.

Healing Ceremonies

Ceremonies are used to help groups of people return to harmony; they are not used for individual healing. The ceremonies used by the tribes vary, and there are differences in the way they practice medicine.

For example, the Navajo heal through their **sand painting** (see **Figure 7.2**). Sitting on the floor of a house, the medicine person begins painting at sunrise using ground-colored rocks and minerals. The paintings depict the gods, elements of the

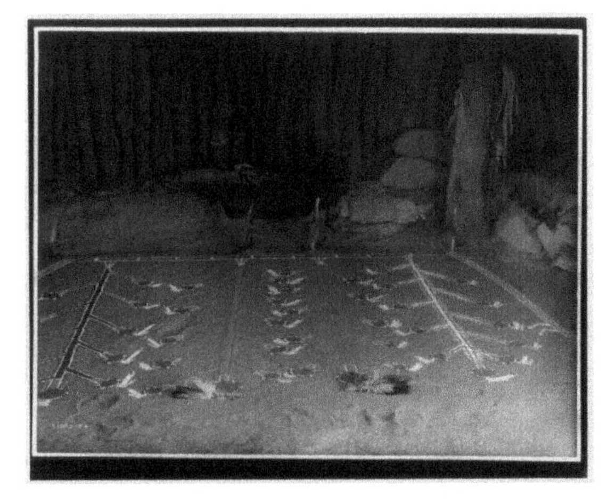

Figure 7.2 Sand painting.

heavens, and religious objects. When the painting, which includes complex forms and designs in great detail, is completed, the patient is placed in the center of the painting and the healing ceremony, which includes rituals and chants, is performed. Before sunset, the medicine person destroys the painting. The sands are sent to the desert and scattered on the four winds.

The Iroquois practice medicine through their False Faces society. Each spring and fall, when most illnesses occur, society members wear strange and distorted masks to drive illness and disease away from the tribe. Wearing these masks and ragged clothes and carrying rattles made from tortoise shells, they perform a dance. After the dance, society members go from house to house to rid the community of evil.

Some tribes use medicine wheels (see **Figure 7.3**), and the medicine wheel's large circle measures 213 feet around. The 28 spokes radiating from its center represent the number of days in the lunar cycle. A medicine wheel is a metaphor or symbol that represents the circle of life and the individual journey everyone must take to find their own path. Within the medicine wheel are the four cardinal directions (north, south, east, and west) and the four sacred colors. Mother Earth is below the wheel and Father Sky is above it. The south (white) represents fire and passion, and the associated animals, such as the eagle and lion, represent pride, strength, and courage. The north (blue) represents air and flight and is associated with winged animals that fly, such as the owl and hummingbird. The west (black) is associated with water and emotions and is associated with animals that work in teams and prepare for winter, such as the snake (because it sheds its skin) and

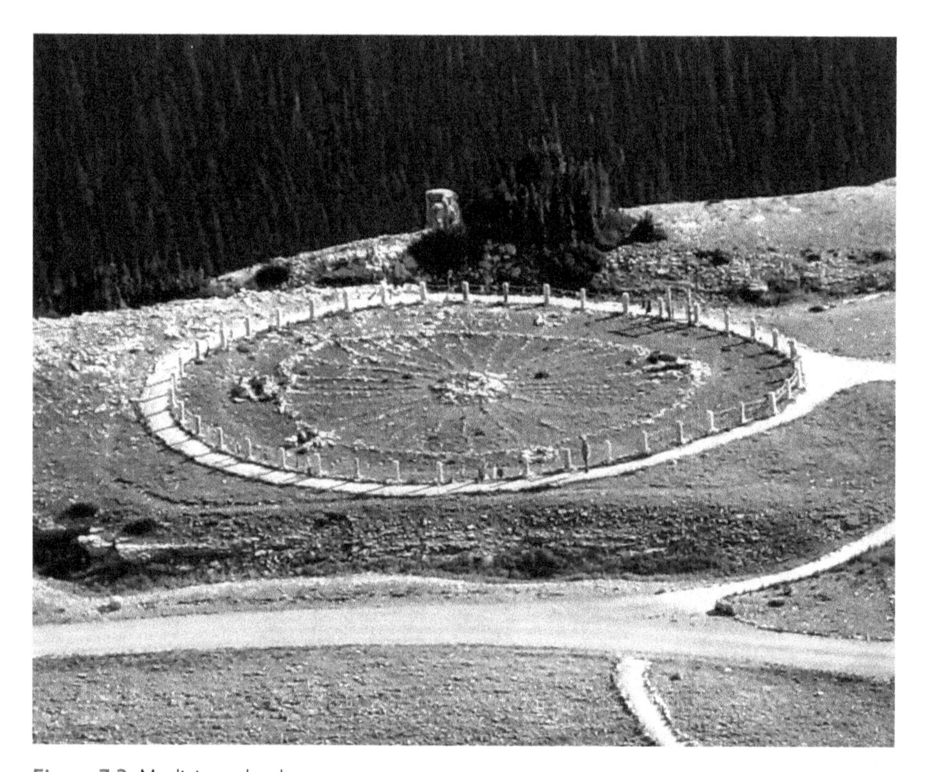

Figure 7.3 Medicine wheel.

the beaver. The east (red) is linked to the earth and wisdom and is related to animals that have layers of fat to sustain them during the winter, such as the buffalo. The wheel helps American Indians see exactly where they are and in which areas they need to develop to realize and fulfill their potential. They see that people are all connected to one another, and by showing the intricacies of the interwoven threads of life, they can envision their role in life. It helps them understand that without their part in the tapestry, the bigger picture is not as it should be. It is a model to be used to view self, society, or anything that one could ever think of looking into.

Healers

Medicine men, who are prominent healers in the American Indian community, can be male or female. They have knowledge about the interrelationships of human beings, the earth, the universe, plants, animals, the sun, the moon, and the stars (Spector, 2017). These healers are in tune with the way human beings interact with the world around them, and they are able to use their environment to help provide treatment. A healer is held in high regard because it has taken many years of training and apprenticeship to be able to heal the community. Many American Indians first consult a medicine man before seeking other health professionals because of their belief that the treatment they receive from the traditional healer is better than treatment from Western health care establishments (Spector, 2017).

Medicine people have power that other members of the tribe do not have. Their power comes from visions that lead them into studying medicine or by being born into a family with many generations of medicine people. In many tribes, both men and women can serve as medicine people, but in some, like the Yurok in California, only women can be medicine people. Some medicine people are also shamans (holy men and women). All medicine people are considered learned and are respected members of the tribe. Many modern medicine people will not discuss their practices or beliefs with non-Native American individuals simply because the rites and rituals are sacred and not to be shared commercially (Wigington, 2020).

Medicine people have naturalistic skills. Some medicine people specialize in herbal medicine, bone setting, midwifery, or counseling. Often the medicine people cure patients simply because they believe in the medicine person (placebo effect). Medicine people bring hope, understanding, and confidence to patients, which are often as powerful as modern medicine could have been. They work in the unseen world of good and bad spirits to restore harmony and health.

American Indians believe that they are related to all forms of life. Medicine people make medicine tools out of materials from nature, including fur, skins, bone, crystals, shells, roots, and feathers. They use these tools to evoke the spirit of what the tool has been made of, which helps strengthen their inner powers. For example, a medicine drum is made of wood and animal skins. When medicine people play the drum, they can call up the assistance of the spirits of the tree and the animal from which the drum was made.

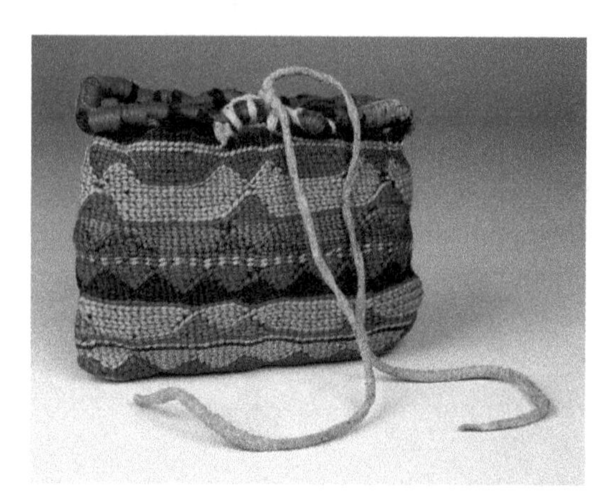

Figure 7.4 Medicine bundle.

Medicine people keep their medicine tools in a **medicine bundle** (see **Figure 7.4**), a large piece of cloth or hide that they tie securely with a thong, piece of yarn, or string. The contents of the medicine bundle are sacred. Each medicine person may own or share different medicine bundles: one's own, the tribe's, and bundles for special purposes, such as seeking visions, hunting, or protection in battle. Some are passed down from one generation to the next. Personal medicine bundles are private, and asking about another person's medical tools is forbidden. Some medicine bundles are small enough to be worn around the neck. Medicine bundles that belong to tribes are often called the "grandmothers" because they have the power to nourish and nurture the tribe and promote continued well-being. Tribal medicine bundles grow stronger with each passing year.

Tribes carefully guard the knowledge of their medicine people. Members of the tribe who want to become medicine people must first serve a long apprenticeship with an experienced medicine person. In many tribes, medicine people cannot charge for their services. Gifts, however, are expected. Some tribes do require payment and have set lists of standard gifts. Nearly all tribes recognize tobacco as a gift of respect.

Healers receive special teachings. Healing traditions are passed from one generation to the next through visions, stories, and dreams. Healing does not follow written guidelines. Healers work differently with each person they help. They use their herbs, ceremony, and power in the best way for each individual. Healing might involve sweat lodges, talking circles, the ceremonial smoking of tobacco, herbalism, animal spirits, or vision quests. Each tribe uses its own techniques. The techniques by themselves are not considered "traditional healing." They are only steps toward becoming whole, balanced, and connected.

Sweat Lodges

Sweat lodges are used for healing and balancing. American Indians consider sweat lodges a good way to clean one's body and sweat out illness or disease (Desy, 2019). The purpose of the sweat ceremony is to spiritually reunite with the Creator and to respectfully connect to the earth and for purging toxins out of the physical body.

The building of a sweat lodge is sacred and symbolic. Willow saplings are bent and tied together to form a square with four sides, which represents the four sacred directions. There is usually a single entryway that faces either west or east. The connected poles create a frame that looks like an overturned basket, which represents items such as the womb or arch of the sky. In some tribes there are 28 poles, which represent either the ribs of a woman, a female bear or turtle, or the lunar cycle. The framework is covered in the skins of buffalo or other animals that represent the animal world (see **Figure 7.5**). The interior of sweat lodges can be created out of many different materials depending on what is available to the community. The interior can be made out of furs, grasses, or various types of bark from trees. A small pit, or altar, is dug in the center of the lodge for the stones. A branch that represents the tree of life is placed in the middle of the altar and is surrounded by small stones. Antlers are used to move the hot stones, and a medicine pipe is placed near the altar.

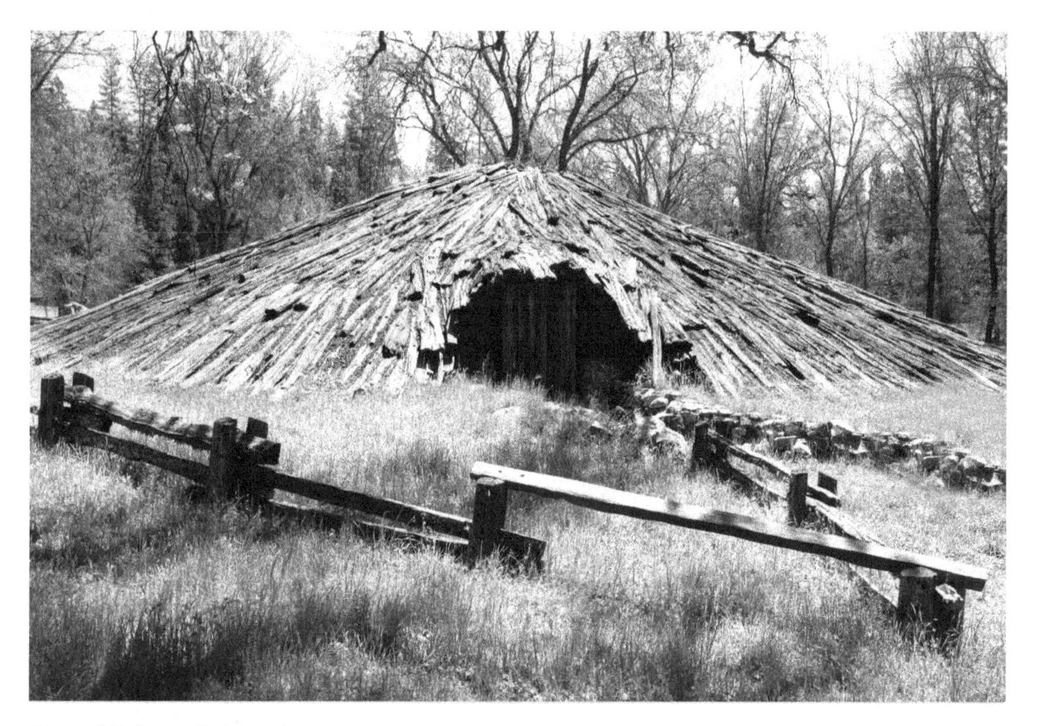

Figure 7.5 Sweat lodge.

Before the sweat lodge is used, "The One Who Pours the Water" purifies the surrounding area by smearing it with sacred herbs to ensure that positive spirits will be present. A stone tender stays outside the lodge, heating stones and passing them inside when summoned by The One Who Pours the Water. One heated stone is not used; it is left for the spirits to sweat with and honors the spirits who have come to the ceremony.

Plants and Herbs

American Indians use herbs to purify the spirit and bring balance to people who are unhealthy in spirit, mind, or body. They learned about the healing powers of herbs by watching sick animals. Only a few of the herbs are discussed here, but a wide variety of plants and herbs are used by American Indians for healing. In fact, many books have been written about them.

Sage is believed to protect against bad spirits and to draw them out of the body or the soul. American Indians use sage for many purposes, such as to heal problems of the stomach, colon, nasal passages, kidneys, liver, lungs, pores of the skin, bones, and sex organs; to heal burns and scrapes; as an antiseptic for allergies, colds, and fever; as a gargle for a sore throat; and as a tea to calm the nerves. Cedar, a tall evergreen tree, is a milder medicine than sage. It is combined with sage and sweetgrass, a plant that grows in damp environments like marshes or near water, to make a powerful mixture used in sacred ceremonies. Cedar fruit and leaves are boiled and then drunk to heal coughs. For head colds, cedar is burned and inhaled. Other herbs often used include acacia, prickly pear, saw palmetto, sunflower, yerba mansa, cliffrose, and cayenne.

Tobacco, often smoked in medicine pipes, is one of the most sacred plants to American Indians, and it is used in some way in nearly every cure. It is smoked pure and is not mixed with chemicals. When American Indians smoke sacred tobacco and other herbs, their breath, which they consider the source of life, becomes visible. When smoke is released, it rises to the Great Spirit carrying prayers. People who share a pipe are acknowledging that they share the same breath. There are many different types of medicine pipes; some are for war, sun, and marriage, and others are tribal, personal, ceremonial, and social pipes. The pipe itself, made of wood with a soft pithy center, is symbolic, and some are shaped like animals. The bowl represents the female aspect of the Great Spirit–Mother Earth. The stem represents the male aspect of the Great Spirit–Father Sky. Together, the bowl and stem represent the union that brings forth life. The bowl in which tobacco is burned also symbolizes all that changes. The stem signifies all that is unchanging. Smoking the pipe is a central component in all ceremonies because it unites the two worlds of spirit and matter.

Peyote, which is a hallucinogenic drug, comes from a spineless, dome-shaped cactus (*Lophophora williamsii*) native to Mexico and the southwest United States. It has button-like tubercles that are chewed fresh or dry. Peyote has a history of ritual religious and medicinal use among certain American Indian and Alaskan Native tribes going back thousands of years. Peyote is legal only on Indian reservations. Because of its spiritual and healing properties, it is viewed by American Indians as an agent that allows one to encounter spirits and receive visions or messages from spirits or Gods.

WHAT DO YOU THINK?

Should the use of peyote for religious purposes be allowed in prisons?

> **Title 42— The Public Health and Welfare, Chapter 21—Civil Rights Subchapter I —Generally, Sec. 1996a**—*Traditional Indian Religious Use of Peyote provides:* (1) *Notwithstanding any other provision of law, the use, possession, or transportation of peyote by an Indian for bona fide traditional ceremonial purposes in connection with the practice of a traditional Indian religion is lawful, and shall not be prohibited by the United States or any State. No Indian shall be penalized or discriminated against on the basis of such use, possession or transportation, including, but not limited to, denial of otherwise applicable benefits under public assistance programs.*

However, this law also provides for possibly limiting this freedom for prisoners by requiring a balancing of personal rights and compelling governmental interest by indicating:

> (5) *This section shall not be construed as requiring prison authorities to permit, nor shall it be construed to prohibit prison authorities from permitting, access to peyote by Indians while incarcerated within Federal or State prison facilities.*

Currently, if a state intends to limit religious rights of a member of an Indian tribe to use peyote, it must confer with tribal religious leaders and narrowly craft a rule that is carefully limited to restrict practice only so much as is required to protect a compelling state interest. With overcrowding and correctional programs designed to end the use of drugs by most inmates, do you think the use of peyote by American Indians is something that should be limited in prisons? Does it create an opportunity for cross-cultural learning? Does it show favoritism for a particular cultural group? If a state allows the smoking of peyote, would it conflict with antismoking laws the state may have adopted to promote health? Does the issue of sincerity come into play when a prisoner claims a right to certain religious practices? What if those practices offend the sensibility of practitioners of another religion?

Dancing

Drumming, dancing, and singing are known to be very powerful sources of healing among Alaskan Natives. The ceremonies incorporate music, movement, and drum rhythms to penetrate within the people involved and aid them in fully expressing emotion, increasing physical energy, making a strong connection with life and one another, and promoting happiness. This also helps promote overall well-being and a sense of love among the community.

Behavioral Risk Factors and Common Health Problems

Due to the great number and diversity of tribes and locations, it is important for health care professionals to gather data about the specific tribe and geographic region prior to developing any individual- or community-based practice. However, some general patterns may be considered.

American Indians and Alaskan Natives have an infant death rate twice as high as the rate for Non-Hispanic Whites (HHS, OMH, 2021g). In 2018, American Indians and Alaskan Natives adults were almost three times more likely than non-Hispanic White adults to be diagnosed with diabetes (HHS, OMH, 2021e). An example is the Pima tribe of Arizona, who has one of the highest diabetes rates in the world. American Indians and Alaskan Natives also have disproportionately high death rates from unintentional injuries and suicide. The rate of tuberculosis (TB) disease in American Indians and Alaska Natives was 4.3 cases per 100,000, which is over eight times higher than the rate of TB disease in non-Hispanic Whites (0.5 cases per 100,000) (CDC, 2018). The 10 leading causes of death among American Indians and Alaskan Natives in 2017 were as follows:

1. Heart disease
2. Cancer
3. Unintentional injuries
4. Diabetes
5. Chronic liver disease and cirrhosis
6. Chronic lower respiratory diseases
7. Stroke
8. Suicide
9. Influenza and pneumonia
10. Alzheimer's disease (National Center for Health Statistics, 2018).

Native youth aged 12 to 17 years and American Indians and Alaskan Natives adults aged 18 years or older had the highest prevalence of current smoking compared with other racial/ethnic populations (CDC, 2019).

American Indians have a high risk of motor vehicle deaths and injuries, which is caused by several factors. One factor is that they have the lowest rate of using seat belts in the nation. The other reason is their high rate of drinking and driving. The lands of American Indians do not impose taxes, and they do not have laws that prevent the sale of alcohol and tobacco products to minors. Because of this, the young population easily uses alcohol and tobacco products. Some American Indian and Alaskan Native populations believe that tobacco is sacred, and it is therefore more often used in ceremonies.

The American Indian and Alaskan Native populations suffer from a high suicide rate. Between 1999 and 2017 the largest increase in suicides among all groups occurred for non-Hispanic American Indian or Alaska Native females (139%) while the increase for American Indian or Alaska Native males was 71% (Curtin, 2019).

Alcohol abuse has been linked to many health problems, both directly and indirectly. Generally, American Indian and Alaskan Native peoples abstain more and have fewer regular drinkers than most other populations, but those who do drink are more likely to drink heavily and have serious problems. Past month alcohol use and alcohol use disorder among the American Indian or Alaska Native population is increasing in ages 12–17 (Substance Abuse and Mental Health Services Administration [SAMHSA], 2019).

Alcohol has caused health problems and behavioral issues in many societies, but Alaskan Natives have been struck much harder than most. There are many theories as to why alcohol is such a major issue in Alaska, but one study conducted by the National Center for American Indian and Alaska Native Mental Health Research goes back to the beginning (Seale et. al., 2006). According to this study, alcohol was not a part of Alaska's culture until it was introduced by the Russians, who used it to abuse the natives and take advantage of them. Alcohol quickly became a problem in small villages. The immediate effect was an increase in spousal abuse and neglect of daily chores. This behavior led to shame and guilt, which was often dealt with by more drinking. This behavior is learned by the children in the home, and the cycle continues. The average starting age for drinking is around 9 years old. The traditional culture for many Alaskan Natives is gone, and they are left to live with limited resources for success. Without adequate health education and easy access to medical or mental health care, it has become a difficult task to fight the problem of alcohol abuse.

Another behavioral risk factor that is prevalent among Alaskan Natives is the use of tobacco. During 2012–2016, 38.6% of Alaska Native adults reported current smoking compared to 17.6% of Alaska non-Native adults, and the difference was statistically significant (Alaska Native Epidemiology Center, 2018). When viewed nationwide, 19.2% American Indian and Alaska Native population smoked in 2017 (National Center for Health Statistics, 2018).

Obesity is a problem among Alaskan Natives, having 1.6 times more obesity compared to Non-Hispanic Whites. However, overall, American Indians and Alaska Natives experience similar levels of being overweight with a body mass index of over 25 (HHS, OMH, 2020).

Serious COVID-19 infection has been associated with many types of underlying health conditions. In 23 states with adequate race/ethnicity data, the cumulative incidence of laboratory-confirmed COVID-19 among American Indian or Alaska Native persons was 3.5 times that among non-Hispanic White persons (Hatcher et al., 2020). The CDC speculated that persisting racial inequity and historical trauma have contributed to disparities in health and socioeconomic factors between American Indian or Alaska Native and White populations that have adversely affected tribal communities. The CDC (2020) has speculated that the elevated incidence within this population might also reflect differences in reliance on shared transportation, limited access to running water, household size, and other factors that might facilitate community transmission.

QUICK FACTS

Health disparities reported by the CDC HHS, and OMH include the following:

- American Indians/Alaska Native adults are more likely to be obese than White adults, more likely to have high blood pressure, and more likely to be current cigarette smokers—all risk factors for heart disease (HHS, OMH, 2021b).
- In 2018, American Indians/Alaska Natives were 50% more likely to be diagnosed with coronary heart disease than their White counterparts (HHS, OMH, 2021b).

(continued)

QUICK FACTS (*CONTINUED*)

- American Indian/Alaska Natives were 50% more likely to be current cigarette smokers, as compared to non-Hispanic Whites, in 2018 (HHS, OMH, 2021b).
- American Indian/Alaska Native adolescents are 10% less likely than non-Hispanic White adolescents to be obese (HHS, OMH, 2021c).
- American Indian or Alaska Native adults are 50% more likely to be obese than non-Hispanic Whites (HHS, OMH, 2021c).
- People who are overweight are more likely to suffer from high blood pressure, high levels of blood fats, diabetes and low-density lipoproteins cholesterol—all risk factors for heart disease and stroke (HHS, OMH, 2021c).
- In 2018, chronic liver disease was the fourth leading cause of death for all American Indians/Alaska Natives, and the third leading cause of death for American Indian/Alaska Native men, ages 35–44 (HHS, OMH, 2021d).
- American Indians/Alaska Natives are 1.6 times more likely to be diagnosed with chronic liver disease as compared to non-Hispanic Whites (HHS, OMH, 2021d).
- The overall death rate from liver disease for American Indians/Alaska Natives is three times higher than the non-Hispanic White population (HHS, OMH, 2021d).
- American Indian/Alaska Native women are 2.3 times as likely to be diagnosed with chronic liver disease and 4.4 times more likely to die from chronic liver disease as compared to non-Hispanic White women (HHS, OMH, 2021d).
- American Indian/Alaska Native adults are almost three times more likely than non-Hispanic White adults to be diagnosed with diabetes (HHS, OMH, 2021e).
- American Indians/Alaska Natives were 2.3 times more likely than non-Hispanic Whites to die from diabetes in 2017 (HHS, OMH, 2021e).
- In 2017, American Indians/Native Americans were 2.4 times more likely to be diagnosed with end-stage renal disease than non-Hispanic Whites (HHS, OMH, 2021e). American Indian/Alaska Native men and women have some lower cancer rates than the non-Hispanic White population. However, disparities still exist in certain types of cancer (HHS, OMH, 2021f).
- From 2014–2018, American Indian/Alaska Native men were almost twice as likely to have liver and inflammatory bowel disease (IBD) cancer as compared to non-Hispanic White men (HHS, OMH, 2021f).
- American Indian/Alaska Native men are 30% more likely to have stomach cancer than non-Hispanic White men and are over twice as likely to die from the same disease.
- American Indian/Alaska Native women are 2.2 times more likely to have, and twice as likely to die from, liver and IBD cancer, as compared to non-Hispanic White women (HHS, OMH, 2021f).
- American Indian/Alaska Native women are 40% more likely to have kidney/renal pelvis cancer than non-Hispanic White women (HHS, OMH, 2021f).

Considerations for Health Promotion and Program Planning

Consider the following concepts when planning and implementing a health promotion program for this target audience:

- American Indian and Alaskan Native peoples use their tribal names when referring to themselves, so it is advised that health care professionals ask individuals or groups how they prefer to be addressed.
- Recognize that there are varying degrees of acculturation levels, so health care professionals need to assess where the patient or client is on the continuum of acculturation.
- Recognize that there is great diversity among the tribes, so do not make assumptions.
- Holistic thinking is common and should be used to identify appropriate and acceptable prevention and treatment plans.
- Try to accommodate complementary and alternative forms of healing.
- Do not be surprised or offended by a handshake that is softer or gentler than you are accustomed to.
- Be patient with silence and give the listener time to reflect on what you said prior to responding.
- Prolonged eye contact should be avoided because it is viewed as being disrespectful.
- Work with the families and remember that elders are respected.
- Do not encourage or try to reward competitive behavior because cooperation is valued.
- Do not appear to be in a hurry; it may give patients a negative impression of you.
- Do not interrupt the person who is speaking as this is considered extremely rude.
- Keep nonverbal communication to a minimum.
- With the exception of a handshake, touch is not usually acceptable.
- Remember that listening is more valued than speaking.
- Be aware that suspicion and mistrust may exist.
- When developing community programs, involve the community members.
- Be aware of superstitions such as unlucky and lucky numbers and colors.

Tips for Working With American Indian and Alaskan Native Populations

Some suggestions developed by the Indian Health Services for working with American Indian and Alaskan Native patients include being warm and friendly so that the patient feels that you genuinely care about them. The first meeting is extremely important because it sets the basis of your relationship. Make the patient feel welcome. Use language the patient can understand (medical terminology may be confusing). If a patient speaks a different language, do your best to explain yourself and to find a staff person who can speak the patient's language.

With the patient's consent, involve the family as they play a crucial role in the patient's outcome and support of family will help speed recovery and raise social well-being. Do not rush the patient. Silence is valued and is not necessarily a negative behavior. Sometimes the patient may require time to think and respond to a comment. Time is viewed more passively, and the people are more task conscious than time conscious. Eye contact is used in varying degrees and should be limited.

Respect traditional healing ways and work to accommodate their beliefs. You can support traditional healing by respecting the people's ways and not degrading their beliefs.

Show great respect to the elderly. Elders are not accustomed to modern health care facilities, the new atmosphere, the noises, the caregivers, or the types of treatment used. For many elders, this may be their first trip to a medical facility. It is important to ease their minds and to explain procedures thoroughly.

Summary

American Indian and Alaskan Native populations have a history of being conquered by other nations, having foreign cultures impose on their way of life, and being the victims of discrimination. Fortunately, they have been able to hold onto their traditional culture in many ways. They continue to express their traditional values within their villages by maintaining close-knit families and using traditional healing modalities to prevent and heal illness. Unfortunately, both groups experience major health disparities, such as a high incidence of suicide, alcoholism, cancer, unintentional injuries, diabetes, and mental illness. Through high-quality, culturally sensitive health promotion programs, perhaps one day better health and access to quality health care can be achieved.

This chapter has described the challenges that these populations encountered historically. These populations do not believe in the germ theory as the cause of disease, although some Alaskan Natives are adopting this belief system now. They have various approaches to healing, such as sweat lodges and ceremonies, and their common behaviors, risk factors, and illnesses are similar. General tips for working with these populations were provided, but we caution that there is a vast amount of diversity within these groups, so it is important not to generalize.

Review

1. Describe the histories of American Indian and Alaskan Native people in the United States.
2. According to American Indian and Alaskan Native beliefs, what are the causes of illnesses?
3. Describe some plants and herbs that are used for healing.
4. Describe what medicine men are and their approach to healing.

Activity

Conduct research on health programs that have been implemented for members of the American Indian and Alaskan Native population. Summarize the literature and identify some best practices.

Review the white bison website (http://whitebison.org/index.php) and reflect on what you learned. Watch the video "The Wellbriety Movement: Journey of Forgiveness" and include comments about it in your paper as well.

Case Study 1

Kerry, a 32-year-old Native American woman from a small reservation in Montana presented to a large urban clinic in the Northwest for care. She was married at age 17 and had contracted HIV from prior IVDU.[1] She has been unemployed for the past 10 years. Her husband, Carlos, a Central American immigrant, had been HIV tested and was negative, although Kerry admitted they occasionally had unprotected intercourse. Her medical history was complicated by periodic alcohol and crack binges, and a history of abnormal Pap smears. Her family and social history revealed childhood physical and sexual abuse, and chemical dependency.

Although she had a brother living nearby in the city, she was adamant that he and family in Montana know nothing about her diagnosis or treatment as she feared family revenge. She did not want her family to try to take her back to the reservation—a place she escaped and it was clear she didn't want to return, even after death. Her husband agreed with her decision not to return to the reservation and noted that her family did not like him, as he was an "outsider."

Kerry knew that her brother Mike often called the primary care doctor for updates on her condition. The patient reminded her physician that she wanted her diagnosis kept confidential, even if that seemed harmful to others.

1 *Editor's Note*: IVDU means intravenous drug use.

She was initially started on antiretroviral therapy, but frequently missed appointments for medical and gynecological care. She occasionally spoke of wanting to see a medicine person through the clinic, but did not follow through on this because the healer was male, and because she occasionally needs drugs. Her CD4 counts continued to decline, with rising viral load, and she was admitted to the hospital's intensive care unit with opportunistic infection and cardiomyopathy.

She had previously expressed a strong desire to be a "no code," but suddenly changed her mind in the intensive care unit just prior to her death. After her death, her brother and elder aunt demanded to know her diagnosis. Then they told her husband that "they were her blood family, and she should be buried at home," regardless of her wishes, and that he had no legal or other rights to make any decisions.

1. What are the barriers to care in this case?
2. What ethical decisions must the health care providers make concerning her diagnosis and treatment?
3. What course of action could the health care providers have taken for more culturally competent care?
4. How can the issue of her burial be resolved?
5. Discuss other cultural competence issues that may impact retention into care and treatment.

Source: AETC-NMC, "Case Study 17: Addressing HIV Care and Latino Model," https://www.aetcnmc.org/documents/case-study-17.pdf.

Case Study 2

Joe, a 35-year-old homeless Iroquois veteran, with no recent family contact and a history of alcohol abuse, receives care in a large urban clinic in the Pacific Northwest. Joe was diagnosed with HIV 4 years ago. He presents at the clinic as a walk-in client and asks to see Maggie Hernandez, the nurse he usually sees in the clinic for his "appointments." After about an hour, Ms. Hernandez escorts Joe to an exam room and asks, "What brings you in today?" Joe likes Ms. Hernandez and seeks her out at the clinic, refusing to receive care from other available staff. He tells Ms. Hernandez that he "just thought it was time to come in."

During the clinic visit, Ms. Hernandez notes that Joe is forgetful and exhibits mental slowing and language problems. He appears disheveled and in need of a shower. His last CD4+ T cell count was 620 cells/mm3, and his viral load was 45,000 copies/mL. Joe says he has difficulty taking his medications; he forgets his schedule, often loses medications, and is generally ambivalent about his need for non-Native drugs. He believes that a traditional Native healer could help him feel more comfortable with his illness. He lives in street camps and continues to drink alcohol on a daily basis.

Joe and Ms. Hernandez discuss an occasion when he received services from a traditional Native healer. The healer refused to continue helping Joe unless he stopped drinking. Joe told the traditional Native healer that he didn't drink and was offended by what he considered the healer's disrespectful behavior. Ms. Hernandez attempts to talk with Joe about his drinking, but he becomes very upset. She shifts her approach and asks if he would consider a referral for a neuropsychiatric assessment. She also presents the possibility of finding a case manager to help Joe with medication adherence and housing. Joe asks, "What type of assessment is that and why do I need a case manager?"

1. How does culture influence Joe's ambivalence regarding HIV medication, his desire to maintain walk-in visits with Ms. Hernandez, and his interest in receiving assistance from a traditional Native healer?
2. How could a provider clarify the need for a neuropsychiatric assessment and assigning a case manager for Joe?
3. Discuss the health literacy implications of Ms. Hernandez's interaction with Joe.
4. Should Ms. Hernandez have made an effort to find out what services or treatment Joe received from the traditional Native healer? Why or why not?
5. What types of veteran services are available for Joe?
6. Based on the case study discussion, what strategies to address health literacy might you include in an action plan for Joe's care?
7. Discuss other cultural competence issues that may impact retention into care and treatment.

Source: AETC-NMC, "Case Study 25: Addressing HIV Care and Health Literacy," https://www.aetcnmc.org/documents/case-study-25.pdf.

References

Alaska Department of Fish and Game. (n.d.). *Subsistence in Alaska.* https://www.adfg.alaska.gov/index.cfm?adfg=subsistenceresearch.main

Alaska Native Epidemiology Center. (2018). *Alaska Native current smoking report.* http://anthctoday.org/epicenter/healthData/factsheets/Adult_Current_Smoking_09_28_2018.pdf

Alexandria, V. (1994). *People of the ice and snow.* Time Life.

American Heart Association. (n.d.). *Is broken heart syndrome real?* http://www.heart.org/HEARTORG/Conditions/More/Cardiomyopathy/Is-Broken-Heart-Syndrome-Real_UCM_448547_Article.jsp

Centers for Disease Control and Prevention. (2018). *Health disparities, American Indian and Alaska Natives.* https://www.cdc.gov/mmwr/volumes/67/wr/mm6747a4.htm

Centers for Disease Control and Prevention. (2019). *American Indian/Alaska Native tobacco use.* https://www.cdc.gov/tobacco/disparities/american-indians/index.htm

Centers for Disease Control and Prevention. (2020). *CDC data show disproportionate COVID 19 impact in American Indian/Alaska Native populations.* https://www.cdc.gov/media/releases/2020/p0819-covid-19-impact-american-indian-alaska-native.html

Curtin, S. (2019). *Suicide rates for females and males by race and ethnicity: United States, 1999 and 2017.* National Center for Health Statistics. https://www.cdc.gov/nchs/data/hestat/suicide/rates_1999_2017.htm

Desy, P. (2019, May 9). *Recounts of the healing benefits of sweat lodge ceremonies.* Learn Religions. https://www.learnreligions.com/sweat-lodge-benefits-1732186

Federal Register. (2020). *Indian entities recognized by and eligible to receive services from the United States Bureau of Indian Affairs.* https://www.federalregister.gov/documents/2020/01/30/2020-01707/indian-entities-recognized-by-and-eligible-to-receive-services-from-the-united-states-bureau-of

Frankis, M. P. (2006). *Picea sitchensis (Bongard).* http://www.conifers.org/pi/pic/sitchensis.htm

Garces, M. (n.d.). *American Indians, diet of.* http://www.faqs.org/nutrition/Met-Obe/Native-Americans-Diet-of.html

Hammerschlag, C.A. (1988) *The dancing healers:A doctor's journey of healing with Native Americans.* San Francisco, CA: Harper.

Hatcher, S. M., Agnew-Brune, C., Anderson, M., Zambrano, L. D., Rose, C. E., Jim, M. A., Baugher, A., Liu, G. S., Patel S. V., Evans, M. E., Pindyck, T., Dubray, C. L., Rainey, J. J., Chen, J., Sadowski, C., Winglee, K., Penman-Aguilar, A., Dixit, A., Claw, E., Parshall, C., Provost, E., Ayala, A., Gonzalez, G., Ritchey, J., Davis, J., Warren-Mears, V., Joshi, S., Weiser, T., Echo-Hawk, A., Dominguez, A., Poel, A., Duke, C., Ransby, I., Apostolou, A., & McCollum, J. & (2020, August 28). COVID-19 among American Indian and Alaska Native persons—23 states, January 31–July 3, 2020 *Morbidity and Mortality Weekly Report, 69*(34), 1166–1169 https://www.cdc.gov/mmwr/volumes/69/wr/mm6934e1.htm

Indian Health Service. (2020). *IHS profile.* https://www.ihs.gov/newsroom/factsheets/ihsprofile/

Jernigan, V. B. B., Peercy, M., Branam, D., Saunkeah, B., Wharton, D., Winkleby, M., Lowe, J., Salvatore, A. L., Dickerson, D., Belcourt, A., D'Amico, E., Patten, C. A., Parker, M., Duran, B., Harris, R., & Buchwald, D. (2015). Beyond health equity: Achieving wellness within American Indian and Alaska native communities. *American journal of public health, 105,* S376–S379. https://doi.org/10.2105/AJPH.2014.302447

National Alliance on Mental Illness. (n.d.). Identity and cultural dimensions. https://www.nami.org/Your-Journey/Identity-and-Cultural-Dimensions/Indigenous

National Alliance on Mental Illness. (2003). *American Indian and Alaska Native resource manual.* https://sprc.org/sites/default/files/resource-program/AI%20AN%20Resource%20Manual.pdf

National Center for Health Statistics. (2018). *Table 6. Leading causes of death and numbers of deaths, by sex, race, and Hispanic origin: United States, 1980 and 2017.* https://www.cdc.gov/nchs/data/hus/2018/006.pdf

Nixon, R. (1970). *Special message on Indian affairs.* Public Papers of the Presidents of the United States. http://www.ncai.org/attachments/Consultation_IJaOfGZqlYSuxpPUqoSSWIaNTkEJEPXxKLzLcaOikifwWhGOLSA_12%20Nixon%20Self%20Determination%20Policy.pdf

Purnell, L. (2021) Transcultural health care. In *Transcultural health care: A culturally competent approach* (p. 164). F. A. Davis.

Roberts, N. F. (2020, November 29). 7 Native American inventions that revolutionized medicine and public health. *Forbes.* https://www.forbes.com/sites/nicolefisher/2020/11/29/7-native-american-inventions-that-revolutionized-medicine-and-public-health/?sh=5a8ef61d1e73

Seale, J., Shellenberger, S., & Spence, J. (2006). Alcohol problems in Alaska Natives: Lessons from the Inuit. *American Indian and Alaska Native Mental Health Research: The Journal of the National Center, 13*(1), 1–31.

Spector, R. E. (2017). *Cultural diversity in health and illness* (9th ed.). Pearson.

Stanford Medicine. (2020). *Traditional healing, ethnogeriatrics.* https://geriatrics.stanford.edu/ethnomed/alaskan/fund/traditional_healing.html

Substance Abuse and Mental Health Services Administration. (2019). *2019 National survey on drug use and health: American Indians and Alaska Natives (AI/ANs).* https://www.samhsa.gov/data/sites/default/files/reports/rpt31098/2019NSDUH-AIAN/AIAN%202019%20NSDUH.pdf

Thornton, R. (2019, February 19). *American Indian Holocaust and survival: A population history since 1492.* Daily Kos. https://www.dailykos.com/stories/2019/2/19/1835704/-Indians-101-Disease-and-Indians-in-the-16th-Century

U.S. Census Bureau. (2015, October). *Detailed languages spoken at home and ability to speak English for the population 5 years and over for United States: 2009-2013.* https://www.census.gov/data/tables/2013/demo/2009-2013-lang-tables.html

U.S. Census Bureau. (2019). *National population by characteristics: 2010–2019.* https://www.census.gov/data/tables/time-series/demo/popest/2010s-national-detail.html

U. S. Census Bureau. (2020). *About the topic of race.* https://www.census.gov/topics/population/race/about.html

U.S. Department of Health and Human Services, Office of Minority Health. (2018). *American Indian/Alaska Native profile.* https://www.minorityhealth.hhs.gov/omh/browse.aspx?lvl=3&lvlid=62

U.S. Department of Health and Human Services, Office of Minority Health. (2021a). *Mental and behavior health, American Indian/Alaska Natives.* https://www.mnortyhealth.hhs.gov/omh/browse.aspx?lvl=4&lvlid=39

U.S. Department of Health and Human Services, Office of Minority Health. (2021b). *Heart disease and American Indians/Alaska Natives.* https://minorityhealth.hhs.gov/omh/browse.aspx?lvl=4&lvlid=34

U.S. Department of Health and Human Services, Office of Minority Health. (2021c). *Obesity, American Indian and Alaska Native.* https://minorityhealth.hhs.gov/omh/browse.aspx?lvl=4&lvlid=40

U.S. Department of Health and Human Services, Office of Minority Health. (2021d). *Chronic liver disease, American Indian and Alaska Native.* https://minorityhealth.hhs.gov/omh/browse.aspx?lvl=4&lvlid=32

U.S. Department of Health and Human Services, Office of Minority Health. (2021e). *Diabetes and American Indian/Alaska Natives.* https://minorityhealth.hhs.gov/omh/browse.aspx?lvl=4&lvlid=33

U.S. Department of Health and Human Services, Office of Minority Health. (2021f). Cancer and American Indian/Alaska Natives. https://minorityhealth.hhs.gov/omh/browse.aspx?lvl=4&lvlid=31

U.S. Department of Health and Human Services, Office of Minority Health. (2021g). *Infant mortality and American Indians/Alaska Natives.* https://minorityhealth.hhs.gov/omh/content.aspx?lvl=3&lvlID=8&ID=3038

Wigington, P. (2020, August 26). *Native American spirituality.* Learn Religions. https://learnreligions.com/native-american-spirituality-2562540

CREDITS

Fig. 7.1: Copyright © by CANFIT, Project of Tides Center.

Fig. 7.2: Source: https://www.loc.gov/pictures/item/2003652721/.

Fig. 7.3: Source: https://commons.wikimedia.org/wiki/File:MedicineWheel.jpg.

Fig. 7.4: Source: https://commons.wikimedia.org/wiki/File:Medicine_Bundle_Bowl_and_Bag_MET_TR.165.34.2011_c.jpeg.

Fig. 7.5: Copyright © 2017 Depositphotos/jeffbanke.

CHAPTER 8

African American Populations

I have a dream that my four little children will one day live in a nation where they will not be judged by the color of their skin, but by the content of their character.

—MARTIN LUTHER KING, JR.

If I'd known I was going to live this long, I'd have taken better care of myself.

—EUBIE BLAKE

KEY CONCEPTS AND TERMS

Candomblé	Tuskegee study
Santeria	Voodoo

LEARNING OBJECTIVES

After reading this chapter, you should be able to do the following:

1. Provide an overview of the social and economic circumstances of African Americans in the United States.
2. Provide an overview of African American beliefs about the causes of illness.
3. Describe at least three African American healing practices.
4. Describe African American health risk behaviors and common illnesses.
5. List at least six tips for working with African American populations.

Introduction

The U.S. Census Bureau racial category "Black or African American" includes people who identify themselves as such and have origins in any of the Black racial groups in Africa. (U.S. Census Bureau, 2020). Culture is not the same as race, but much data is correlated and available under the racial label. In this chapter we focus on the culture derived from the original Africans brought to America as slaves, which forms the foundation of the somewhat vague term *African American culture.*

Many people who classify themselves as Black or African American do not trace their history back to the early American experience. With many immigrants from African nations, the Caribbean, Central America, and other countries, African American communities across the United States are more culturally diverse now than at any other time in history. For instance, former President Obama self-identifies as African American and falls within the Census Bureau definition. However, his father was from Kenya, and his paternal family members still reside there. Under Census Bureau guidelines, former President Obama could just as well self-defined as mixed race because his mother was White, and he was raised by her and his White grandparents. Certainly, Obama lives in a society in which the majority population still imposes assumptions and bias on Black people of any origin. However, in this chapter we distinguish African Americans from Black people who can come from any culture. We are looking at the culture that derived from people who were captured and forced to America by Europeans as individuals torn from their families and communities and compelled to reestablish their lives within a new culture created by White people who wanted the slaves for their labor but not their social company. These Africans had to individually learn a new language, new lifestyle, new eating habits, and live among Whites and other slaves from various African locations in essentially a random mix of peoples. They forged a new adapted slave culture, and Michelle Obama, former President Obama's wife and first lady, is a descendant of these original African slaves. More recently, Kamala Harris, as vice president, symbolized the progress of African Americans, although her parents are from India and Jamaica.

This chapter begins with the unique history of African Americans in the United States. This history plays a role throughout the chapter, which includes a discussion about their current socioeconomic position within the United States, beliefs about the causes of illness and how to treat it, health behaviors, and common health problems. Then we discuss how to create a successful community health program that takes these factors into consideration.

Terminology

Historically, African Americans were identified by a number of terms (*Negro, colored, Black*). The correct current term to refer to anyone who has roots in any of the African countries is *African American*. In the literature, both African American and Black are used, but the latter term incorporates a broader population. For example, Black Caribbean Islanders fall within the category of "Black" but not necessarily "African American." In this chapter, the focus is on African Americans who are descended from slaves, but when referring to research, the terminology found in the original source is used.

History of African Americans in the United States

What is now considered African American culture is a mixture of the oral traditions brought to this country from Africa with modifications developed within a context of slavery, prejudice, discrimination, and poverty. With the massive reduction in potential workers caused by the death of most of the original Indigenous population in the Americas due to war and disease, the Europeans in America needed labor and turned to slavery to develop commerce. The African Americans are unique in that they were forced here to be exploited for their labor. To understand the African American culture, it is important to realize this fundamental fact that carries over to the present day.

Slavery has existed throughout the world for thousands of years. Even though some pre-Columbian Indigenous American tribes enslaved their captors, and European settlers did not come to America to intentionally become slave owners, the practice became a significant part of the American economy. With the increasing need for labor to raise rice, sugar cane, and cotton, slavery was soon seen to be acceptable and was imposed on Africans not only for their lifetimes, but also for generations of their descendants.

The slave trade, which was called the "transatlantic slave trade," was the forced transportation of Africans to the New World, which occurred in or around the Atlantic Ocean. Spain increased the number of enslaved Africans it brought to the Caribbean after 1518 because the Native people it had previously enslaved there were dying from European disease and colonial violence (U.S. National Park Service, n.d.).

The introduction of sugarcane as a cash crop was another factor motivating the Spanish to enslave Africans. Spanish planters needed a large, controllable work force, so they turned to Africa for laborers (U.S. National Park Service, n.d.). It lasted from the 16th century to the 19th century. An estimated 12 million men, women, and children were transported by force to the Americas from their homeland of Africa. Approximately 500,000 were brought to what is today the United States.

The majority of the ancestors of African Americans came from a part of Africa bounded by the Senegal River in the north and by Angola in the south. This area also was called the area of catchment (Perry, 1998). Africans were taken by force, made to be slaves, and shipped to other countries against their will. Under these circumstances, it was very unlikely that families stayed intact. Men were separated from women and accounted for about two thirds of the slave population. Most slaves were captured in wars, with some wars conducted specifically to capture people and sell them as slaves. Although the survival and health of the slaves were important to slave traders from an economic point of view, sanitation and health conditions on slave ships were simply filthy and disease ridden, resulting in a death rate of about 20% of the cargo. There was no interest at all in keeping families and groups together, and slaves suffered and struggled to survive individually among strangers of different cultures. One of the first challenges was simply to stay alive and not die of disease.

There was an ongoing difference of opinion among ship captains as to whether to keep the cargo load limited to improve health conditions or to pack as many people on as possible so that after attrition the net load was still very profitable. The trip generally took 30 to 90 days, and up to 290 slaves per ship were keep naked in chains two by two on floors and platforms below deck at night with 3 feet or less between the floor and the next level up so that it was impossible to sit up.

If the weather was good, slaves were allowed on deck during the day but remained chained. The ship's crew would require slaves to have some exercise, including forcing them to dance. There were usually four buckets, shaped 1 foot wide at the top and 2 feet wide at the bottom, for toilets, which were dumped once a day. Although accessible to the slaves nearest the buckets at night, most captives gave up the struggle at night to crawl past other complaining captives in tight quarters to reach the buckets and just relieved themselves where they lay, mixing their waste with the vomit and waste from the hundreds of others. Each slave was issued a spoon to dip in and eat from a bucket of food shared by five to 10 others at once. If the spoon was not available, many were simply left to dip in and eat with their hands, even after crawling around on the filthy decks. Disease and illness were rampant. There were more than 200 slave rebellions, and some suicides in response to the experience. Many surviving slaves suffered skin lesions from crawling around on bare wet floors and platforms, and were cleaned up by the sellers with special cosmetic coloring and grease to make them presentable for sale once delivered (Falconbridge, 1788).

Having been captured, kidnapped, dispossessed, removed from their countries and countrymen, and held in filthy unsanitary conditions, the Africans came to a new culture and a new way of life for themselves and their descendants. At home in Africa, culture was passed between generations through an oral tradition rather than in writing. In America, the slaves relied on their individual memory and continued to transfer and adapt their culture, one person at a time, among each other, through oral traditions despite being forced to learn a new language and living a life of confinement and forced labor. Some slaves led stable lives with long-term worksites, but many were sold from place to place. Relationships, both personal and social, were often broken and needed to be redeveloped among strangers.

African enslaved laborers were instrumental in the European colonial expansion in North America, clearing the land, erecting shelters, and constructing forts. They raised commercial and subsistence crops, gathered lumber, raised cattle and hogs, and harvested and produced exports that supported the colonial economies. In some places, such as South Carolina, the population of African American slaves outnumbered the people of European descent. African Americans, free and bound, helped defend the colonies against Indians and against other European colonial powers' attempts at territorial expansion. After the British colonies established territorial dominance along the Atlantic coast, people of African descent—many second- and third-generation Americans, some free or near-free indentured servants, but most bound in slavery—participated in the American Revolution, on both sides, and in the birth and growth of the United States.

The U.S. Constitution framed the divided view of freedom and slavery, demonstrating that the problem of slavery could not be resolved even among men who were seeking freedom themselves. A House of Representatives was established to provide for representation according to population, including women, each of whom counted as a person.

But in areas with substantial slave populations that sometimes outnumbered the possible voters, African American slaves were constitutionally defined each as counting as three fifths of a person (U.S. Constitution, Article I, Section 2). The issues were contentious, and the compromise that allowed movement forward provided that the slave issue could not be addressed further until 20 years after its adoption (Article I, Section 9, Clause 1). In the meantime, the states, free or not, were constitutionally required to return escaped slaves (Article IV, Section 2). The count of the number of slaves was part of establishing the basis for setting the number of representatives in Congress. It would be well over 100 years before the right to vote for those representatives was gradually extended to African Americans, as well as to women, American Indians, Chinese, Asian Indians, and others.

Even as African Americans made great contributions to North America, they faced horrific acts of mistreatment, sexual assault, lynching, and other forms of violent acts and discrimination. During the time of slavery, slave overseers were authorized to whip and brutalize noncompliant slaves. Each state had laws (known as slave codes) that defined the status of slaves and the rights of masters; the codes gave slaveowners near-absolute power over the rights of their slaves and even made it illegal to teach slaves to read.

DID YOU KNOW?

The combination of both jail and flogging was at one time the official punishment for free African Americans who tried to educate slaves:

> *Passed by the state of North Carolina in 1830—1831,*
>
> AN ACT TO PREVENT ALL PERSONS FROM TEACHING SLAVES TO READ OR WRITE, THE USE OF FIGURES EXCEPTED
>
> Whereas the teaching of slaves to read and write, has a tendency to excite dis-satisfaction in their minds, and to produce insurrection and rebellion, to the manifest injury of the citizens of this State:
>
> *Therefore,*
>
> *Be it enacted by the General Assembly of the State of North Carolina, and it is hereby enacted by the authority of the same,* That any free person, who shall hereafter teach, or attempt to teach, any slave within the State to read or write, the use of figures excepted, or shall give or sell to such slave or slaves any books or pamphlets, shall be liable to indictment in any court of record in this State having jurisdiction thereof, and upon conviction, shall, at the discretion of the court, if a white man or woman, be fined not less than one hundred dollars, nor more than two hundred dollars, or imprisoned; and if a free person of color, shall be fined, imprisoned, or whipped, at the discretion of the court, not exceeding thirty nine lashes, nor less than twenty lashes.
>
> II. *Be it further enacted,* That, if any slave shall hereafter teach, or attempt to teach, any other slave to read or write, the use of figures excepted, he or she may be carried before any justice of the peace, and on conviction thereof, shall be sentenced to receive thirty-nine lashes on his or her bare back. **(Legislative Papers, 1831)**

These codes indemnified abusers and even required the use of violence. They were condemned by people who opposed slavery as being evil. In addition to physical abuse and murder, slaves were at constant risk of losing members of their families if their owners decided to trade them for profit or punishment or to pay debts. A few slaves retaliated by murdering owners and overseers, burning barns, killing horses, or staging work slowdowns. After slavery and the Civil War ended, Black codes continued to regulate the freedom of former slaves. The Black codes outraged some people in the North, because it seemed that the South was creating a form of quasi-slavery to evade the results of the war. After winning the 1866 elections, the Republicans put the South under military rule. The new governments repealed most of the Black codes, but segregation laws were enforced for the next 100 years. Even with the changes in laws, African Americans still faced informal unequal treatment and discrimination, which continues into the present day despite mixed efforts to end it. Once freed in the South, many African Americans migrated to the urban North to seek greater opportunities. Yet even there they met segregation and discrimination, ironically many times from new immigrants from Europe competing for opportunities in the newly industrializing United States.

After the Civil War, the United States adopted the 13th Amendment of the Constitution, which gave government the power to root out all attributes of slavery and discrimination, yet the U.S. Supreme Court in *Plessy v. Ferguson* (1896) decided to establish "separate but equal" as a legitimate practice. It took the World War II experience to show that separate "minority" units of African American and Japanese service members performed as well or better than White units. President Truman ended segregation in the military in 1948.

However, separation of the races and cultures was legally authorized until the 1954 U.S. Supreme Court decision in *Brown v. Board of Education of Topeka* declared "separate but equal" inherently discriminatory. This has had profound effects on education and the provision of health care. Problems continued even after passage of the U.S. Civil Rights Act of 1965, major race riots occurred in the late 1960s, and demonstrations for racial justice continue to this day. The historical manifestation of racial prejudice and history of slavery continues in various ways and influences both public policy and social interactions. While the Confederacy lost the Civil War, monuments to its leaders are still visible; the prejudice inherent in policies in the Reconstruction and Jim Crow laws still emerge in White supremacy movements and have been argued to continue to negatively impact the health and well-being of African Americans through the focus on the war on drugs, disparate patterns of incarceration, as well as policing patterns. Of note, street demonstrations protesting the killing of unarmed African Americans contribute to the suspicion of government in the face of apparent lack respect for African Americans and has become known as the Black Lives Matter movement.

It is difficult to separate the acculturation effect of people living in poverty and aspiring for a better life from actual cultural features of African Americans. The development of what we can consider African American culture did not evolve in one clear locality or uniform manner. Over a period of 150 years, generations of slaves passed oral history and culture along by word of mouth. Music and allegorical stories were shared among people from different African origins and between generations. This resulted in a new

African American culture that embodied fundamental characteristics unique to America. Churches and schools, and many other places, were segregated, which inadvertently provided opportunities for African American culture to flourish.

Characteristics of African music made it into church choirs, and allegorical styles became axiomatic for preaching in southern African American churches, but completely new culture forms such as jazz also emerged. Much of what is considered African American culture evolved from simple poverty. "Soul food" involving greens and all parts of farm animals, which were essentially subsistence and survival food, became associated with African Americans. Yet the African culture added its own parts to the picture with items such as okra and red peas from Africa. Africans adapted "soupikandia," a Senegalese stew, to create gumbo, which is now associated with southern Louisiana.

The concept of family evolved to include people not related by biology as "cousin"' or "brother" or "sister" due to affinity of experience and in place of any traceable actual family. The African tradition of respect for elders in an extended family survives in many families to this day.

Despite these hardships, African Americans have demonstrated their capacity to excel in every area of society. Political leaders, Olympic and other sports champions, entertainment figures, scientists, astronauts, Supreme Court justices, military leaders, civic leaders and mayors, religious leaders, award-winning authors and poets, members of the president's cabinet, newscasters, university presidents, and even a vice president of the United States have emerged from people sharing the African American culture.

African Americans in the United States

In July 2019, African Americans were the second largest minority population, following the Hispanic/Latino population, totaling about 40.6 million people and 12.8% of the total population. In 2019, most Blacks or African Americans lived in the South (58.7%). About 60% of the Black population were in Texas, Georgia, Florida, New York, North Carolina, California, Illinois, Maryland, Virginia, and Louisiana (HHS, OMH, 2021a [see **Figure 8.1**]).

In 2017, the average African American family median income was $43,771 compared to $71,664 for non-Hispanic White families. It was reported that 21.2% of non-Hispanic Blacks in comparison to 9.0% of non-Hispanic Whites were living at the poverty line (HHS, OMH, 2021a). For 2019, the unemployment rate for African Americans was twice that for non-Hispanic Whites (7.7% versus 3.7%) (HHS, OMH, 2021a).

African Americans often have strong religious affiliations, especially with Christian denominations, notably Baptist and Church of God in Christ. When the slave trade began, Christianity was only starting to spread in Africa due to European explorers. However, Islam had a much larger influence in Africa at the time, and it is estimated that about 20% of the transported slaves were Muslims. Once in America, there was some debate about whether Christianity should be taught, because it might imply some kind of affinity among peoples. Nevertheless, many slaves were taught Christianity, and many continued to follow Islam as well.

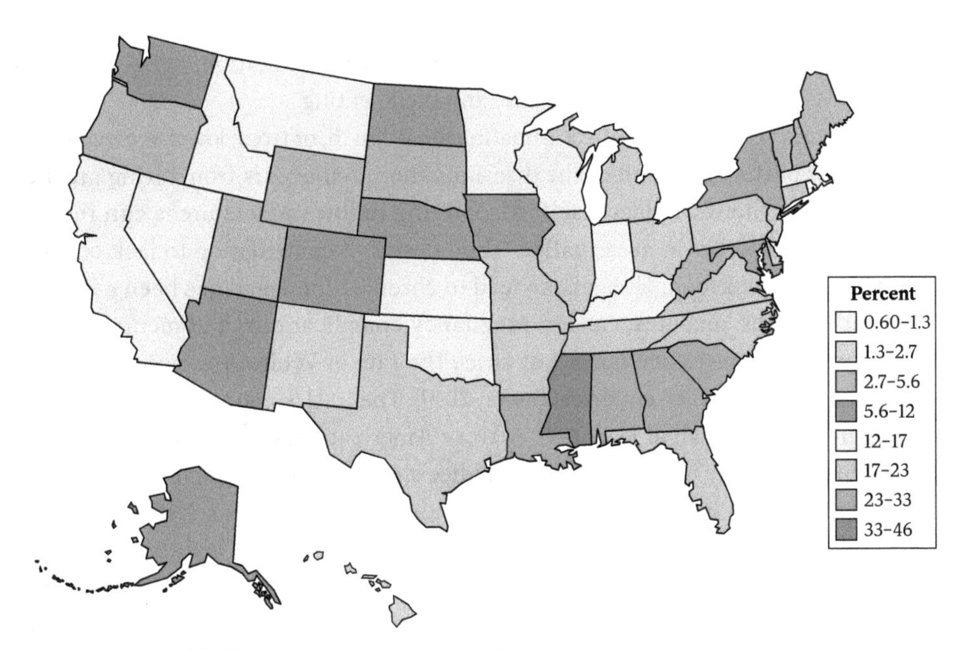

Figure 8.1 U.S. Black population percentage by State.

Due to historic practices of subjugation, African Americans experience discrimination in many settings, including within the health care system. Subtle insults and comments make African Americans feel inferior in health care settings. This mistrust is what leads some African Americans to rely on traditional healing methods or not to seek care until it can no longer be avoided.

People who are constantly treated unfairly tend to have more stress, which can lead to emotional, physical, and behavioral problems. When people face discrimination during adolescence, they tend to have behavioral problems that lead to antisocial behavior. Teens can feel out of place among their peers, and because they choose not to talk about it, they may act out their unspoken frustrations. They may engage in aggressive or illegal acts, such as fighting and shoplifting. Young teens may feel that there is nowhere to turn, which may push them to consider suicide.

When adults go through depression because of racial discrimination, they often develop behaviors such as being irritable and hostile toward others for no reason, having insomnia, and discriminating against others around them. Growing up around discrimination often causes adolescents to have a hard time concentrating in school and or achieving their goals. Dealing with discrimination and confronting people of other races who think they are better than African Americans can lead to low self-esteem and less satisfaction in their adult lives. When people have had interaction with racial discrimination, they sometimes believe the world is out to get them. Everywhere they go, they think there is racial discrimination—even when there is no sign of discrimination.

The physical effects of discrimination-induced stress can also lead to problems such as high blood pressure and a weakened immune system. Another physical effect of racial discrimination is obesity and diabetes. Due to racial discrimination, many unhealthy behaviors arise, such as drinking, drug use, and binge eating.

People who experience racial discrimination are often in, or from, lower socioeconomic status, which is partially a result of the discrimination that occurs from hiring practices and conditions in the workplace itself. Also, living in low-income areas can result in African Americans living in areas called "food deserts," contributing to lack of access to affordable nutritious food. Hunger can lead to chronic illness and has been associated with low birthweight, diabetes, cancer, pregnancy complications, and mental distress. African Americans experience hunger at twice the rate of White Americans, including one in four African American children (Taylor, 2019). The 10 U.S. counties with the highest food insecurity rates are all at least 60% African American (Taylor, 2019).

The disparities in treatment and the prejudice shown have resulted in African Americans having the worst health profile of any population in the United States. This is not to say that individuals are not responsible to take care of their own health and to follow well-known wellness practices. However, individual efforts to maintain health within the African American community do exist within a historical and societal context that present significant challenges to individuals and exist within a context of major health disparities.

General Philosophy About Disease Prevention and Health Maintenance

Many African Americans mistrust the U.S. health care system. This distrust is not a paranoid reaction. It has been fueled by incidences such as the Tuskegee study, in which the U.S. Public Health Service conducted a study from 1932 to 1972 on hundreds of African American men with syphilis. The men were not treated with antibiotics that would have cured the disease, and indeed most of them died (Clarke-Tasker, 1993). The scientific and medical communities reacted with shock when the study was exposed, but most African Americans saw the study as a blatant act of genocide perpetrated against Blacks by Whites. The study was only part of a long history of abusive conduct within the medical field. During the early 1800s African American bodies were sought for dissection in medical schools; later, medical texts such as English biologist Dr. Richard Owen's "The Gorilla and the Negro," were accepted as authoritative, graves were dug up at night by "night doctors" to provide cadavers to medical schools, and the human HeLa cell line, used extensively for genetic research, resulted from cells taken from African American patient, Henrietta Lacks, in 1951 without her permission or knowledge (Lee et al., 2018).

Over time such stories have been told via African American oral folklore, warning generations of African Americans of the abusive nature of the medical profession and public health programs. As a result, many people in the African American community believe that health care professionals simply do not value their lives.

Health differences are often due to economic and social conditions that are more common among African Americans than Whites. For example, African American adults are more likely to report they cannot see a doctor because of cost (CDC, 2017a).

Worldview

Many African Americans believe that health is a gift from God; illness is a result of something that was not pleasing to God or may be determined by fate (Sadler & Huff, 2007). African Americans have historically believed that illness may be due to their failure to live according to God's will. Some African Americans even believe that illness comes directly from the devil. Although most African American communities rely on religion and their relationship with God as a main reason for illness, some community members do not. Sometimes the belief that one's health is in God's hands, a fatalistic perspective, can prevent engagement in preventive measures or treatment.

In general, African Americans are present oriented. Some are rather relaxed about time and may be late for appointments. Time is viewed as circular; showing up for their appointment is more important than being on time (Purnell & Fenkl, 2021). Older persons tend to be more punctual.

Some African Americans use a form of standard English referred to as African American English (AAE), also called Black English or Ebonics. Non-African Americans who hear this dialect may have the impression that the speaker is uneducated; this can be erroneous as it is a legitimate and rule-governed language system spoken by many African Americans unrelated to level of education. African Americans tend to speaker louder than those from other cultures, and it is important not to interpret that as being angry. Many tend to prefer close personal space and are comfortable with touching and hugging. Highly animated nonverbal communication methods are sometimes misinterpreted as being aggressive. Eye contact is viewed as a sign of respect.

Pain is often expressed openly, but this can vary. With the exception of family members, organ donations usually are not acceptable.

WHAT DO YOU THINK?

African Americans, as well as members of other cultures, believe that their health is in God's hands. How can medical providers and public health professionals encourage preventive efforts while respecting this worldview?

Pregnancy, Birth, and Child Rearing

Little has been documented in the literature about African American women's preparation for childbirth. Like other African American patients, pregnant and new mothers are often made to feel marginalized, stigmatized, and stereotyped because of racism practiced against them.

Like all cultures, traditional beliefs may continue into the present, and many of these beliefs are not supported by medical research. African American beliefs and traditions surrounding pregnancy and birth include the following:

- A pregnant woman holding her hands up over her head will strangle the unborn baby.
- A pregnant woman crossing her legs when sitting will cause hemorrhoids.

- A pregnant woman should indulge her food cravings. If she does not, the baby will have unpleasant physical or personality traits that match the characteristics of the food.
- Babies are not named until it is known they will survive. It is believed that spirits of the dead cannot see and therefore cannot harm a child who does not have a name.
- The placenta has a spirit of its own and must be secretly buried where it will never be disturbed and negatively affect the child.
- Pregnant women should not have their pictures taken, because it will cause a stillbirth.
- A small portion of the umbilical cord should be wrapped in paper and put away to ensure the infant will not get colic.
- Henna body art is used during the postpartum period. The henna wards off depression, eliminates spirits that cause disease, helps prevent poor bonding with the infant, and signifies the mother's new and higher social status.
- Talismans, also called amulets, are used for protection and to connect the child to ancestral powers and the spirits of nature.
- New mothers are to rest and be cared for by their family and the community. This care should take place during the 4 to 8 weeks after birth.

Nutrition and Exercise

A family tradition of soul food may be problematic for some African Americans. Soul foods traditionally have been characterized by added fats, fried food, eggs, organ and processed meats, and sugar-sweetened beverages (Shikany, 2015).

Many American-born African Americans consume pork products with high salt content, fried foods, and heavy gravy. Common ways that African Americans prepare foods include frying, barbequing, and using gravy and sauces (Purnell & Fenkl, 2021). Their diets are typically high in fat, sodium, and cholesterol, with more animal fat, less fiber, and fewer fruits and vegetables than the rest of American society (Purnell & Fenkl, 2021). Studies have shown that African American diets stress the consumption of meat and eggs, which results in a high-cholesterol and saturated fat diet. African American foods also tend to be lower in complex carbohydrates and dietary fiber. This may contribute to their high incidence of being overweight.

A food guide pyramid was developed to reflect the cultural foods historically eaten by African Americans and to help them improve their nutrition status (see **Figure 8.2**). The African American food pyramid had a foundation of biscuits, corn (corn breads, grits, and hominy), pasta, and rice. In urban communities, store-bought breads have replaced biscuits. Vegetables (green leafy vegetables—chard, collard, kale, mustard greens—and corn, okra, sweet potatoes, and yams) and fruits (apples, bananas, berries, peaches, and watermelon) make up the middle of the pyramid. Fruit consumption by today's African Americans is considered low compared to other groups.

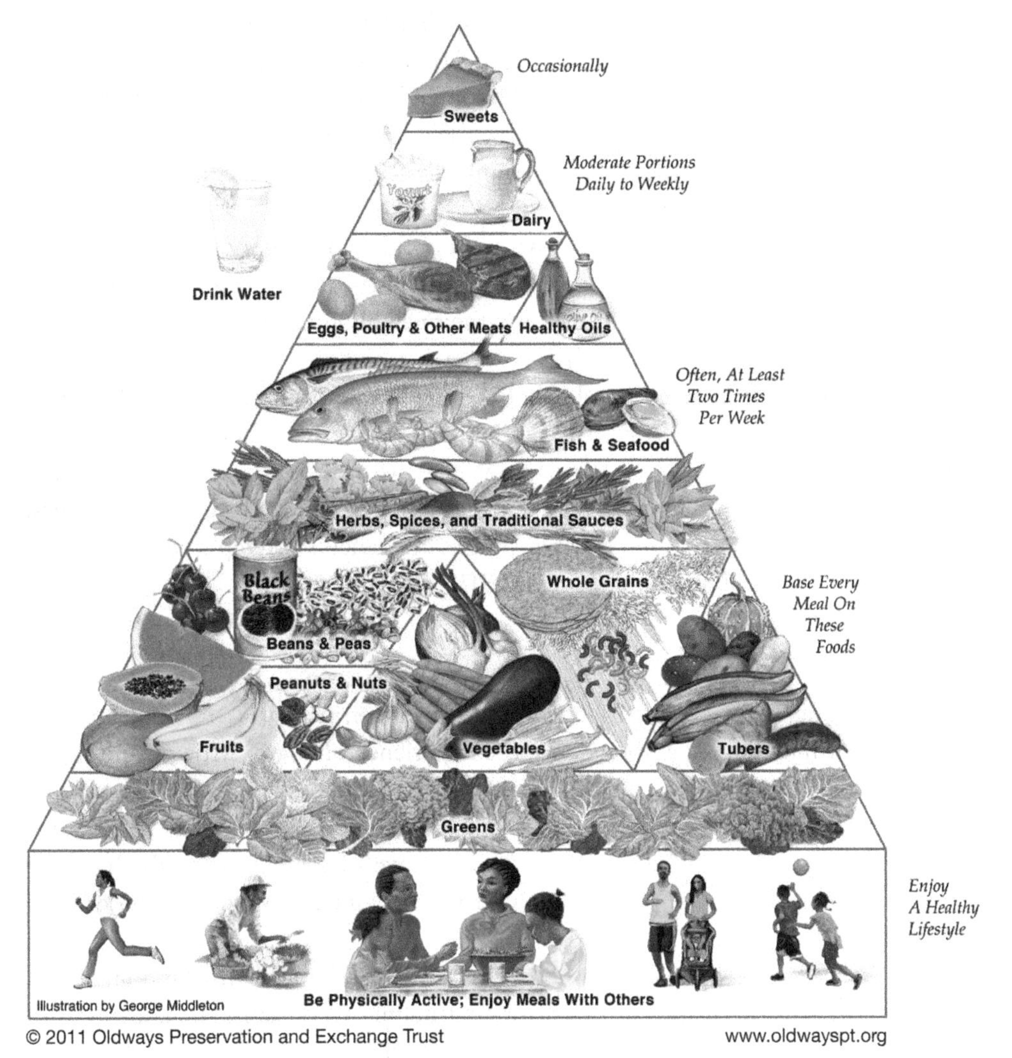

Figure 8.2 African American food pyramid.

Mental Health

African Americans have about the same degree of mental health issues, or even less, than non-Hispanic Whites. This may be because African Americans often rely on family, church, and community to cope. The level of religious participation among African Americans is high.

The rate of substance use among African American is lower than for other ethnicities, and alcohol and drugs are responsible for a lower percentage of deaths among African Americans than among non-Hispanic Whites (Monnat, 2017). Some adverse behaviors that particularly affect the African American community are drug use, smoking, poor nutritional habits, and limited physical activity. The consumption and trafficking of drugs, such as alcohol and cocaine, in the African American community is market driven and stimulated by unemployment, poverty, despair, alienation, depression, hopelessness, and dependency (addiction). Homicide rates for African Americans are more than other races and ethnicities. In 2016, there were 38 homicide deaths per 100,000 population among male African Americans, but only five such deaths per 100,000 population for White males. Firearm-related deaths of African American men is more than double that of White males (Statista, 2019).

Despite years of protest from African Americans, their communities are still targeted by billboards with positive messages about alcohol. This means African American youth are exposed to more alcohol advertisements in their neighborhoods than any other youth groups in the United States (Hill, 2007).

African Americans have a remarkably low suicide rate compared to non-Hispanic Whites. According to the CDC, in 2018, both African American men and women had a suicide rate only 40% that of non-Hispanic Whites. However, there has been a noted increase in suicide deaths and attempted suicides among African American teenagers, with a suicide rate of 60% of non-Hispanic Whites and suicide attempts at 150% of that of non-Hispanic White high school students (HHS, OMH, 2021b).

Death and Dying

Generally speaking, in the African American experience, spirituality is a fundamental part of how many people process and reconcile the experience of death. African Americans tend to believe in the sanctity of life and rely on a strong sense of community and family at times of loss. Family-centered consensus is valued in decision-making, and there is often a strong need for extended family to gather at times of death. The family should be informed of an impending death so that extended family members who live out of state can be notified.

Many African Americans have a holistic view of death and dying, and birth and death are understood to be part of a cycle or continuum. At the same time, many older African Americans, who believe that death is God's will, may also tend to believe that life support should be continued as long as necessary. Cremation is generally avoided in this community, and organ donation may be viewed by some as a desecration of the body.

In medical settings, so much emphasis is placed on the physical care of the dying that spirituality is often overlooked. Health care providers do not always recognize that this should be an integral part of the continuum of care. In hospital settings, one way to accomplish this is to suggest the support of the hospital chaplain. It would be ideal to involve clergy from the individual's own faith community, but if that is not possible, be sure that the hospital chaplain is available as an integral part of the care team. Overall, African Americans prefer more aggressive treatment, conduct less advanced care planning, and "are more likely to informally discuss end of life care than to formally document wishes" (Lee et al., 2018, p. 25).

Cultural-Bound Illnesses

There are no specific culture-bound illnesses attributed to the African American culture. While sickle cell anemia is often associated with African Americans it is actually a genetic condition that has a high incidence in African Americans, with 1 in 12 having this trait, but it is not exclusive to African Americans. The disease occurs in about one out of every 365 African American births, but it also affects Hispanic Americans, occurring in about one out of every 16,300 Hispanic American births (CDC, 2020a).

DID YOU KNOW?

There were 25,665 sickle cell disease–related deaths reported among Blacks in the United States from 1979 through 2017. During that period, the annual sickle cell disease–related death rate declined in children and increased in adults, and the median age at death increased from 28 to 43 years (Payne et al., 2020).

Healing Traditions

African American healing traditions encompass a variety of beliefs and practices. Some of them were brought through slavery and ancestral roots. The ancestral roots from West Africa brought many herbal and spiritual healing techniques. Types of healers that African Americans use include faith or spiritual healers. African American healers may choose to use rituals, charms, and herbs. Today, African Americans can choose whether they want to be seen by a biomedical doctor or a traditional healer. Although they have the freedom to choose their practitioner, certain factors can affect their choice, such as trust, access to care, and insurance, as well as other socioeconomic factors.

Prayer is the most common treatment for illness among people who believe that illness is caused by God's will. Spiritual beliefs form a foundation for the health belief systems of many African Americans. Instead of going to the doctor when they are ill, some African Americans will pray for their actions that caused them to get sick, asking God to make them healthy before seeking the help of Western medicine. The belief in God tends to be with absolute certainty and includes belief in miracles (Komen, 2020).

Herbs and remedies are other important aspects of the healing traditions of African Americans. Some herbs and remedies that are used include the following (Spector, 2017):

- St. John's wort is used for scrapes, strains, and burns. Today it is known for being a mild treatment for depression.

- Petals from an African plant called okra are used to cure boils.
- Wild yam is used to cure indigestion.
- Rectified turpentine with sugar is used to treat a cough.
- Nine drops of turpentine 9 days after intercourse may act as a contraceptive.
- Sugar and turpentine are used to get rid of worms.
- Dried snake ground up and brewed as tea is used to treat blemishes.
- Cool baths, isopropyl alcohol (applied topically), warming the feet, and cool drinks or popsicles are used to treat fever.
- Catnip, senna extract, chamomile, cigarette smoke, and walking are used to treat colic.
- Whiskey, pennies, eggs, and ice cubes or popsicles alleviate teething pain.

The goal of treatment for unnatural illness is to remove evil spirits from the body. Traditional healers, who are usually women, are consulted. These women possess knowledge about use of herbs and roots as well as mystical voodoo-like powers.

Voodoo (from *vodoun*, meaning spirit) originated in Africa nearly 10,000 years ago. Although its origins remain mysterious and elusive, scholars are fairly certain that its birthplace was somewhere in West Africa. It is recognized as one of the world's oldest religions (Dakwar, 2004). Voodoo was brought to this country in 1724 with the arrival of slaves from the West African coast (Spector, 2017). Historian Sharla Fett identified four themes that link the medical practices of southern slaves to those of the West and Central African cultures: a belief that medicine possesses a spiritual force, that preparing medicine brings the healer closer to spiritual power, that healing maintains relationships between the living and the world of ancestors, and that power can be used for healing and harming (Savitt, 2002). Voodoo is divided into two types: white magic and black magic. White magic is known to be harmless and includes the use of powders and oils that are pleasantly scented. Black magic is quite rare but dangerous and includes the use of oils and powders with a foul and vile odor (Spector, 2017). The practice involves candle-lit rituals and spiritual ceremonies, most commonly held by women.

During the 19th and 20th centuries, voodoo suffered persecution in both the Americas and the Caribbean. The practice of voodoo was illegal, and the spiritual tools of voodoo—fetishes, rods, and sculptures—were confiscated and destroyed (Dakwar, 2004). Simultaneously, a campaign to discredit and disparage voodoo in the public eye began; this led to the popular understanding of voodoo as being malicious, dark, foolish, primitive, dangerous, and violent—ideas that continue to resonate today. Despite this campaign, voodoo is still practiced by millions of people in Africa, the Americas, and the Caribbean (Dakwar, 2004).

Santeria is practiced by some African Americans. It is based on West African religions that were brought to the New World by slaves imported to the Caribbean to work on the sugar plantations. These slaves carried with them their own religious traditions, including a tradition of possession trance for communicating with the ancestors and deities, the use of animal sacrifice, and the practice of sacred drumming and dance. Those slaves who landed in the Caribbean and Central and South America were nominally converted to Catholicism. However, they were able to preserve some of their traditions by fusing various Yoruban beliefs and rituals with elements from the surrounding Catholic culture. In Cuba this religious tradition has evolved into what we know today as Santeria, the Way of the Saints. Today, hundreds of thousands of Americans participate in this ancient religion. Many are of Hispanic and Caribbean descent, but as the religion moves out of the inner cities and into the suburbs, a growing number of followers are of African American and European American heritage.

Another religion tied to the days of slavery is **Candomblé**, which was developed in Brazil by enslaved Africans who attempted to re-create their culture on the other side of the ocean. The rituals involve animal sacrifices, healing, dancing, drumming, and the possession of participants by orishas, which are religious deities said to represent human characteristics such as bravery, love, and honor. Today, Candomblé is widely practiced in Brazil, but because of its secrecy it is unknown how widespread it is in the United States. Attempts at spiritual healing may be concealed from Western health care providers to avoid the stigma attached to such practices, which may be labeled as devil worshipping or mumbo jumbo by the mainstream European American culture.

Behavioral Risk Factors and Common Health Problems

Discrimination, poverty, and poor nutrition and exercise habits have resulted in serious health problems for African Americans. The poverty rate is higher among African Americans than any other racial/ethnic groups except American Indian/Alaska Natives (Kaiser Family Foundation, 2021). As a group, African Americans lead all other racial/ethnic groups in low birthweight, infant mortality, obesity, diabetes, asthma, hepatitis B, HIV/AIDS, sexually transmitted diseases, waiting list for organ transplants, and cancer deaths. In 2017, the death rate for African Americans was higher than Whites for heart diseases, stroke, cancer, asthma, influenza and pneumonia, diabetes, HIV/AIDS, and homicide (HHS, OMH, 2019a). Yet African Americans had only 40% the suicide rate as non-Hispanic Whites (HHS, OMH, 2021b). This held true for all ages, but a serious problem seems to be developing regarding attempted suicide among high school students in grades 9–12 where the attempted suicide rate was 1.5 times the rate of non-Hispanic Whites in 2018 (HHS, OMH, 2021b).

The 10 leading causes of death among African American in 2018 were as follows:

1. Heart disease
2. Cancer
3. Unintentional injuries

4. Stroke
5. Diabetes mellitus
6. Chronic lower respiratory disease
7. Homicide
8. Nephritis, nephrotic syndrome, and nephrosis
9. Alzheimer's disease
10. Essential hypertension and hypertensive renal disease (Elfein, 2021)

In 2017–18, obesity among African Americans men aged 20 and over was 41.1% and was 56.9% among women of the same age range (Hales, 2020). African American women have the highest rates of obesity or being overweight compared to other groups in the United States. About four out of five African American women are overweight or obese. In 2018, African American women were 50% more likely to be obese than non-Hispanic White women, and non-Hispanic Blacks, in general, were 1.3 times more likely to be obese as compared to non-Hispanic Whites. In addition, in 2018, African Americans were 20% less likely to engage in active physical activity as compared to non-Hispanic Whites (HHS, OMH, 2020a).

Obesity among African Americans contributed to excess risk during the COVID-19 pandemic. Having obesity, defined as a body mass index (BMI) between 30 kg/m^2 and < 40 kg/m^2 or severe obesity (BMI of 40 kg/m^2 or above), increases risk of severe illness from COVID-19. Being overweight, defined as a BMI > 25 kg/m^2 but less than 30 kg/m^2 might also increase risk of severe illness from COVID-19 (CDC, 2022a).

Associated with obesity is the fact that African American adults are diagnosed with diabetes at a rate 60% higher than non-Hispanic White adults. In 2017, non-Hispanic Blacks were 3.5 times more likely to be diagnosed with end-stage renal disease as compared to non-Hispanic Whites and were 2.3 times more likely to be hospitalized for lower limb amputations as compared to non-Hispanic Whites (HHS, OMH 2021b). In 2017, African Americans were twice as likely as non-Hispanic Whites to die from diabetes (CDC, 2019a).

In 2019, African Americans had an infant mortality rate more than twice that of non-Hispanic Whites. In 2020, African Americans had 2.3 times the infant mortality rate as non-Hispanic Whites, were 4.0 times more likely to die from low birthweight, and had twice the sudden infant death syndrome mortality rate as non-Hispanic Whites. In addition, during 2019, African American mothers were 2.1 times more likely than non-Hispanic White mothers to receive late or no prenatal care (HHS, OMH, 2021c).

African Americans have the highest mortality rate of any racial and ethnic group for all cancers and for most specific major types of cancers. From 2014–2018, African American men had 1.2 times the rate for colon cancer and 1.5 times the rate of prostate cancer, as compared to non-Hispanic White men. The disparity for having stomach cancer for African American men was similar to that of prostate cancer, but while

African American men die at a rate 1.8 times that of non-Hispanic men from prostate cancer, they are 2.5 times as likely to die from stomach cancer (HHS, OMH, 2021e). On the other hand, from 2012–2016, African American women were just as likely to have breast cancer as non-Hispanic White women; however, they were almost 40% more likely to die from breast cancer. African American women were twice as likely to be diagnosed with stomach cancer, and they were 2.2 times as likely to die from stomach cancer as compared to non-Hispanic White women (HHS, OMH, 2021d). African American men still have the highest rate of lung cancer among all demographics (77.7 versus 62.6/100,000 for non-Hispanic Whites) the incidence in young Black/African Americans has declined to now match young Whites but is increasing in Black/African American women (Jemal et al., 2020).

Despite high incidence of lung cancer, when it comes to smoking African American youth and young adults have significantly lower prevalence of cigarette smoking than Hispanics and Whites, and smoking among African American and White adults is similar. However, African Americans smoke fewer cigarettes per day. In addition, African Americans generally begin smoking at a later age compared to Whites (CDC, 2020b).

African Americans are the group most affected by HIV, with the 2019 rate of new HIV infection in African Americans 8.1 times that of Whites based on population size. African Americans represented about 42.1% of infections in 2019 although being only 13% of the overall population. African American men had 8.4 times the AIDS rate as White men in 2019, while African American women were about 15 times more likely to have of HIV/AIDS as White women. African American men were almost 6.4 times as likely to die from HIV/AIDS as non-Hispanic White men while African American women are almost 14.5 times as likely to die from HIV/AIDS as non-Hispanic White women (HHS, OMH, 2021a).

In 2018, the primary HIV transmission category for African American men was sexual contact with other men, followed by injection drug use and high-risk heterosexual contact. For African American women, the primary transmission category was high-risk heterosexual contact followed by injection drug use (CDC, 2021).

Another problematic issue is the number of teenage pregnancies among African Americans. Although the number of teenage pregnancies has declined over the years, teen pregnancy rates vary widely by race and ethnicity. In 2017, a total of 194,377 infants were born to women aged 15–19 years, resulting in a birth rate of 18.8 per 1,000 women in this age group. This continued a decline to a record low for U.S. teens and represented a 7% decrease from 2016. While non-Hispanic African Americans and American Indians both showed a 6% reduction from 2016, they trailed reductions by non-Hispanic Whites (8%), Hispanics (9%), and non-Hispanic Asians (15%) (CDC, 2019b). African Americans experience higher rates of other sexually transmitted infections (STIs) compared with other racial/ethnic groups in the United States (CDC, 2021). The higher rates are not caused by ethnicity or heritage, but by social conditions affecting minority groups. Poverty, large gaps between the rich and the poor, fewer jobs, and low education levels can make it more difficult for people to stay sexually healthy (CDC, 2020c). Of particular significance is that from 2014 to 2018 the rate of congenital syphilis increased 126.7% among Blacks (38.2 to 86.6 cases per 100,000 births). In 2018, the rate of among Blacks was 6.4 times the rate among Whites (86.6 versus 13.5 per 100,000 live births, respectively) (CDC, 2020d).

In 2017, African Americans were 1.5 times as likely to die from viral hepatitis compared to non-Hispanic Whites, and they were 2.6 times as likely to die from hepatitis B in 2016 than the White population (HHS, OMH, 2020b). Among African Americans, chronic liver disease is a leading cause of death. Although the cause is not always known, some cases can be initiated by conditions such as chronic alcoholism, obesity, and exposure to hepatitis B and C viruses. In 2018, chronic liver disease was the ninth leading cause of death for non-Hispanic Blacks 45–64 years old (HHS, OMH, 2020c).

Poverty level affects mental health status. Poor African Americans compared to those double the poverty level are twice as likely to report psychological distress. African Americans are 20% more likely to report having serious psychological distress than non-Hispanic Whites, but Whites are more than twice as likely to receive antidepressant treatments.

Remarkably, African American men have a suicide rate 60% lower than non-Hispanic White men. Even more significantly, African American women have a suicide rate only one quarter that of African American men and less than a third that of non-Hispanic White women (HHS, OMH, 2021b).

Heart disease is the leading cause of death for African Americans. In 2018, African Americans were 30% more likely to die from heart disease than non-Hispanic Whites (HHS, OMH, 2021e). African American men and women are more likely than people of other races to have heart failure and to suffer from more severe forms of it. Heart disease develops at a younger age in African Americans, and about 48% of African American women and 44% of African American men have some form of heart disease (The Heart Foundation, 2021).

Overall, African American death rates are higher than those of non-Hispanic Whites. The pre-COVID-19 life expectancy in 2015 for Blacks at birth was 76.1 years, with 78.9 years for women and 72.9 years for men. For non-Hispanic Whites the projected life expectancies were 79.8 years, with 82.0 years for women and 77.5 years for men (HHS, OMH, 2019a).

African Americans were disproportionately impacted by the COVID-19 pandemic. While the infection rate was about 1.1 times that of non-Hispanic Whites, the hospitalization rate was 2.9 and death rate 1.9 times that of non-Hispanic Whites (CDC, 2022b). While the pandemic impacted all populations, and actually led to a reduction in the calculated life expectancy for the overall population by 1 year, life expectancy for African Americans declined the most from 2019—by 2.7 years to 72 years—its lowest level since 2001 (Rodrigues, 2021).

From its onset COVID-19 attacked and spread rapidly among people of all types but particularly affected people with preexisting conditions. Many of these conditions were widespread in the African American population and included old age, obesity, heart disease, liver disease, lung conditions, and a number of others. In addition, after a year of the national COVID-19 experience, according to the CDC, in 2021 some of the multiple inequities in social determinants of health that put African Americans and other racial and ethnic minority groups at increased risk of contracting and possibly dying from COVID-19 included the following:

- *Discrimination.* Discrimination exists in systems meant to protect well-being or health, including health care, housing, education, criminal justice, and finance. Discrimination, which includes racism, can lead to chronic and toxic stress and shapes social and economic factors that put some people from racial and ethnic minority groups at increased risk for COVID-19.
- *Health care access and utilization.* African Americans and some racial and ethnic minority groups are more likely to be uninsured than non-Hispanic Whites. Health care access can also be limited for these groups by many other factors, such as lack of transportation, childcare, or ability to take time off from work; communication and language barriers; cultural differences between patients and providers; and historical and current discrimination in health care systems. African Americans and people from racial and ethnic minority groups may hesitate to seek care because they distrust the government and health care systems responsible for inequities in treatment.
- *Occupation.* African Americans and members of other minority groups are disproportionately represented in essential work settings such as health care facilities, farms, factories, grocery stores, and public transportation. People employed in these settings have more chances to be exposed to the virus that causes COVID-19 due to several factors, such as close contact with the public or other workers, not being able to work from home, and not having paid sick days.
- *Educational, income, and wealth gaps.* Inequities in access to quality education for some African Americans and other minority groups can lead to lower high school completion rates and barriers to college entrance. This leads to low-paying and more unstable employment. People with limited job options likely have less flexibility to leave jobs that may put them at a higher risk of exposure to the virus that causes COVID-19. People in these situations often cannot afford to miss work, even if they are sick, because they do not have enough money saved up for essential items like food and other important living needs.
- *Housing.* Some African Americans and other minority groups live in crowded conditions that make it more challenging to follow prevention strategies. In addition, growing and disproportionate unemployment rates for African American and other minority groups during the COVID-19 pandemic may lead to greater risk of eviction and homelessness or the sharing of housing.

These factors and others are associated with more COVID-19 cases, hospitalizations, and deaths in areas where African Americans and other minority groups live (CDC, 2022a).

QUICK FACTS

Health disparities reported by the CDC include the following:

- Age-adjusted death rates for non-Hispanic White and non-Hispanic Black adults aged 25 and over declined from 2000 to 2011–2012 but remained stable through 2017 (Curtin & Arias, 2019).
- African Americans ages 18–49 are **two times** as likely to die from heart disease than Whites (CDC, 2017a).
- African Americans age 35–64 years are **50%** more likely to have high blood pressure than Whites (CDC, 2017a).
- In 2018, African Americans/Blacks represented 43% of all deaths of people diagnosed with HIV (CDC, 2020d).
- Although African American adults are 40% more likely to have high blood pressure, they are less likely than non-Hispanic Whites to have their blood pressure under control (HHS, OMH, 2021e).
- African American women are 60% more likely to have high blood pressure compared to non-Hispanic White women (HHS, OMH, 2021e).
- African American women were 50% more likely to be obese than non-Hispanic White women in 2018 (HHS, OMH, 2020a).
- In 2017, African Americans were twice as likely to die from diabetes as non-Hispanic Whites (HHS, OMH, 2019c). African Americans are more likely to die at earlier ages than all other racial groups from all causes (CDC, 2017a).

Considerations for Health Promotion and Program Planning

Consider the following concepts when planning and implementing a health promotion program for this target audience:

- Be aware and sensitive to the distrust of the medical community and the government that may exist among African American community members.
- Be aware that peer educators have not been shown to be effective in developing health programs for African American audiences.
- Until invited otherwise, greet African Americans with formal titles.
- Be aware of different terminology because there are various regional terms used to describe medical conditions. Among immigrants from Haiti, Jamaica, and the Bahamas, and among many Southern African Americans, for example, blood may be characterized as *low* or *high*, referring to anemia as opposed to hypertension. *Spells*, also

called *falling outs,* are perceived to be a result of *low blood;* elderly African Americans especially may refer to *having had a spell. Shock* is a common term for a stroke. Other common terms include *having sugar, sweet blood,* or *thin blood,* referring to diabetes.

- Understand that occasional outbursts of laughter that may appear inappropriate for the situation are in fact appropriate because African Americans find solace in laughter and playfulness.
- Maintaining good health is often correlated with good religious practice. Many churches maintain a health ministry through which congregations and parish nurses support good health with flu shots, blood pressure checks, and health education (Carteret, 2011). Therefore, health screening programs may best be initiated through community and church activities.

Tips for Working With the African American Population

To improve communication, which enhances the building of a trusting relationship, acknowledge and respect your patients' meaning for their illness. Spend time with your patients and ask about their health beliefs. Listen carefully.

Acknowledging and respecting your patient's understanding of their illness will help improve communication, which is a cornerstone of a trusting caregiver-patient relationship. If there is a mismatch, many African American patients will rely on their own explanations before those of medical professionals. Making one medically neutral suggestion that fits your patients' belief system builds rapport quickly.

Assess and acknowledge the significance of spirituality; avoid dominating the content of the discussion, and offer choices for treatment options. Be available to consult with your patient's family, minister, and friends in cases of serious or terminal illness, especially at the time the illness is being explained.

Include your patients in the decision-making process. Answer your patients' questions and concerns about diagnosis and treatment plans. Expand the decision-making process to include social decisions.

Show respectful behavior. Your patients may include many people as part of their extended family, some related, and others who may be friends of the family or part of the patient's wider social networks. What is unique about this patient and family that you will not learn from tips or information about their culture?

Before touching patients, always explain what will be done and why. Your patients may prefer that family members of the other gender leave the room.

In addition, it is important to remember that the culture of poverty, discrimination and lack of education has been inflicted upon African Americans and is not original to them, nor unique. The basic African American culture reflects a fatalistic worldview, the value of religious faith, respect for traditions, and family, even if family members are informally "invented."

Summary

African Americans were originally brought forcibly to the United States through the slave trade. African Americans experience high levels of poverty, discrimination, and violence. The overall health of the population is worse than any other group in the United States. The many underlying conditions that made hundreds of thousands of Americans more likely to die from COVID-19 were prevalent conditions among the African American population resulting from generations of subjugation and discrimination that contributed to poverty, lack of food security, limitations on access to health care, and suspicion of governmental health programs. Heart disease, high blood pressure, cancer, diabetes, and liver disease are each leading serious health problems, even without COVID-19. The main behavioral risks associated with African Americans are smoking, alcohol consumption, weight management, and lack of physical activity. Some of their beliefs about causes of illness and treatment approaches are related to their religious practices and ancestral roots, so some African Americans will choose to use faith or spiritual healers rather than a biomedical doctor. In some ways, African Americans have developed some capacity to cope with stress in a way that results in their having a low incidence of suicide compared to other groups.

In this chapter we described the unique aspects of the history of African Americans and how their history has had a negative impact on their trust in the medical system. We learned that religion plays a central role in this community and how that is integrated into their health belief system and practices. General tips for working with these populations were provided, but as usual we caution that there is a vast amount of diversity within this community, so it is important not to generalize.

Review

1. Explain the history of African Americans in the United States.
2. Provide an overview of African Americans' socioeconomic situation.
3. Why is there is general mistrust of the medical system by African Americans?
4. What are some of the behavior risk factors and common diseases that African Americans experience?

Activity

Conduct research on health programs that have been implemented for members of the African American population. Summarize the literature and identify some best practices.

Watch the video "Miss Evers' Boys" on YouTube by following the link provided here: (https://www.youtube.com/watch?v=JVmV0cWFG6g.) Write a reaction paper to the video. What surprised you? Should the nurse or physician have done anything differently? How does ethics play a role? How do you think this study influences the interactions between African Americans and the health care system?

Case Study 1

The number of infants who die before their first birthday is much higher in the United States than in other countries, and for African Americans the rate is nearly twice as high as for White Americans. Even well-educated African American women have birth outcomes worse than White women who have not finished high school. Why?

Meet Andrea Jackson, a successful lawyer, executive, and mother. When Andrea was pregnant with her first child, she, like so many others, did her best to ensure a healthy baby; she ate right, exercised, abstained from alcohol and smoking, and received good prenatal care. Yet 2.5 months before her due date, she went into labor unexpectedly. Her newborn weighed less than 3 pounds. Andrea and her husband were devastated. How could this have happened?

We know that, in general, health follows wealth; on average, the higher on the socioeconomic ladder you are, the lower your risk of cancer, heart disease, diabetes, infant death, and preterm deliveries. For highly educated African American women like Andrea, the advantages of income and status do make a difference in health, but something else is still in play: racism.

There are several issues to consider about this case:

1. How may have Andrea's race and culture played a role in her having a low-birthweight baby?
2. Are there any culture-specific protective factors that may have helped Andrea cope with the racism she has faced?

Case Study 2

Emma is a homeless 35-year-old African American mother of four children between the ages of 4–10 and was diagnosed with HIV 3 months ago. Her most recent HIV test was 5 years ago, and she did not return for the results. Emma has a 15-year history of intravenous drug use. She stated that her last use of drugs was 12 hours ago. Emma has only a 10th-grade education, and she has a history of schizophrenia. Emma has had several close friends die of AIDS. She receives care at an urban community clinic where all her providers are of European descent. She is very cautious about starting any drug therapy for HIV because of the stories she has heard of other African Americans being used in an experimental way without their consent. She has not expressed her concerns to her provider.

1. What do you do next?
2. What barriers to care are present in this case?

3. How can these barriers be overcome?
4. How can the encounters between Emma and her provider be improved?
5. Should Emma's children be tested? How would you approach this topic with her?
6. Based on the case study, what strategies to address health literacy might you include in an active plan for Emma's care?
7. Discuss other cultural competence issues that may impact retention in care and treatment (AETC-NMC Aids Education and Training Center, n.d).

References

AETC-NMC Aids Education and Training Center. (n.d.). *Case studies: African Americans.* https://www.aetcnmc.org/studies/african_americans.html

Brown v. Board of Education of Topeka, 347 U.S. 483 (1954)

Carteret. M. (2011). *Health care for African American patients/families.* https://www.dimensionsofculture.com/2011/05/health-care-for-african-american-patientsfamilies/

Centers for Disease Control and Prevention. (2017a). *African American health, creating equal opportunities for health.* https://www.cdc.gov/vitalsigns/aahealth/index.html

Centers for Disease Control and Prevention. (2019a). *National Vital Statistics Report, 68*(9). https://www.cdc.gov/nchs/data/nvsr/nvsr68/nvsr68_09-508.pdf

Centers for Disease Control and Prevention. (2019b). *About teen pregnancy.* https://www.cdc.gov/teenpregnancy/about/index.htm

Centers for Disease Control and Prevention. (2020a). *Data & statistics on sickle cell disease.* https://www.cdc.gov/ncbddd/sicklecell/data.html

Centers for Disease Control and Prevention. (2020b). *African Americans and tobacco use.* https://www.cdc.gov/tobacco/disparities/african-americans/index.htm

Centers for Disease Control and Prevention. (2020c). *STD health equity.* https://www.cdc.gov/std/health-disparities/default.htm#ftn4

Centers for Disease Control and Prevention. (2020d). *African Americans/Blacks.* https://www.cdc.gov/nchhstp/healthdisparities/africanamericans.html

Centers for Disease Control and Prevention. (2021). *HIV and African American People.* https://www.cdc.gov/hiv/group/racialethnic/africanamericans/index.html

Centers for Disease Control and Prevention. (2022a, January 25). *Health equity considerations and racial and ethnic minority groups.* https://www.cdc.gov/coronavirus/2019-ncov/community/health-equity/race-ethnicity.html

Centers for Disease Control and Prevention. (2022b, February 16). *Health of Black or African American Non-Hispanic Population.* https://www.cdc.gov/nchs/fastats/black-health.htm

Centers for Disease Control and Prevention. (2022c, February 9). *Risk for COVID-19 infection, hospitalization, and death by race/ethnicity.* https://www.cdc.gov/coronavirus/2019-ncov/covid-data/investigations-discovery/hospitalization-death-by-race-ethnicity.html

Centers for Disease Control and Prevention. (2022d, February 9). *People with certain conditions.* https://www.cdc.gov/coronavirus/2019-ncov/need-extra-precautions/people-with-medical-conditions.html#obesity

Clarke-Tasker, V. (1993). Cancer prevention and detection in African Americans. In M. Frank-Stromburg & S. J. Olsen (Eds.) Cancer prevention in minority populations: Cultural implications for health care professionals. St. Louis, MO: Mosby.

Curtin, S. C., & Arias, E. (2019, July). *Mortality trends by race and ethnicity among adults aged 25 and over: United States, 2000–2017.* https://www.cdc.gov/nchs/products/databriefs/db342.htm

Dakwar, E. (2004). *Voodoo therapy.* Creighton University Medical Center. http://altmed.creighton.edu/voodoo/

Elfein, J. (2021). *Leading causes of death among black U.S. residents in 2018.* Statista. https//www.statista.com/statistics/233310/distribution-of-the-10-leading-causes-of-death-among-african-americans/

Falconbridge, A. (1788). *An account of the slave trade on the coast of Africa.* J. Phillips.

Hales, C. M., Carroll, M. D., Fryar, C. D., & Ogden, C. L. (2020) Prevalence of obesity and severe obesity among adults: United States, 2017–2018. NCHS Data Brief, no 360. Hyattsville, MD: National Center for Health Statistics.

Hill, P. J. (2007). Legacy of addiction, incarceration feeds itself. *Call & Post,* 9–11.

Jemal, A., Miller, K. D., Sauer, A. G., Bandi, P., Fidler-Benaoudia, M. M., Culp, M., Islami, F., Fedewa, S. A., & Ma, J. (2020). Changes in Black-White difference in lung cancer incidence among young adults. *JNCI Cancer Spectrum, 4*(4). https://doi.org/10.1093/jncics/pkaa055

Kaiser Family Foundation. (2021). *State health fact: Poverty rate by race/ethnicity.* https://www.kff.org/other/state-indicator/poverty-rate-by-raceethnicity/?currentTimeframe=0&sortModel=%7B%22colI d%22:%22Location%22,%22sort%22:%22asc%22%7D

Komen, S. G. (2020). *Education toolkit: Applying culturally-responsive communication in Black and African American communities.* https://komentoolkits.org/wp-content/uploads/2015/03/Applying-Culturally-Responsive-Communication-in-Black-and-African-American-Communities-B-AA-Comm.pdf

Lee, J. H. M., Lee, Reddy, K., Chowdhury, J., Kumar, N., Clark, P. A., Ndao, P., Suh, S. J., & Song, S. (2018). Overcoming the legacy of mistrust: African Americans' mistrust of medical profession. *The Journal of Healthcare Ethics and Administration, 4*(1). https://philarchive.org/archive/LEEOTL-2

Legislative Papers, (1830) Session of the General Assembly (1830-31), A Bill to Prevent All Persons from Teaching Slaves to Read or Write, the Use of Figures Excepted (1830), https://www.ncpedia.org/anchor/bill-prevent-all-persons

Monnat, S. M. (2017). *Drugs, alcohol, and suicide represent growing share of U.S. mortality.* https://lernercenter.syr.edu/wp-content/uploads/2018/05/completed_Drugs-Alcohol-and-Suicide-Represent-Growing-Share-of-US-Mortality.pdf

Payne, A. B., Mehal, J. M., Chapman, C., Haberling, D. L., Richardson, L. C., Bean, C. J., & Hooper, W. C. (2020). Trends in sickle cell disease-related mortality in the United States, 1979 to 2017. *Annals of Emergency Medicine, 76*(3S), S28-S36. https://pubmed.ncbi.nlm.nih.gov/32928459/

Perry, J. A. (1998). *African roots of African-American culture.* Black Collegian Online. https://www.thefreelibrary.com/African+roots+of+African-American+culture.-a053643733

Plessy v. Ferguson, 163 U.S. 537 (1896)

Purnell, L., & Fenkl, E. (2021). *Textbook for transcultural health care: A population approach. Cultural competence concepts in nursing care* (5th ed.). Springer Nature.

Rodrigues, A. (2021, February 18). The U.S. lost a whole year of life expectancy—and for Black people, it's nearly 3 times worse. *USA Today.* https://www.usatoday.com/story/news/health/2021/02/18/covid-us-life-expectancy-record-low-blacks-latinos-most-affected/6778474002/

Sadler, C., & Huff, M. (2007). *African-American women: Health beliefs, lifestyle, and osteoporosis.* Lippincott Nursing. Center. http://www.nursingcenter.com/prodev/ce_article.asp?tid=710316

Savitt, T. L. (2002). *Medicine and slavery: The diseases and healthcare of blacks.* University of Illinois Press.

Shikany, J. M., Safford, M., Newby, P. K., Durant, R. Brown, T., P. K. Newby, P.K., Juddet, S. (2015). Southern dietary pattern is associated with hazard of acute coronary heart disease in the reasons for Geographic and Racial Differences in Stroke (REGARDS) study. *Circulation, 132*(9), 804–814.

Spector, R. E. (2017). *Cultural diversity in health and illness* (9th ed.). Pearson.

Statista. (2019). *Distribution of the 10 leading causes of death among Black US residents in 2017.* https://www.statista.com/statistics/233310/distribution-of-the-10-leading-causes-of-death-among-african-americans/

Taylor, J. (2019, December 19). *Racism, inequality, and health care for African Americans.* The Century Foundation. https://tcf.org/content/report/racism-inequality-health-care-african-americans/?agreed=1

The Heart Foundation. (2021). *African Americans and heart disease.* https://theheartfoundation.org/2018/09/07/african-americans-and-heart-disease/

U.S. Census Bureau. (2020). *About the topic of race.* https://www.census.gov/topics/population/race/about.html

U.S. Department of Health and Human Services, Office of Minority Health. (2019a). National Vital Statistics Reports, *Death Final Data 2017,* 68(9), https://www.cdc.gov/nchs/data/nvsr/nvsr68/nvsr68_09-508.pdf

U.S. Department of Health and Human Services, Office of Minority Health. (2020a). *Obesity and African Americans.* https://minorityhealth.hhs.gov/omh/browse.aspx?lvl=4&lvlid=25

U.S. Department of Health and Human Services, Office of Minority Health. (2020b). *Hepatitis and African Americans.* https://minorityhealth.hhs.gov/omh/browse.aspx?lvl=4&lvlid=20

U.S. Department of Health and Human Services, Office of Minority Health. (2020c). *Chronic liver disease and African Americans.* https://minorityhealth.hhs.gov/omh/browse.aspx?lvl=4&lvlid=17

U.S. Department of Health and Human Services, Office of Minority Health. (2021a). *Profile: Black/African Americans.* https://minorityhealth.hhs.gov/omh/browse.aspx?lvl=3&lvlid=61

U.S. Department of Health and Human Services, Office of Minority Health. (2021b). *Mental and behavioral health, African Americans.* https://minorityhealth.hhs.gov/omh/browse.aspx?lvl=4&lvlid=24#1

U.S. Department of Health and Human Services, Office of Minority Health. (2021b). *Diabetes and African Americans.* https://minorityhealth.hhs.gov/omh/browse.aspx?lvl=4&lvlid=18

U.S. Department of Health and Human Services, Office of Minority Health. (2021c). *Infant mortality and African Americans.* https://www.minorityhealth.hhs.gov/omh/browse.aspx?lvl=4&lvlid=23

U.S. Department of Health and Human Services, Office of Minority Health. (20219d). *Cancer and African Americans.* https://www.minorityhealth.hhs.gov/omh/browse.aspx?lvl=4&lvlid=16

U.S. Department of Health and Human Services, Office of Minority Health. (2021e). *Heart disease and African Americans.* https://minorityhealth.hhs.gov/omh/browse.aspx?lvl=4&lvlid=19

U.S. National Park Service. (n.d.). *African American heritage and ethnography: The transatlantic slave trade.* https://www.nps.gov/ethnography/aah/aaheritage/histContextsC.htm

CREDITS

CHAPTER 9

Asian American Populations

Keeping your body healthy is an expression of gratitude to the whole cosmos—the trees, the clouds, everything.

—THICH NHAT HANH

Always aim at complete harmony of thought and word and deed. Always aim at purifying your thoughts and everything will be well.

—MAHATMA GANDHI

Sickness is a thing of the spirit.

—JAPANESE PROVERB

KEY CONCEPTS AND TERMS

aAma and aDuonga
Hmong
Karma
Kior chi force
Shintoism
Timbang

LEARNING OBJECTIVES

After reading this chapter, you should be able to do the following:

1. Discuss the social and economic circumstances of the various Asian Americans in the United States.
2. Describe the beliefs about the cause of illness for Asian American cultures.
3. Discuss risk factors and illnesses that particularly affect Asian Americans.
4. Describe beliefs about healing practices for Asian Americans.

Introduction

This chapter addresses the cultural health attributes of the approximately 5.7 % of the U.S. population who trace their origins from the original peoples of the Far East, Southeast Asia, or the Indian subcontinent. These areas are the home of about 60% of the world's population of 7 billion people. The 2017 Census Bureau population estimates included 18.9 million Asian people, alone, living in the United States (HHS, OMH, 2021a).

Race is not the same as culture, and this is particularly true when speaking of Asians in America who come from the most populous and diverse countries in the world, including China, with more than 1.4 billion people, India with 1.3 billion people, and Indonesia with 275 million people (U.S. Census Bureau, 2021). The people of China alone speak many different languages and dialects, and it was necessary to establish Mandarin as a language to be learned and used in addition to local languages to enable nationwide communication. All the major religions of the world are practiced by Asians, including Hinduism, Buddhism, Islam, and Christianity.

The people of Asia are not one homogeneous culture, and many groups have been in major conflict with one another over the centuries. Vietnam fought wars with China for thousands of years, Japan inflicted major destruction and inhumane treatment on the Chinese during World War II, and India and China continue to have border disputes. However, there are many cultural aspects of people from Asia that transcend national boundaries.

This chapter provides a brief history of the Asian population in the United States, along with information about their demographic information, their beliefs about the causes of illness and healing practices, behavioral risk factors, and the common health problems that they face.

Terminology

Asia is the largest land mass on the planet, and referring to a person as an Asian is not particularly descriptive due to the great variety of its peoples and cultures. Some analysts break the continental reference into South Asia, Southeast Asia, and the Far East, and the many Asian countries organized into these categories are depicted in **Table 9.1**.

TABLE 9.1 Asian American Origins

Far East. China, Japan, Korea, Mongolia, Okinawa, Taiwan
Southeast Asia. Borneo, Brunei, Burma, Cambodia, Philippines, Indonesia, Laos, Malaysia, Singapore, Thailand, Vietnam
South Asia (Indian subcontinent). Afghanistan, Bangladesh, Bhutan, India, Maldives, Nepal, Pakistan, Sri Lanka, Tibet

Source: U.S. Census Bureau (n.d.).

The U.S. Census combines people who describe their heritage as "Asian." Hawaiian and Pacific Islander had been included in this group until 2000. To complicate the matter, much of the analysis of historical trends and even current literature often refers to "Asian and Pacific Islanders." Including Pacific Islanders adds about one half of the world geography but a very small part of the world population. In this chapter we refer to Asian Americans in the same way as the current Census terminology but try to make some distinction among the very different populations and cultures included in the term *Asian.*

History of Asian Americans in the United States

The experience of Asian Americans in the United States is similar to Whites and Hispanics, because, in general, Asians came to the United States voluntarily seeking to prosper or to avoid persecution in their homeland. Cultural practices within these groups vary greatly depending on country of origin, culture, and when they arrived in this country. The historical background for many of these groups is discussed in this section.

Asian Indian Americans

Asian Indians have generally immigrated to the United States voluntarily seeking economic opportunity. In 1965, the U.S. Congress altered laws that restricted Asian immigration after which the Asian Indian population grew significantly. The Immigration Reform Act of 1965 was an amendment to the 1952 McCarran-Walter Act, under which a quota system gave preference to skilled laborers and relatives of U.S. citizens.

Chinese Americans

Although agreement cannot be reached on when the first Chinese people arrived in North America due to lack of records, there is little disagreement about when their immigration exploded. When gold was discovered in California in 1849, word spread to China, and immigrants voluntarily flooded the West Coast. During the gold rush era, Chinese worked, and sometimes succeeded, in the gold fields. Many started businesses to service and support the gold miners who came from around the world to seek riches. When the gold rush diminished, Chinese immigrants began working on the transcontinental railroad. They settled in great numbers in California and established businesses and farms and worked as farm laborers and in factories.

Nevertheless, they were met with strong discrimination. Chinese Americans, as well as other minorities, tended to live in racially segregated areas and established enduring social structures that continue to the present day. Immigration restrictions targeted various Asian populations. The Chinese Exclusion Act of 1882 restricted the admission of unskilled Chinese workers. In 1907 and 1908, an informal arrangement known as the "Gentlemen's Agreement" placed similar limits on Japanese and Koreans, and in 1917 the Immigration Act of 1917 restricted the entry of Asian Indians. In response to a growing population of Filipino immigrants who worked as daily wage laborers in California agriculture, the Tydings-McDuffie Act of 1934 denied entry to Filipinos.

These discriminatory practices continued until the McCarran-Walter Act of 1952 made naturalization available to all races. After the reforms of the Immigration and Naturalization Act of 1965, immigration of Asian people increased dramatically.

During the COVID-19 pandemic, a disparaging message was promulgated by many against Chinese people because it was thought the virus originated in Wuhan, China. In March 2021, a House of Representatives Judiciary subcommittee hearing called for a shift in public rhetoric surrounding COVID-19 and foreign policy as well as passing new hate crime legislation to address rising discrimination and violence against Asian Americans. Testimony highlighted the impact of public officials blaming China for the Covid crisis and using offensive terms such as *kung flu* and *China virus* to describe the coronavirus, particularly by former President Donald Trump. The hearing had been called in part because of a dramatic increase in assaults and hate crimes against Asian Americans and particularly the Chinese Americans (Miao, 2021). The Anti-Asian hate crime in 16 of America's largest cities increased 149% in 2020 compared to 2019, with the first spike occurring in March and April amidst a rise in COVID cases and negative stereotyping of Asians relating to the pandemic. This rise for Asian related hate crimes occurred amidst an otherwise overall decline in hate crimes likely caused by a lack of interaction at frequent gathering places liked transit, commercial businesses, schools, events, and houses of worship. Yet, hate crimes overall declined by 7% in 15 of major U.S. cities, including the 11 largest ones (California State University, San Bernardino, Center for the Study of Hate & Extremism, 2021).

Japanese Americans

Many Japanese began immigrating to the United States in the 19th century. At first, they moved to Hawaii and the western United States to work on plantations, farms, and in the fishing and canning industries. During World War II, in an act later found unconstitutional by the U.S. Supreme Court, Japanese Americans were interned in concentration camps because of their race and concerns that they would collaborate with the Imperial Japanese government. Even in the face of this discrimination, many Japanese Americans enlisted to assist the country in the war effort. In fact, the U.S. Army's 442nd Regimental Combat Team was composed of Japanese Americans who fought in Europe and was the most decorated unit in U.S. military history. Since the end of World War II, Japanese Americans have grown in their influence on American culture, and currently the U.S. government is engaged in a program of reparations for the suffering endured by Japanese Americans in the camps during World War II.

Korean Americans

Korean immigration to the United States began in the early 20th century when Koreans immigrated to Hawaii to work on the plantations. Thereafter, a significant wave of immigration was related to the Korean War in the 1950s. That immigration brought many more Koreans to the U.S. mainland, and most settled in the western states (Beller et al., n.d.).

Vietnamese Americans

The Vietnamese presence in the United States occurred in waves primarily resulting from the U.S. involvement in the Vietnam War. Continuing conflicts in Southeast Asia led to the immigration of Laotians and Cambodians to the United States as well. Vietnamese people who worked with the United States during that conflict fled to the United States when the Thieu government lost power in 1975. It is believed that 130,000 Vietnamese came to the United States in 1975 alone. Most of those immigrants were young, well-educated, English-speaking city dwellers.

Other waves of immigrants were from the invasion of Laos and Cambodia by Vietnamese troops. Between 1979 and 1983, 455,000 Vietnamese, Laotian, and Cambodian refugees came to the United States. These refugees were made up of different ethnic groups and were more rural, less educated, and not as familiar with American ideas as the first wave of immigrants (LaBorde, 1996).

A third group of refugees from Southeast Asia arrived from 1985 to 1991. This group tended to include both Vietnamese and Chinese who were admitted to the country in family reunification programs (LaBorde, 1996).

Asian Americans in the United States

According to the 2019 Census Bureau population estimate, Asian Americans represent about 5.6% of the U.S. population and number about 18.2 million (HHS, OMH, 20219a). The states with the top 10 largest Asian populations are shown in **Figure 9.1**.

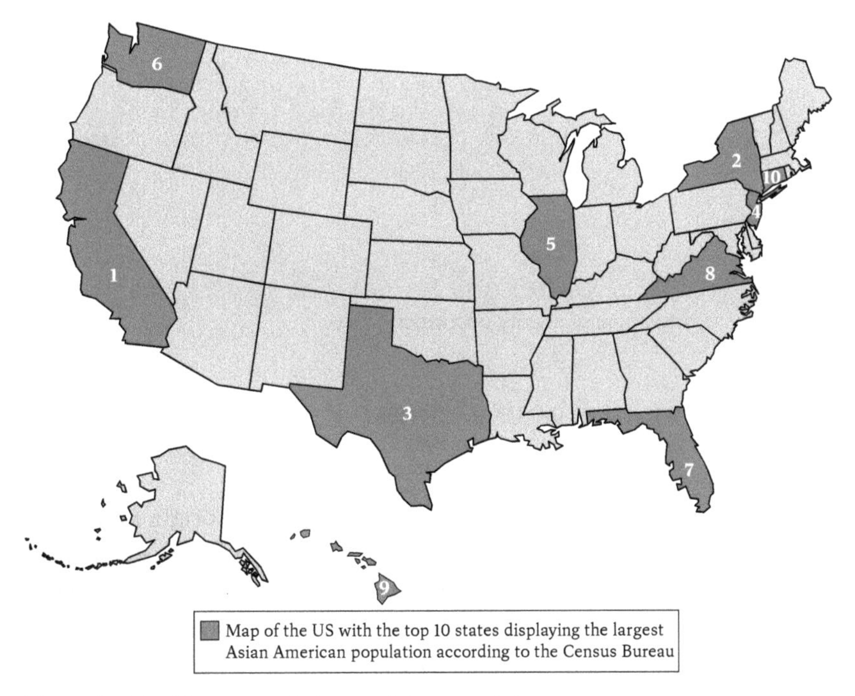

Figure 9.1 Top 10 states with largest Asian populations.

The percentage of people 5 years or older who do not speak English at home varies among Asian American groups; 48.2% of Vietnamese, 42.0% of Chinese, 19.8% of Filipinos, and 17.7% of Asian Indians are not fluent in English. In 2019, 73.5% of Asian Americans spoke a language other than English at home (HHS, OMH, 2021a). In 2019, U.S. Census data showed the median household income of Asian Americans was $93,759 compared to $ 71,664 for non-Hispanic Whites. Yet 9.6% of Asian Americans, compared to 9.0% of non-Hispanic Whites, live at the poverty level. Economic status varies widely among Asian populations in the United States, with the poverty rate for Filipinos at 5.8%, compared to 14.0% for the Hmong (HHS, OMH, 2021a). **Figure 9.2** depicts the distribution of Asians as a percentage of the population as reported in the 2010 Census (U.S. Census Bureau, 2012).

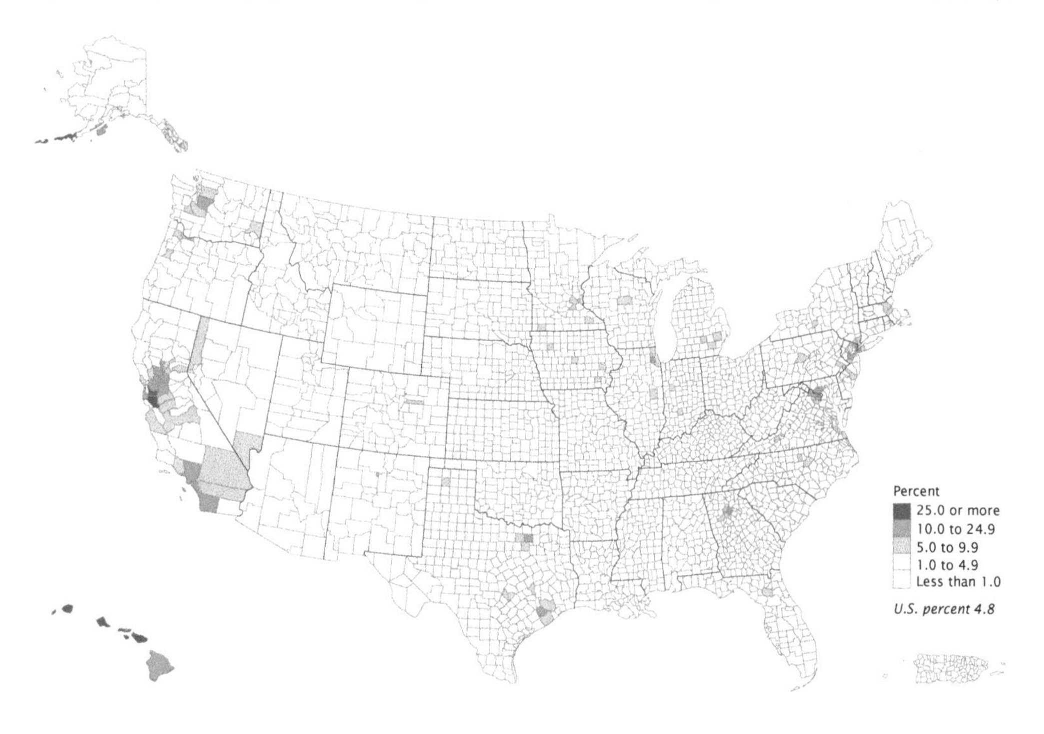

Figure 9.2 Asians as a percentage of county population, 2010.

General Philosophy About Disease Prevention and Health Maintenance

Asian beliefs regarding health and illness vary by country of origin and often among districts within the country of origin. However, a common thread through many Asian health practices is the belief that the body must remain balanced to remain healthy.

Traditional Chinese beliefs about health and illness stem from the vital energy that flows through the body. Maintaining harmony is essential to health, and restoring the harmony of the energy is necessary to overcome illness. The balance of yin and yang, hot and cold, are often employed in traditional health practices. Yin accounts for "cold" problems such as depression, hypoactivity, hypothermia, abdominal cramps, and indigestion. Health problems influenced by yang include hyperactivity, hyperthermia, stroke, and seizures. The treatment of hot and cold illnesses is accomplished through the use of the opposite force to regain balance (Beller et al., n.d.).

Vietnamese theories of illness and health vary greatly by ethnic groups. The Hmong, who originated as mountain-dwelling people, believe in the interrelatedness of medicine and

religion. They believe sickness is due to being cursed by the wrath of the gods. A traditional healer is a priest who exorcises bad spirits or intercedes with the gods to remove disease. Amulets are also employed for good health. For example, babies often wear *bua*, an amulet of cloth containing a Buddhist verse, that is worn on a string around the wrist or neck.

Urban Vietnamese people utilize a health system very similar to traditional Chinese medicine. These beliefs are based on maintaining the balance of *aAma* and *aDuonga*, similar to yin and yang theory. They believe that living things are made of the four elements: fire, air, water, and earth. The characteristics associated with the elements are hot, cold, wet, and dry. Treating an illness requires employment of the opposite characteristic to the one that is causing the sickness. Like Chinese medicine, herbal remedies, massage, thermal treatments, and acupuncture are utilized to treat illness (LaBorde, 1996).

For traditional Koreans, illness is often seen as one's fate, and hospitalization may be seen as a sign of impending death. Illness is often attributed to yin and yang, just as in Chinese medicine. Also, the *Kior* chi force, the life force similar to chi in traditional Chinese medicine, is important in maintaining health, and efforts are made to balance this force and not to engage in activities that could diminish it. Herbal remedies are utilized for illness.

Filipino health practices incorporate a number of ideas, such as *timbang*:

> This is a key indigenous health concept that includes a complex set of fundamental principles. A range of "hot" and "cold" beliefs regarding humoral balances in the body, food, and dietary balances includes the following:
>
> - Rapid shifts from "hot" to "cold" lead to illness.
> - "Warm" environment is essential to maintain optimal health.
> - Cold drinks or cooling foods should be avoided in the morning.
> - An overheated body (as in childbirth or fever) is vulnerable; and heated body or muscles can get "shocked" when cooled suddenly.
> - A layer of fat ("being stout") is preferred to maintain "warmth" and protect vital energy.
> - Heat and cooling relate to quality and balance of air in the body.
> - Sudden changes in weather patterns, cool breezes or exposure in evening hours to low temperature, presence of hot sun immediately after a lengthy rain, or vapors rising from the soil, all may upset the body balance by simply blowing on the body surface. (McBride, 2010)

Physical and mental illnesses among Filipino immigrants are considered to be caused by different factors:

1. *Mystical* causes are often associated with experiences or behaviors such as retribution from ancestors for unfulfilled obligations. Some believe in soul loss and that sleep related to the wandering of the soul out of body, known as *bangungot*, or nightmares after a heavy meal may result in death.

2. *Personalistic* causes may be attributed to social punishment or retribution by supernatural beings such as an evil spirit, witch, or *mankukulam* (sorcerer). A stronger spirit, such as a healer or priest, may counteract this force. For protection, using holy oils, wearing religious objects, or wearing an anting (amulet or talisman) may be recommended.
3. *Naturalistic* causes include a range of factors from nature events (thunder, lightning, drafts, etc.), excessive stress, incompatible food and drugs, infection, or familial susceptibility.

Asian Indians often practice ayurvedic medicine. This ancient practice is based on the theory that the five great elements—ether, air, fire, water, and earth—are the basis for all living systems. The five elements are in constant interaction and are constantly changing. Asian Indians also employ Western medicine.

Worldview

Islam and Christianity have significant influence for some Asians who view time as linear, comprised of a current life and a hereafter. Most of the world's Muslims live in Asia and believe that guidelines for a successful, even perfect life, have been laid down by religious teachings. Personal life can therefore be enhanced by individual decisions to follow the rules. Christians generally hold a similar perspective, although they may not believe that individual conduct can help avoid illness and other troubles due to the imperfection of man.

Many other Asian Americans hold a worldview framed by the great religions of Hinduism and Buddhism. The worldview of these religions is that time and history are eternally circular or cyclical, and individuals are involved in a "cycle of rebirths" or "reincarnation." The current life of a person is probably just the most recent of many previous lives and will be followed by many more in the future. Rebirths will continue until the person reaches "liberation" from the cycle of rebirths based on dealing with the universal law that governs rebirths known as **karma**. Unless liberation is achieved by conduct in this life, rebirth will occur, in some form, as required by a universal impersonal and indescribable force. This worldview can include the belief that a main goal in life is to rid oneself of all cravings and desires. These beliefs can result in a communication style that may perplex Westerners due to its emphasis on intuition, direct experience, and silence (Kete et al., 2014).

Japanese **Shintoism** takes a different perspective and is based on a belief that spiritual powers exist in the natural world. It is somewhat external and pantheistic, and individuals can ask for help by turning to divine beings or spirits (Kami) for assistance.

Perspectives on time vary among Asians. Punctuality is highly valued in the Japanese culture. Hmong born in Laos have a different sense of time because there are no clocks or calendars in Laos, so the concept of time may be new to them. Therefore, appointment times for the Hmong are challenging, and they may arrive early in the morning even though their appointment is in the afternoon. This contrasts with Filipino time, which often means arriving one or several hours after the appointment time (Purnell, 2021).

Regardless of differences in worldview of time, most Asians hold a humanistic view that places responsibility on themselves to follow guidelines or work to develop personal perfection. This makes them likely conducive to learning and following guidance from medical professionals. God and spirits may play some role, but personal accountability also plays a role in many cultural beliefs.

When communicating with Asian Americans, a gentle touch may be appropriate. Respect for those of a higher status is shown by avoiding eye contact. Respect also is shown by bowing the head slightly. Personal space is generally more distant than what is preferred by Euro-Americans. Tone of voice is generally soft. For some, such as those of Japanese descent, self-disclosure is made after trust is established and usually occurs only after it has been elicited.

Modesty and personal hygiene are important. Organ donation is generally not done due to respect given to the body. For this same reason, autopsies are not favored.

DID YOU KNOW?

Beliefs in spirituality and afterlife are strong in Asian culture. Ghost money, also known as Joss or spirit money, is one of the gifts that can be given to deceased relatives. The ghost money is burned at funerals of some Asian subcultures, particularly the Chinese, to ensure that the spirit of the deceased has ample good things in the afterlife. The Joss paper is typically made from bamboo or rice. The paper is white to represent mourning. The foil typically has a silver or golden shade that represents wealth or money. The sheets are placed carefully and respectfully in the fire.

Pregnancy, Birth, and Child Rearing

Specific practices vary considerably among the various Asian cultures. The Chinese may believe in "lying in" before birth and practicing a "sitting month" after birth when the body is allowed to come back into balance and during which time strict drinking and eating guidelines accompany a prohibition against bathing. Other cultures expect normal activity up to the day of birth, a stoic response to pain, and a rapid return to normal chores shortly after birth. Contact with a child may be limited so as not to make the baby too dependent. In Vietnamese culture, touching may be seen as inviting too much attention to the baby and must be avoided to protect the child from dangerous spirits.

Many Asians look to Buddhist and Confucian beliefs that infants are born as clean slates and only learn improper behavior while growing up. Although some children may be given minor chores and be taught reading and arithmetic earlier, children are expected to begin serious efforts at development and family participation at about 6 or 7 years old. The time is not specific, because it is understood that children mature at different paces, but children are expected to exert effort when ready. Generally, they are seen as important parts of the continuum of the family and its history and not fully independent. Harmony of the family is highly encouraged, and dishonor or disgrace to one's self or the family is to be avoided. Traditional Asian parents define the rules, and children must comply, because respect for elders is critical. Generally, parents expect that they will be judged by the achievements of their children, and they take great interest in their achievements.

Parents make a strong effort to have close involvement and direct and even demand the effort expected of the child. Rules of conduct encourage self-control, and inner stamina is expected when dealing with a crisis. Asian patients may not express strong emotion, grief, or pain due to their cultural values (Dewar, 2012).

Nutrition and Exercise

As a group, Asian Americans are not as concerned with nutrition as people from Western cultures. The texture, flavor, color, and aroma of food is much more important in Chinese cooking. The balance of yin and yang, hot and cold, is much more important than food groups.

Because many Asian Americans are lactose intolerant, dairy products are not a large part of their diet. Soy milk and tofu are the staples that provide protein and calcium. The primary food groups for Asian Americans are grains, vegetables, fruit, and meat or fish, and rice and noodles are daily staples (see **Figure 9.3**).

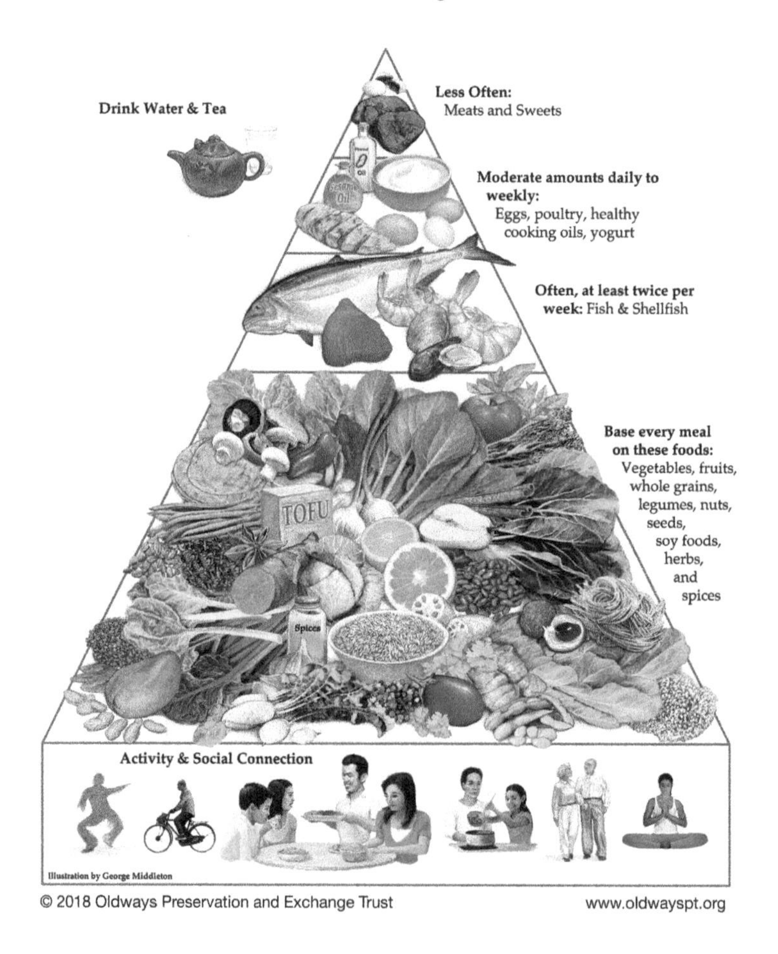

Figure 9.3 Asian food pyramid.

The Asian Indian diet and cooking involves the use of aromatic spices. Asian Indian dietary practices have religious influences from the Hindu and Muslim traditions. Many Hindus are vegetarians and believe that food was created by a Supreme Being for the benefit of man. Muslims have several dietary restrictions.

Mental Health

Asian Americans as a group have similar perspectives on mental health issues. Many traditional Asian cultural and religious beliefs view mental health problems as shameful and disgraceful. Such problems often are not discussed and, consequently, seeking help is often avoided. These views also instruct Asians' view of the world and the differences between Asian cultures and Western societies. **Table 9.2** presents a comparison of the differing approaches to society, family, and behavioral issues between Asian and Western societies.

Many Asians believe that mental illness in a family reflects negatively on family reputation and lineage and on the family member's suitability for marriage. Asians may deny the experience and expression of emotions. These factors make it more acceptable for psychological distress to be expressed through the body rather than the mind (Office of the Surgeon General, 2001).

TABLE 9.2 Comparison of Eastern and Western Values

Values	Eastern/Traditional	Western/Modern
Societal orientation	Family	Individual
Family makeup	Extended	Nuclear
Primary relationship	Parent–child	Marital
Family values	Well defined	Flexible
Relationship emphasis	Interpersonal and harmony	Self-fulfillment and development
Gender roles	Male dominant	Opportunity for females
Control	Authoritative	Democratic
Emotional expression	Suppressive	Expressive
Beliefs	Fatalism/karma	Personal control
	Harmony with nature	Control of nature
	Cooperation	Competition
	Spiritualism	Materialism

Source: Carrasco and Weiss (2005).

Death and Dying

Asian culture may affect behavior related to telling the truth to ill persons about their health state, using life-prolonging technology, and decision-making styles. Although there is a great variety of beliefs, Asians often do not like to tell a person who is ill of impending death, and many believe even speaking of it may bring bad luck or a poor outcome. Decisions and communication are often considered the responsibility of the oldest male in the family and can be seen as a moral obligation for that person to act in that capacity. Some of these beliefs can be attributed to Confucian philosophy, which emphasizes perfecting oneself during the current life, including honoring your ancestors, that death is simply another natural challenge to be dealt with in life, and that the afterlife has its own complexity that is not something to focus on or try to fully understand.

WHAT DO YOU THINK?

In the Asian culture, there is a belief that terminally ill patients should not be informed about their prognosis. As a provider, would you respect the cultural practice and not inform the patient about the prognosis? Is there a way for providers to balance the patient's right to know with respect for the cultural practices and beliefs of the family? Is not fully disclosing information to the patient an ethical breach?

Cultural-Bound Illnesses

The Chinese recognize a disorder called neurasthenia. This is a condition characterized by physical and mental exhaustion, including headaches, insomnia, and irritability. It may result from other conditions such as depression, stress, or conflict. Although Chinese Americans may experience neurasthenia, health professionals using the standard U.S. diagnostic system may not identify their need for care.

Koreans may have *hwa-byung*, with both somatic and psychological symptoms. *Hwa-byung*, or suppressed anger syndrome, is characterized by sensations of constriction in the chest, palpitations, sensations of heat, flushing, headache, anxiety, irritability, and problems with concentration (Prince, 1989).

Healing Traditions, Healers, and Healing Aids

Many Asian Americans use traditional Chinese medicine and ayurvedic medicine. Cambodians use coining, cupping, and pinching to treat many problems associated with "wind illness," which are forms of respiratory illness. Coining is rubbing or scratching the skin of the back, neck, upper chest, and arms with a coin. Cupping and pinching function in the same manner to bring blood to an area of the body. Before or during rubbing, they apply Tiger Balm, herbal liquid medicine, skin lotion, or water on the skin. The technique helps smooth the skin and is believed to improve the coining outcome.

Behavioral Risk Factors and Common Health Problems

In 2015 life expectancies at birth for Asian Americans was 79.9 years, with 82.0 years for women and 77.5 years for men, which was the same for non-Hispanic Whites with projected life expectancies at 79.8 years, with 82.0 years for women and 77.5 years for men. Asian Americans contend with numerous factors which may threaten their health. The 10 leading causes of death among Asian Americans in 2017 were as follows (Statista, 2021):

1. Cancer
2. Heart disease
3. Stroke
4. Unintentional injuries
5. Diabetes mellitus
6. Alzheimer's disease
7. Influenza and pneumonia
8. Chronic lower respiratory disease
9. Nephritis, nephrotic syndrome, and nephrosis
10. Suicide

Asian Americans also have a high prevalence of chronic obstructive pulmonary disease, hepatitis B, HIV/AIDS, smoking, tuberculosis, and liver disease. In 2017, tuberculosis was 35 times more common among Asians, with an incidence rate of 17.7 compared to 0.5 for the White population (HHS, OMH, 2021).

Some health risk factors include infrequent medical visits due to the fear of deportation and language/cultural barriers. Most Asian Americans can afford health care, but foreign-born Asian Americans have been found to have below-average access to both routine care and sick care. In 2019, insurance coverage among Asian American subgroups varied, with the following rates of coverage: 65.7% for Cambodian, 78.8% for Filipino, 73.3% for Chinese, and 62.0% for Hmong. Public insurance coverage rates also varied, with 31.8% for Vietnamese, 26.2% for Filipino, 27.0% for Chinese, 35.9% for Hmong, and 25.6% for all Asian groups (HHS, OMH, 2021a).

Most Asian American adults have never smoked; however, for those who do, the highest rate of smoking was among Korean American and Vietnamese American adults (CDC, 2019). Asian American men are four times more likely to smoke cigarettes compared to Asian American women (HHS, OMH, 2021b).

Asian American adults are less likely to report being diagnosed with hypertension and high blood pressure than African American, White, or Hispanic adults. Among Asian American populations, Filipino Americans and Japanese Americans are more likely to be diagnosed with hypertension than Chinese Americans, Korean Americans, or Asian Indian Americans. Asian Americans are also less likely to have diabetes than African American or Hispanic Americans. However, within the Asian American population, Asian Indian Americans had a significantly greater incidence of diabetes than Chinese or Japanese Americans.

Compared to White, African American, and Hispanic Americans, Asian Americans are less likely to suffer from migraines. Among the Asian American population, Vietnamese Americans and Filipino Americans have the highest incidence of migraines (Barnes et al., 2008).

Immunization rates for Asian American populations are lower than for the other groups overall. Asian Americans are less likely to have received a pneumonia vaccine. They receive the hepatitis B vaccine at the same rate as White and African American adults, but they are less likely to obtain HIV testing. However, in 2018 Asians made up 6% of the American population and accounted for only 2% of new HIV diagnoses (CDC, 2020). Although heart disease occurs less frequently among Asian Americans than any other minority group, it is still a leading cause of death among Asian Americans. Asian Americans are at risk for silent heart attacks, a painless form of the disease that can lead to a fatal outcome.

During the COVID-19 pandemic, minority populations of color, the aged, and people with underlying health conditions, such as obesity or heart conditions, were the highest risk populations. While the overall Asian American death rate from COVID-19 was similar to that of White Americans, significant disparities emerged among Asian subgroups. For example, Pacific Islanders were likely to be diagnosed with the virus two to three times more as compared with the average population in three states. In San Francisco, Asian Americans accounted for 13.7% of cases but 52% of deaths. In Nevada, Asian Americans died at more than twice the rate of White Americans (McKinsey & Company, 2020).

However, when vaccinations were authorized, recipients were prioritized by age category and high-risk activities such as medical personnel and first responders. Minority populations were not specifically prioritized for the nationwide COVID-19 vaccination campaign that was developed after the remarkable development of an effective vaccine with a year of the outbreak. Yet, when people became eligible, many refused or hesitated to receive the vaccine. Just prior to the onset of the vaccination campaign in December 2020, Asian Americans were the most open to be vaccinated. A Pew Research survey in November 2020 found 83% of Asian Americans said they would “definitely or probably get vaccinated,” leading all other racial or ethnic groups, White and Latino respondents answered about the same, with 63% and 61%, respectively, saying they definitely or probably would get the vaccine, but only 42% of African Americans said they would do so (Booker, 2020).

QUICK FACTS

Asian Americans represent the extremes of both health outcomes and socioeconomic status:

- In 2017, tuberculosis was 35 times more common among Asians, with an incidence rate of 17.7 as compared to 0.5 for the White population.
- The 2015 life expectancies at birth for Asian Americans was 79.9 years.
- In 2018, high blood pressure was an issue for 49.4% of Asian American men over 20 and 43.6% for Asian American women over 20 (CDC, 2021).
- In 2018, obesity was an issue for 14.2% of Asian American men and 16% of Asian American women over the age of 20 (CDC, 2021).
- In 2018, only 7.4% of Asian Americans under 65 years did not have health insurance (HHS, OMH, 2019a).
- From 2013–2016, Asian Americans were twice as likely to develop chronic hepatitis B when compared to Whites (HHS, OMH, 2020).
- In 2018, Asian Americans were almost eight times more likely to die from hepatitis B than non-Hispanic Whites (HHS, OMH, 2020).
- In general, in 2021, Asian American adults have lower rates of being overweight or obese and lower rates of hypertension, and they are less likely to be current cigarette smokers (HHS, OMH, 2021). In 2018, Asian Americans were about 50% less likely to die from heart disease than non-Hispanic Whites (HHS, OMH, 2021).
- In 2017, Asian American men were four times more likely to smoke cigarettes compared to Asian American women (HHS, OMH, 2021).
- In 2019, Asian American infants were 40% more likely to die from maternal complications compared to non-Hispanic White mothers (HHS, OMH, 2019c).
- In 2017, 53.8% of Asian Americans, in comparison to 35.8% of the total non-Hispanic White population, had earned at least a bachelor's degree (HHS, OMH, 2019a).

Considerations for Health Promotion and Program Planning

Health promotion for Asian Americans creates a unique challenge given the varied cultures and traditions involved. Points to consider when developing Asian American programs include the following:

- Ensure good communication by thorough explanation and language translation where necessary.
- Show respect for family relationships and their needs and include family in discussions.

- Provide dietary-appropriate meals.
- Inquire about other treatments used for health problems and obtain specific information regarding herbs and other substances being used.

Tips for Working with the Asian American Population

Asian Americans, and particularly Chinese Americans, hold strong allegiance to their families, are reluctant to express emotions, show great respect for authority, and prefer direct and immediate solutions to problems. It is important to remember that the oldest male may need to be included in communication and decision-making. Younger family members, particularly women, may feel they must confer with older family members before making a decision. In addition, the oldest male may believe it is his obligation to make important decisions for the family, particularly for single female members.

In communicating, deference to authority or politeness may result in questions being answered in the affirmative to avoid offending the person asking questions. Asian Muslim women may have a heightened sense of personal privacy and may prefer to be fully clothed during medical exams.

Summary

This chapter provided an introduction to the varied cultures and health practices that comprise Asian Americans through a discussion of their heritage, history in the United States, traditional health practices, and common health risks. The term *Asian American* is a generality for many people who trace their heritage to numerous countries, cultures, and traditions across Asia. They continue the traditions of their ancestors and experience health care issues unique to their heritage. Asians represent about 6% of the U.S. population, are less likely to be in poverty, and are more likely to be well educated, hold good jobs, be higher paid, have better health, and live longer than other ethnic groups.

Review

1. Discuss Asian Americans' history in the United States and the influence it has had on their health.
2. What cultural influences affect the health of Asian Americans?
3. Discuss the health behaviors of Asian Americans and how those behaviors affect their health.
4. Discuss some differences among the different populations that are referred to as Asian Americans.

Activities

Conduct research on health programs that have been implemented for members of the Asian American population. Summarize the literature and identify best practices.

Visit, virtually or in person, a store or website that sells Asian health products. What products did you see that were new to you? What role in health did they have (e.g., to prevent colds, to treat stomachaches)? Write a paper on your findings.

Case Study 1

An elderly Japanese American woman lived alone in her apartment. Recently it was noted that she was not keeping her apartment and garden up as she did in the past: She has locked herself out of her apartment four times this year, she has forgotten to pay the rent, and last week she left the stove on and burned a pot.

Her friends and family made an appointment for her with a geriatric consultant through her health care provider. She was evaluated by a social worker, and a Caucasian caregiver was hired to assist her with activities of daily living. Since the caregiver has been cooking, the woman has been experiencing diarrhea, cramping, and abdominal pain. She has been using over-the-counter medications for the problem and is being evaluated at the hospital for her symptoms.

Among the issues for doctors to consider is the possibility that the woman is lactose intolerant, which is prevalent among Japanese people. Because a non-Japanese caregiver now cooks her meals, she may be eating food she is not used to that possibly contains lactose, and she may not be able to discuss this with the caregiver due to communication problems.

1. What can be done to assist this Japanese American woman in a manner more appropriate to her traditions?
2. What issues should the provider consider in addition to the elder Asian woman's diet that may be contributing to her health issues?

Case Study 2

A middle-aged Chinese patient refused pain medication following cataract surgery. When asked, he replied his discomfort was bearable and that he could survive without any medication. Later the nurse found him restless and uncomfortable. Again the nurse offered pain medication. Again he refused, explaining that her responsibilities at the hospital were far more important than his comfort and he did not want to impose. Only after she firmly insisted that the patient's comfort was one of her most important responsibilities did the patient finally agree to take the medication.

1. Chinese are taught self-restraint. The needs of the group are more important than those of the individual.

2. Another factor that may be involved in Asians' refusal of pain medication is courtesy. They generally consider it impolite to accept something the first time it is offered.
3. The safest approach for the nurse is to anticipate the needs of an Asian patient for pain medication without waiting for requests. Nurses should be aware of Asian rules of etiquette when offering pain medication, food, or other services.
4. If the patient continues to refuse medication, their wish should be respected.
5. Discuss other cultural competence issues that may impact retention into care and treatment.

Source: AETC-NMC, "Case Study 9: Addressing HIV Care and Asian American Model," https://www.aetcnmc.org/documents/case-study-9.pdf.

References

Barnes, P., Adams, P., & Powell-Griner, E. (2008). Health characteristics of the Asian Adult population: United States, 2004–2006. *Vital and Health Statistics* (no. 394). National Center for Health Statistics.

Beller, T., Pinker, M., Snapka, S., & Van Dusan, D. (n.d.). *Korean-American health care beliefs and practices*. Baylor University. http://bearspace.baylor.edu/Charles_Kemp/www/korean_health.htm

Bhungalia, S., Kelly, T., VanDeKeift, S., & Young, M. (n.d.). *Indian health care beliefs and practices*. Baylor University. http://bearspace.baylor.edu/Charles_Kemp/www/korean_health.htm

Booker, B. (2020, December 4). *Survey finds Asian Americans are racial or ethnic group most willing to get vaccine*. NPR. https://www.npr.org/sections/coronavirus-live-updates/2020/12/04/943213216/survey-finds-asian-americans-are-racial-or-ethnic-group-most-willing-to-get-vacc

California State University, San Bernardino, Center for the Study of Hate & Extremism. (2021). *Fact sheet: Anti-Asian prejudice March 2020*. https://www.csusb.edu/sites/default/files/FACT%20SHEET-%20Anti-Asian%20Hate%202020%203.2.21.pdf

Carrasco, M., & Weiss, J. (2005). *Asian American and Pacific Islander outreach resource manual*. NAMI. https://www.naminys.org/images/uploads/pdfs/Asian%20American%20Outreach%20Resource%20Manual.pdf

Centers for Disease Control and Prevention. (2019). *Asian Americans, Native Hawaiians, or Pacific Islanders and tobacco use*. https://www.cdc.gov/tobacco/disparities/asian-americans/index.htm

Centers for Disease Control and Prevention. (2020). *Asians*. https://www.cdc.gov/nchhstp/healthdisparities/asians.html

Centers for Disease Control and Prevention. (2021). *Health of Asian or Pacific Islander population*. https://www.cdc.gov/nchs/fastats/asian-health.htm

Dewar, G. (2012). *What research says about Chinese kids and why they succeed*. Parenting Science. http://www.parentingscience.com/chinese-parenting.html

Howard University College of Medicine, AIDS Education and Training Center, National Multicultural Center. (n.d.). *Case study adapted from addressing HIV care and Asian American model*. https://www.aetcnmc.org/documents/case-study-9.pdf

Kete, M., Miike, Y., & Yin, J. (Eds.). (2014). *The global intercultural communication reader* (2nd ed.). Taylor & Francis.

LaBorde, P. (1996, July). *Vietnamese cultural profile.* https://ethnomed.org/culture/vietnamese/ http://www.ethnomed.org/ethnomed/cultures/vietnamese/vietnamese_cp.html

McBride, M. (2010). *Health and health care of Filipino American Older Adults.* https://geriatrics.stanford.edu/wp-content/uploads/downloads/ethnomed/filipino/downloads/filipino_american.pdf http://www.stanford.edu/group/ethnoger/filipino.html

McKinsey & Company. (2020). COVID-19 and advancing Asian American recovery. https://www.mckinsey.com/industries/public-and-social-sector/our-insights/covid-19-and-advancing-asian-american-recovery#

Miao, H. (2021, March 18). *Lawmakers call for change in covid rhetoric amid rise in violence against Asian Americans.* CNBC. https://www.cnbc.com/2021/03/18/lawmakers-call-for-change-in-covid-rhetoric-amid-violence-against-asian-americans.html

Office of the Surgeon General (US), Center for Mental Health Services (US), & National Institute of Mental Health (US). (2001). *Mental Health: Culture, Race, and Ethnicity: A Supplement to Mental Health: A Report of the Surgeon General.* Substance Abuse and Mental Health Services Administration (US).

Prince, R. (1989). Somatic complaint syndromes and depression: The problem of cultural effects on symptomatology *Mental Health Research, 8,* 104–117.

Purnell, L. (2021). *Transcultural healthcare: A culturally competent approach* (5th ed.). F. A. Davis.

Statista. (2021). *Distribution of the 10 leading causes of death among Asians and Pacific Islanders in the United States in 2017.* https://www.statista.com/statistics/233363/leading-causes-of-death-among-asians-and-pacific-islanders

U.S. Census Bureau (2012) Census, Briefs The Asian Population 2010., (2012) https://www.census.gov/content/dam/Census/library/publications/2012/dec/c2010br-11.pdf

U.S. Census Bureau. (2021). *US and world population clock.* https://www.census.gov/popclock/

U.S. Department of Health and Human Services, Office of Minority Health. (2018). *HIV/AIDS and Asian Americans.* https://www.minorityhealth.hhs.gov/omh/browse.aspx?lvl=4&lvlid=51

U.S. Department of Health and Human Services, Office of Minority Health. (2020). *Hepatitis and Asian Americans.* https://www.minorityhealth.hhs.gov/omh/browse.aspx?lvl=4&lvlid=50

U.S. Department of Health and Human Services, Office of Minority Health. (2021a). *Profile: Asian Americans.* http://minorityhealth.hhs.gov/omh/browse.aspx?lvl=3&lvlid=63

U.S. Department of Health and Human Services, Office of Minority Health. (2021b). *Heart disease and Asian Americans.* https://www.minorityhealth.hhs.gov/omh/browse.aspx?lvl=4&lvlid=49

CREDITS

Fig. 9.1: Source: Adapted from https://www.minorityhealth.hhs.gov/omh/browse.aspx?lvl=3&lvlid=63.

Fig. 9.2: Source: https://www.census.gov/prod/cen2010/briefs/c2010br-11.pdf.

CHAPTER 10

European and Mediterranean American Populations

Sometimes God calms the storm, but sometimes God lets the storm rage and calms his child.
—AMISH PROVERB

May God give you luck and health.
—ROMA (GYPSY) BLESSING

KEY CONCEPTS AND TERMS

Drabarni	*Gadje*	*Wuzho*
Ellis–van Creveld syndrome	*Marime*	*Rumspringa*
	Romany	

LEARNING OBJECTIVES

After reading this chapter, you should be able to do the following:

1. Describe the cultural impact on health for the Amish, Roma, and Arab Americans.
2. Discuss the common health risks for European populations in the United States.
3. Describe the behavioral health challenges for these groups.

Introduction

Europeans "discovered" America and made it their own but created a new lifestyle that became the dominant model for the modern United States. This population brought a mix of cultural practices and fundamental beliefs in part based on Christianity, Judaism, and Islam. The current health system in the United States reflects many of the views of this population. Because of its diversity, three subcultures are described in some detail to demonstrate the complexity of this cultural group.

Terminology

This chapter addresses the dominant culture of the United States that can generally be described as European Mediterranean. This cultural group is generally aligned with what the U.S. Census Bureau terms "White" and applies to persons having origins among any of the original peoples of Europe, the Middle East, or North Africa. This is a very broad area that encompasses numerous ethnic and cultural groups. Much has been written about the dominant European groups that inhabit the United States. These cultural groups have fundamentally shaped life throughout the United States and, as a result, have shaped the delivery of health care.

History of European and Mediterranean Americans in the United States

Europeans purposefully came to North America to gain wealth and opportunity and to avoid harassment or economic hardship. Early settlers included Spanish, French, and English in what is now the lower 48 states, and Russians in the area that would become Alaska. None came to integrate and adapt to the peoples already on the continent. Compared to the population of Europe, North America seemed empty and wild. In this setting, all came prepared to be self-sufficient and focused on establishing communities of their own kind, eventually free from the control of European countries. In part due to the limited ability to communicate, but primarily due to a culture of self-reliance and initiative, challenges and hardships were addressed locally without particular guidance from leaders in Europe. Settlement was occurring shortly after the onset of the "Age of Enlightenment" in Europe, and rational practical problem solving and the eventual development of the scientific method reinforced a belief that problems could be understood and solutions found by individuals applying their own intelligence, although the help and guidance of a Christian God was often sought and welcomed. A persistent belief in the righteousness of their acts and entitlement as free persons to exploit essentially free natural resources contributed to spread of the population throughout the continent with confidence and self-assurance despite physical and often financial hardship. Indigenous populations were displaced to make room for the new European arrivals. In the initial contact, particularly in the interior by the French fur traders, some measure of coexistence and commercial relations existed, but the westward expansion of the Europeans was ultimately opposed by the Indigenous peoples. Of course, other Europeans were also subject to displacement and conquest. The French and English and eventually the Spanish and English Americans engaged in wars to settle territorial claims. Throughout the country's development, but particularly in the late 1700s and after, significant numbers of people immigrated to North America to what is now the United States to escape economic hardship and war. The Scots were driven off their rural lands in their native home by the English, the Irish fled famine due to crop failure, and war drove many Europeans, including Jewish, German, and Armenian populations, to find better opportunities and safety. Like other immigrant populations, the Europeans settled in America generally among peoples of the same or similar cultures. They did not come to change themselves but to have better opportunities to become safer or more economically successful. Concentrations of European subcultures have resulted in regions reflecting these settlement patterns. The Germans in Pennsylvania, the Irish in New York and Boston, the Scots in the Carolinas, and the Scandinavians in the upper Midwest are just a few examples of areas that continue to reflect early settlement concentrations.

During the expansion of the European population in America, a new nation was born that reflected the values of the immigrants. A national government was created to protect against outside intrusion, especially against European rule. Government was not trusted, and states retained much of their autonomy and right to protect local public safety and health. Free enterprise and the autonomy of individuals led to the development of health care systems primarily delivered through private businesses. Government services were—and for many still are—suspect and viewed as inefficient. Self-reliance and autonomy have forged the health care system based on individual insurance coverage and the belief that individuals should take proper steps to take care of themselves and their families without interference from others and without burdening others.

In addition, the development of the scientific method and the Industrial Revolution contributed to a belief that humankind could analyze nature and identify or invent solutions to almost any problem, from curing diseases such as yellow fever to developing ways to sustain biologic organisms in outer space. Overlaying this, however, was a predominant and fundamental Christian belief in charity and taking care of the truly needy. Originally, charity hospitals served this purpose, and eventually led to universal emergency medical care by local governments. The structure of the Affordable Care Act is still fundamentally influenced by the free-enterprise, self-reliant view of European Americans with private health insurance available through health exchanges operated by states or the federal government.

Although not participating in the initial territorial conquest and political development of the United States, the peoples of the Middle East and North Africa immigrated, seeking opportunities in the new country. These peoples brought a culture based on a third major religion, Islam, which traces its beliefs to Abraham, as does Judaism and Christianity. Islam focuses on the teaching of Muhammad, who revealed the lessons of the Quran, establishing rules that must be obeyed according to disciplined daily submission to an all-powerful God. This culture has contributed to both the science and the ethics of health care in the United States.

DID YOU KNOW?

Jakob Amman, a Swiss Anabaptist leader, is the namesake of the Amish. Their religion can be traced back through a branch of the Anabaptists to 16th-century Europe during Martin Luther's Protestant Reformation. The Anabaptists would experience subdivision, resulting in groups we know today as the Amish, Mennonites, Church of the Brethren, Hutterites, and many more. The Amish have five religious orders: Old Order, New Order, Andy Weaver, Beachy, and Swartzentruber, with Old Order being the most traditional.

European and Mediterranean Americans in the United States

Data on Whites or non-Hispanic Whites generally applies to European Americans. The population estimate on July 1, 2019, for White alone, non-Hispanic or Latino, was 60.1% of the population of the United States (U.S. Census Bureau, n.d.). It is projected that the nation will become "minority White" in 2045 (Frey, 2018). During that year, Whites will comprise 49.7% of the population (Frey, 2018). European Americans comprise a rich complexity of cultures scattered throughout the country, with the highest proportions in the Midwest and Northeast, especially in Maine, New Hampshire, Vermont, Iowa, North Dakota, Kentucky, West Virginia, Montana, Idaho, and Wyoming (Roney, 2016). These cultural groups dominate the political process at all levels of government and control the government regulation of health care in the United States, but that is changing with growing diversity in leadership positions.

Overall, non-Hispanic Whites fared better during the COVID-19 pandemic than other races and ethnicities, even when income levels were similar among the groups (Henry, 2020). Among younger people in the lowest poverty quartile, non-Hispanic Black and Hispanic/Latinx people had mortality rates nearly three times that of non-Hispanic Whites. For the older population, the mortality rate among non-Hispanic Whites in the highest poverty quartile was less than that of lowest poverty non-Hispanic Black and Hispanic populations (Feldman & Bassett, 2020).

According to the CDC (2021), health equity considerations that may help explain different experiences with COVID-19 between non-Hispanic Whites and other groups include discrimination, health care access and use, occupation, education, and housing:

> These factors and others are associated with more COVID-19 cases, hospitalizations, and deaths in areas where racial and ethnic minority groups live, learn, work, play, and worship. They have also contributed to higher rates of some medical conditions that increase one's risk of severe illness from COVID-19. In addition, community strategies to slow the spread of COVID-19 might cause unintentional harm, such as lost wages, reduced access to services, and increased stress, for some racial and ethnic minority groups.

General Philosophy About Disease Prevention and Health Maintenance

Middle-class European American cultures (the cultures of origin and training for most U.S. health researchers and providers) tend to associate health and well-being with independence, individuality, uniqueness, and control (Kitayama et al., 2010). The European and Mediterranean populations generally view disease prevention and health maintenance based on the germ theory view that scientific methods and physical or chemical treatments can be used to prevent and cure illness. Health can be developed and maintained by making advances in understanding biology and science. Science can and must discover cures, and it is just a matter of time before proper preventive practices and medical interventions will be developed to address most health issues.

Worldview

Generally, the European worldview holds that time is linear. Although individuals are autonomous, they are responsible to account for their behavior to a higher being. Self-reliance and free will are important aspects of life, and a great deal of flexibility is allowed within the rules laid down by religious teachings. Informality of expression and dress reflect achievement, and tangible assets are valued over social status alone.

In general, European Americans are a low-touch culture. This has been reinforced by the guidelines and policies related to sexual harassment. Touching should be avoided until people get to know each other as it generally carries a sexual overtone. People of the same sex, especially men, generally do not touch one another unless they are close friends.

Personal space is important, and European Americans generally do not stand or sit close to one another. If health care providers physically distance themselves from a patient who is culturally programmed for close personal space, the provider may be viewed as cold.

Disclosure of personal information is common. European Americans may share very personal information, such as sex or drug use, with people they do not know very well.

Punctuality is important. European Americans do not like to wait as it wastes time. "Time is money" is the common philosophy. People in this culture generally believe that they have control over their future, and hence, do not adhere to the fatalistic belief. People in these cultures are generally future oriented, but they do not like to wait, so it has become a fast and "on-demand" culture.

Pregnancy, Birth, and Child Rearing

Generally, self-reliance and autonomy lead to a view that children are raised to be adults and "leave home." Although family relationships continue, association between generations is looser than that of extended families in other cultures. Similarly, parents have independent authority over their own children, and grandparents are not necessarily as influential as in extended families.

Children are generally free to grow up and marry who they wish and earn a livelihood of their own choosing. They are expected to become independent. Even with implementation of the Affordable Care Act, children are expected to be fully independent from family health responsibilities up to age 26 when children can no longer be on covered on their parent's health plan.

Culture affects the administration of public health programs. For instance, rules requiring immunizations that have been scientifically proven for effective against common illnesses such as measles must confront challenges from parents based on parental rights to self-determination in raising their own children. Thus "opt out" procedures have been established in several states.

WHAT DO YOU THINK?

It is often difficult to see cultural influences when viewed from within a culture. The three great religions of the European population include Judaism, Christianity, and Islam; each recognizes Abraham as a key figure in history. One common cultural practice, circumcision, derives from Abraham's teaching. Research on the health benefits of circumcision is mixed, but it is such a common practice that it is generally accepted as normal. When the practice is examined from a neutral point of view and is termed "involuntary genital surgery on children," perhaps this culture-bound custom can be viewed for what is—the most common elective surgery in the United States. A majority of infant boys in the United States are circumcised for either religious or hygienic reasons (Owings et al., 2013). In 2012, the American Association of Pediatrics (APP, 2012) said that despite potential medical benefits of newborn male circumcision, the decision for this elective surgery should be left to parents based on their religious, ethical, and cultural beliefs. The Jewish culture holds the procedure of circumcision to be of high importance to bind a covenant with God, and a formal ceremony on the 8th day of a boy's life honoring the event is called *Brit milah*.

Alternatively, many Egyptians and others believe in practicing Pharaonic circumcision, known in the United States as female genital mutilation, on girls during childhood, believing that the girls will be more acceptable for marriage. However, there is a vast difference between that procedure and simply cutting a little skin in the case of boy's circumcision. In this procedure, the girl's exterior genitals are cut in a way that damages the sex organs, inhibits pleasure, and causes severe pain and complications for women's sexual and reproductive health. This procedure is usually performed at the request of mothers outside clinical settings or on "medical vacations" to their home country. In the United States, efforts to stop families from sending their daughters to their home countries to be cut led to a 2013 law making it illegal to knowingly transport a girl out of the United States for the purpose of cutting (Mather & Feldman-Jacobs, 2016).

The CDC (2020) published indirect estimates of the number of U.S.-resident women potentially affected by or at risk for FGM/C, indicating that as many as 513,000 girls and women could have experienced female genital mutilation or be at risk of experiencing it in the future. Should this "involuntary genital surgery on children" practice be seen as any different from "harmless" male circumcision? The procedure has been a specific crime in the United States since 1996, and there is a growing international movement to stop female genital mutilation. What do you think? Is involuntary genital surgery okay for boys but not for girls?

Nutrition and Exercise

The worldview of the majority culture in the United States contributes both to improve health and to harm it. The self-sufficient and autonomous individuals are free and are expected to take care of their own health. The values supporting individual achievement lead many to be highly active in pursuing health through nutrition regimens, physical fitness routines, and commercial programs. For those without discipline, the "problem solving through science" approach has resulted in commercial health care providing cosmetic surgery to enhance beauty, sex appeal, and weight loss through such cosmetic procedures such as lip enhancement, breast implantation, liposuction, and intestinal bands to reduce weight and improve appearance. On the other hand, cultural emphasis on autonomy allows for self-neglect and abuse such as smoking and drinking to excess. This cultural perspective is always present in public health and medical care provider efforts to encourage good health practices.

Mental Health

Mental health, as in other cultures, carries stigma and misunderstanding. However, the focus on individual rights and self-determination is evident in the care and treatment of mental illness. For instance, only if the state can show that people are likely to be harmful to themselves or others are they compelled to receive treatment. Even if clearly marginally functional in daily living, the culture supporting autonomy and free will allows people to avoid treatment or live without medical care. In addition, the Christian cultural value of charity and assisting others often leads to establishment of charitable programs, such as homeless shelters and meal programs for the poor, which include many mentally ill persons.

Death and Dying

The great variety of subcultures within the European population results in a variety of beliefs and rituals associated with death. Overall, the philosophy of being autonomous transfers to death as well. This is demonstrated by the use of advance directives, hospice programs, and other end-of-life care procedures. Mentally competent patients have the right to refuse medical care and make decisions on life-extending treatments such as artificial life support. The Death With Dignity Act is another example of this end-of-life autonomous decision-making.

A great many Christians associate death with old age and something that will be handled later; it is not necessary to think about this today. Muslims, on the other hand, are taught to believe death may occur any day, and this idea is reflected in the importance of five daily prayers. Many deaths that occur in hospitals are possibly due to the "anything can be solved" self-reliant autonomous scientific perspective.

Upon death most will be cremated or buried. Some, such as the Irish, celebrate life with wakes, and others, such as Jewish and Muslims, express various degrees of seriousness and sadness. After death some Christian-based believers may establish elaborate burial events and monuments, whereas Muslims conduct prompt simple and modest burials.

The 1st year after death is often seen as a year of mourning and remembrance. Muslims especially honor the dead for 40 days after death. Muslim women are not allowed to visit cemeteries. Significant variations in burial and death rituals exist within the European American cultural groups.

History, Healing Practices, and Risk Factors for Three Subcultures

The European and Mediterranean American cultural groups are remarkably diverse, and it is probably misleading to suggest that even admitted generalizations are accurate for all. You may already have a general sense of differences between the Italian and English cultures or between Spanish and Scandinavian peoples. Here we describe just three subcultures in this population to provide a sense of the diversity in this group. Included is a brief summary of two small populations, the Amish and the Roma, and a general profile of a large subgroup, the Arabs. Within each group description, culture-bound syndromes and tips for working with the culture are summarized.

Amish Americans

Religious persecution forced the Amish and Mennonites to find safe haven in the New World. In the 1730s, a group of Amish immigrants joined Mennonite colonists who had already established a community in Lancaster, Pennsylvania. Lancaster houses the oldest Amish community in North America.

The Amish social environment, including the family structure, child-rearing practices, religion, communication, and pregnancy beliefs, greatly influences the health of this population. The Amish live a simple lifestyle that abstains from material luxuries; it resembles the lifestyle of 16th-century European peasants. For example, they still utilize horses and buggies for transportation, and their lifestyle is agriculturally based. Their unique heritage is ingrained in a belief system that seeks to retain traditional values while avoiding the influences of the dominant culture. The two most valued aspects of their lives include their family and their church district.

The Amish generally have large families, because they do not routinely practice birth control and because babies are a welcomed gift from God. Children are believed to be economic blessings; they help maintain the farm and the household. It is not unusual for generations of family members to live in the same house and operate as one unit. Single people and single-parent homes are rare.

The gender roles within the family are traditional; the males are the dominant figures within the household, directing the farming operations and overseeing their children's work in the fields. Many husbands assist in childcare, lawn care, and gardening, but they usually do not assist in other household work. Wives are responsible for washing, cooking, canning, sewing, mending, and cleaning. Church leaders teach that wives must submit to the authority of their husbands according to religious doctrine. Women are not usually employed outside of the home. Their main duties revolve around raising the children, gardening, and assisting with barn chores. The Amish religion is deeply integrated with their family structure. The Amish believe that the Bible is a guide for parents to teach their children the values of their religion while training them to conform to the Amish ways. Cultural beliefs are passed down through the generations in such a way that young Amish children are not exposed to the great variety of cultural practices that modern youth outside of the Amish community accept as normal.

Amish culture is focused on community, and health care expenses are usually covered by the community. The Amish generally do not have commercial health insurance. Purchasing insurance shows a lack of faith in God (Ohio's Amish Country, 2021). The Amish believe that medicine helps, but God alone heals. The motivation for being healthy is to be able to work and provide for family (Ohio's Amish Country, 2021).

A unique part of the Amish culture is **Rumspringa**, which means "running around." This practice was the focus of the documentary *Devil's Playground*. Rumspringa is a time when adolescents are free to explore the world outside the Amish culture. Rumspringa is practiced by young males and females between the ages of 16 and 21 years. During this period, individuals may partake in activities of their choosing, which may include drinking alcohol, using illicit drugs, and experimenting with sexual activities. Rumspringa ends when the young person makes the decision to either live in the outside world or become baptized within the Amish community (Cantor & Walker, 2002).

Beliefs About Causes of Health and Illness Among Amish Americans

The Amish believe that sin is the cause of illness. Their body is viewed as the temple of God, and they believe they should be good stewards of their bodies, which are given as a gift to do God's work. Good health is also a gift from God (Ohio's Amish Country, 2021).

Health care practitioners should be sensitive to the unique perspective of their Amish patients. For example, considering that the Amish have little contact with medical professionals and technology, health care practitioners should convey descriptions of treatment procedures carefully, avoiding complex medical language. Moreover, health care professionals should expect to talk to spouses and family members who are likely to gather in support of the patient. Finally, as much treatment as possible should take place in one visit due to transportation difficulties, as the traditional horse and buggy transportation is inconvenient for appointments and visitations.

Healing Traditions Among Amish Americans

The Amish prefer to self-medicate or remedy an ailment by recommendation from family and friends before seeing health professionals. Some approaches are considered folk medicine and include faith healing, herbal treatments, and other nontraditional medical remedies. The use of folk remedies for minor ailments is based on the need of the Amish to remain self-sufficient (Ohio's Amish Country, 2021). Natural products and remedies include honey, comfrey, aloe vera, tee tree oil, vitamin E oil, cloves, and vinegar (Altepeter,

2017). Additionally, the Amish have been known to utilize reflexology and chiropractic procedures (Altepeter, 2017).

Amish women try to limit their use of technology, even during pregnancy and while giving birth. For example, amniocentesis and other invasive prenatal diagnostic tests are not acceptable. Amish women prefer to use nurse midwives and lay midwives, and to have home deliveries, because it limits the use of technology as well as reduces the number of visits to the doctor, which may be costly.

Women practice certain folk traditions during pregnancy to prepare themselves for giving birth. These practices include not walking under a clothesline because that is believed to cause a stillbirth. Another practice includes not climbing through a window or under a table because both can cause the umbilical cord to wrap around the baby's neck (Lemon, 2006). Women use a medley of herbs, called 5-W, 5 weeks before their pregnancy ends. These herbs include a mixture of red raspberry leaves, black cohosh root, butcher's broom root, dong quai root, and squaw vine root. The formula is believed to ease the labor by quieting the nerves, easing pain, and relaxing the uterus. In addition, it has been known to help with menstrual disorders, morning sickness and hot flashes (NursingAnswers.net, 2018).

Behavioral Risk Factors and Common Health Problems Among Amish Americans

The Amish have few behavioral risk factors due to various health-promoting behaviors, which, among the adult population, include low rates of tobacco use and alcohol consumption, and high levels of physical activity. However, the Amish are cautious and conservative and may refuse health care services. With the emphasis on communal care rather than individual care, the decision is often made to forgo a procedure that is deemed too costly as it is a burden the community due to the expense (Ohio's Amish Country, 2021). Amish children and adolescents live in nontechnological farming communities, which results in a population that is physically active and that has a low rate of obesity and Type 2 diabetes (Kluger, 2018). Amish adults also show very high levels of physical activity, which includes consistently walking at moderate to vigorous levels and farming daily. This type of lifestyle, one that promotes physical activity, results in the low prevalence of obesity and positive health outcomes in general for the Amish community (Kluger, 2018).

The Amish do not completely prohibit the use of modern medical technology, but they tend to be extremely cautious and may refuse intervention if it is not approved by community leaders. For example, Amish families vary in receptivity to the practice of immunizations for communicable diseases, leading to increased vulnerability to those illnesses. Moreover, the lack of immunizations puts the Amish at risk when they travel outside of their communities because they may not be protected against diseases to which they become exposed.

Certain Amish communities live by laws and precepts that have been passed down for generations. Such customs include marrying within their own community and allowing first cousins to marry. Consequently, a growing number of distinctive recessive genetic disorders have arisen among the Amish. Individuals who have a recessive genetic disorder, such as Ellis–van Creveld syndrome (EVC), receive a defective recessive gene from each parent. EVC, a form of dwarfism, is an autosomal recessive disorder in which individuals exhibit an extra digit located next to the fifth digit. In addition, EVC is characterized by individuals having short forearms and legs as well as congenital heart failure.

Cartilage-hair hypoplasia, another form of dwarfism, is a genetic disorder that is rarely seen outside of Amish communities. This rare disorder was not recognized until the mid-1960s when Amish children began to present with features similar to, but more pronounced than, EVC. These signs include fine and underdeveloped hair (hypoplasia of the hair) and underdeveloped cartilage (hypoplasia of the cartilage), resulting in skeletal abnormalities and an inability to fully extend the upper limbs.

The Amish tend to prefer natural home remedies; however, they may seek health care services from medical doctors and complementary health providers, such as reflexologists and chiropractors. Due to a relatively stress-free and active lifestyle, positive health outcomes among the population include low rates of obesity, smoking, and cancer. As a result of the lack of vaccinations among the Amish, they are more susceptible to communicable diseases.

Considerations for Health Promotion and Program Planning for Amish Americans

When working with members of the Amish community, the following recommendations should be considered to improve cultural understanding:

- Be cognizant of the cultural differences this group has with society as a whole.
- Recognize the importance of privacy.
- Recognize that Amish people might not understand lifestyle activities and events you consider everyday occurrences.
- Be cognizant of the formality of family relationships.
- Explain all procedures and instructions to ensure understanding.
- Be aware that many Amish do not have health insurance.
- Transportation can be challenging, as many travel via horse and buggy.
- Telephones are not permitted in the home, which may delay communication (Purnell, 2013).

Roma Americans

Romas, commonly known as Gypsies, a term considered pejorative by these people, are properly termed Roma or the Romani. They are an isolated group who maintains a strong social and cultural bond separate and apart from everyday American society. There are approximately 1 million Romani people who live in the United States (FXB Center for Health and Human Rights, Harvard University, 2020).

The Roma are originally from northern India. They migrated throughout Middle and Eastern Europe beginning around 1000 CE. They immigrated to the United States in two stages: in the 18th century as a result of being deported from various European countries and at the end of the 19th century primarily from Eastern Europe.

The Roma primarily speak **Romany**, a wholly spoken language derived from Sanskrit, and English as a second language. Most older Roma are not literate, but some younger members have some education. Written forms of the Romany language have been developing with the education of the younger generations.

Roma Americans have a very complicated social structure based on four loyalties: to their nation, clan, family, and vista. They are first divided into nations; the most common nations are the Machwaya, Kalderasham, Churara, and Lowara. The nations are further divided into clans. A clan is a group of families united by ancestry, profession, and historic ties. Each clan has a leader, but there is no such thing as "Gypsy kings," as characterized in popular lore. Some clans are further divided into tribes, but most are composed of families. It is the family that is the most important social group for the Roma. A *vista* is extended family (Ryczak et al., n.d.).

Roma Americans purposely isolate themselves from the larger community and tend to be ethnocentric. They maintain separation from people and things that are **gadje**, non-Roma, who are considered unclean. The strict code that they live by limits acculturation.

Beliefs About Causes of Health and Illness Among Roma Americans

Roma Americans' beliefs regarding health and illness stem from two concepts: impurity and fortune. The first concept is related to the ideas of ***wuzho*** (pure) and ***marime*** (impure). Roma Americans have very strict traditions about what is polluted and how items and the body are to be kept clean. Secretions from the upper half of the body are not polluted, but secretions from the lower half of the body are polluted. Therefore, separate soap and towels are used for the upper and lower halves of the body. Failing to keep the two secretions separate can result in serious illness. Also, because *gadje* (non-Romas) do not practice body separation, they are considered impure and diseased.

Fortune also plays a role in health. Good fortune and good health are thought to be related. Illness can be caused by actions that are considered contaminating and, therefore, create bad fortune.

Roma Americans distinguish between illnesses that are of a *gadje* cause and those that are part of their beliefs. *Gadje* illnesses can be cured by *gadje* doctors. Roma Americans avoid hospitals because they are unclean and are separate from Roma society. Illness is a problem to be dealt with by the entire clan. Therefore, if a clan member is hospitalized, family and clan members are expected to stay with them and provide curing rituals and protect them. An exception to the aversion to hospitals is childbirth. Women are considered unclean during pregnancy and for a number of weeks after delivery. Childbirth should not happen in the family home because it can cause impurity in the home. Therefore, delivery in hospitals is accepted in the culture.

Finally, older members of a family are very important in health care decision-making. They are considered the authorities in the family and carry great weight in all decisions.

Healing Traditions Among Roma Americans

As previously discussed, illnesses can be characterized as those of the Roma or those that are *gadje*. Roma health treatment is the prerogative of the older women of the clan who are known as ***drabarni***, women who have knowledge of medicines. Roma diseases are not connected to *gadje* diseases; they can only be cured by Roma treatments. Some diseases are caused by spirits or the devil. One spirit, called Mamioro, spreads disease in dirty houses, so keeping a clean home is imperative. The devil has been known to cause nervous diseases. Herbs and rituals are utilized to address these problems.

Behavioral Risk Factors and Common Health Problems Among Roma Americans

In Romani culture, the larger people are, the luckier the luckier they are considered to be. A fat person is considered healthy and fortunate, and a thin person is considered ill and to have poor luck. This belief and other cultural beliefs are sources of health concerns for this group.

As a group, Roma Americans are resistant to immunization, because it does not comport with their beliefs regarding purification. Thus, they are at risk for many communicable diseases.

The Roma American diet is high in fat and salt. A great percentage of Roma Americans smoke and are obese. These practices place them at risk for cardiovascular disease, hypertension, and diabetes. The closeness of living conditions leads to an increased risk of infectious diseases such as hepatitis. Romani children are more likely to be born prematurely or with low birth weight, and the increased incidence of consanguineous marriages has led to an increased risk of birth defects (Ryczak et al., n.d.).

Considerations for Health Promotion and Program Planning for Roma Americans

In working with Roma Americans, the following issues should be considered:

- Understand that illness is an issue for the entire society, and the entire clan will be involved in visiting the sick person in the hospital.
- Recognize the primacy of the elders in the family and the clan in making decisions.
- Always remember the importance of what is considered clean and unclean and provide separate soap, washcloths, and towels for the upper and lower body parts.
- Understand that this population is mistrustful of non-Roma people and things.
- Understand that Roma Americans are ethnocentric and believe that they must be provided with the best doctors and treatment even if such treatment is not indicated.

Arab and Middle Eastern Americans

Being Arab is not based on race. Arabs are usually associated with the geographic area extending from the Atlantic coast of northern Africa to the Arabian Gulf. The people who descend from this area are classified as Arabs based largely on a common language (Arabic) and a shared sense of geographic, historic, and cultural identity. Arabs include peoples with widely varied physical features, countries of origin, and religions.

Persons of Arab and Middle Eastern descent are a growing demographic in American society and, not unlike the Amish and Romani, are not well understood by the larger society. This cultural group has also experienced increased discrimination and suspicion since the September 11, 2001, terrorist attacks.

Arabs immigrated to the United States in three waves. The first migration occurred between the late 1800s and World War I; this group was from the area of Palestine and moved for economic reasons. Many of these immigrants were Christians, and their descendants have become firmly acculturated. The second wave began after 1948 with establishment of the state of Israel. This group included many professionals and Muslims. This wave tended to settle in the Midwest and accounts for the large concentration of Arab descendants in the Detroit and Chicago areas. The third wave began with the 1967 Arab–Israeli War and continues today. This group fled political instability.

Because the vast majority of Arabs are Muslim, the tenets of the Islamic religion are very influential in Arab Americans' lives. Arab American culture is centered around family relationships. The basic relationship is the nuclear family, but each Arab American belongs to a large, extended family and often to an even more extended clan that is related by blood kinship (Purnell, 2013).

The Arab American family is the center of Arab American culture. It is a paternalistic structure, but women are respected, especially mothers. Marriage is highly valued and is considered the basic structure of society. Divorce is discouraged. Having children is very important in the Arab American culture, and a marriage with many children is considered highly blessed. Therefore, the use of reversible birth control is undesirable and irreversible birth control is forbidden (Purnell, 2013). Sickness, birth, and death are events that involve participation by the community.

Cleanliness is a basic tenet of Islam. The Quran, the Islamic holy book, proscribes eating certain foods, including pork or pork products, meat of dead animals, blood, and all intoxicants. Fasting from dawn to dusk every day during the month of Ramadan is required by the religious tenets.

Beliefs About Causes of Health and Illness Among Arab and Middle Eastern Americans

Middle Eastern health beliefs arise from the long-standing traditions of the great Islamic healers of the 7th and 8th centuries. Western theories from Hippocrates and Galen came to Arab medicine through trading routes and were incorporated into the Arabs' knowledge base. They advanced human knowledge of anatomy, physiology, and medical treatments. Thus, the tenets of allopathic medicine form the basis of most Arab beliefs about health and illness. Muslims consider an illness atonement for their sins, and they receive illness and death with patience and prayers. Death is part of their journey to meet Allah (God) (Athar, n.d.).

Healing Traditions Among Arab and Middle Eastern Americans

Almost all Middle Eastern people believe in maintaining good health through hygiene and a healthy diet. Women and men are modest and may refuse treatment by practitioners of the opposite gender. This modesty of women contributes to low rates of screening such as with Pap smears and mammograms (Purnell, 2013).

Iraqis have a significant history of traditional healing practices. Some common practices include the following (Iraqi Refugees, 2002):

- Cumin, in conjunction with various other ingredients, is used to treat fever, abdominal pain, and tooth pain.
- Respiratory complaints are treated with honey and lemon.
- Infertility can be treated by a placenta being placed over the doorway of the infertile couple's home.
- Henna is believed to have magic healing properties and will be painted on the body to protect against the evil eye and spirits.
- Pregnant women should satisfy their cravings; otherwise, they will develop a birthmark in the shape of the food that they crave (Purnell, 2013).
- Middle Eastern diets have the following characteristics (Nolan, 1995):
    - *Dairy products.* The most common dairy products are yogurt and cheese; feta cheese is preferred. Milk is usually used only in desserts and puddings.
    - *Protein.* Pork is eaten only by Christians and is forbidden by religion for Muslims and Jews. Lamb is the most frequently used meat. Many Middle Easterners will not combine dairy products or shellfish with the meal. Legumes, such as black beans, chickpeas (garbanzo beans), lentils, navy beans, and red beans, are commonly used in all dishes.
    - *Breads and cereals.* Some form of wheat or rice accompanies each meal.
    - *Fruits.* Fruits tend to be eaten as dessert or as snacks. Fresh, raw fruit is preferred. Lemons are used for flavoring. Green and black olives are present in many dishes, and olive oil is most frequently used in food preparation.
    - *Vegetables.* Vegetables are preferred raw.

The Mediterranean diet pyramid is shown in **Figure 10.1**.

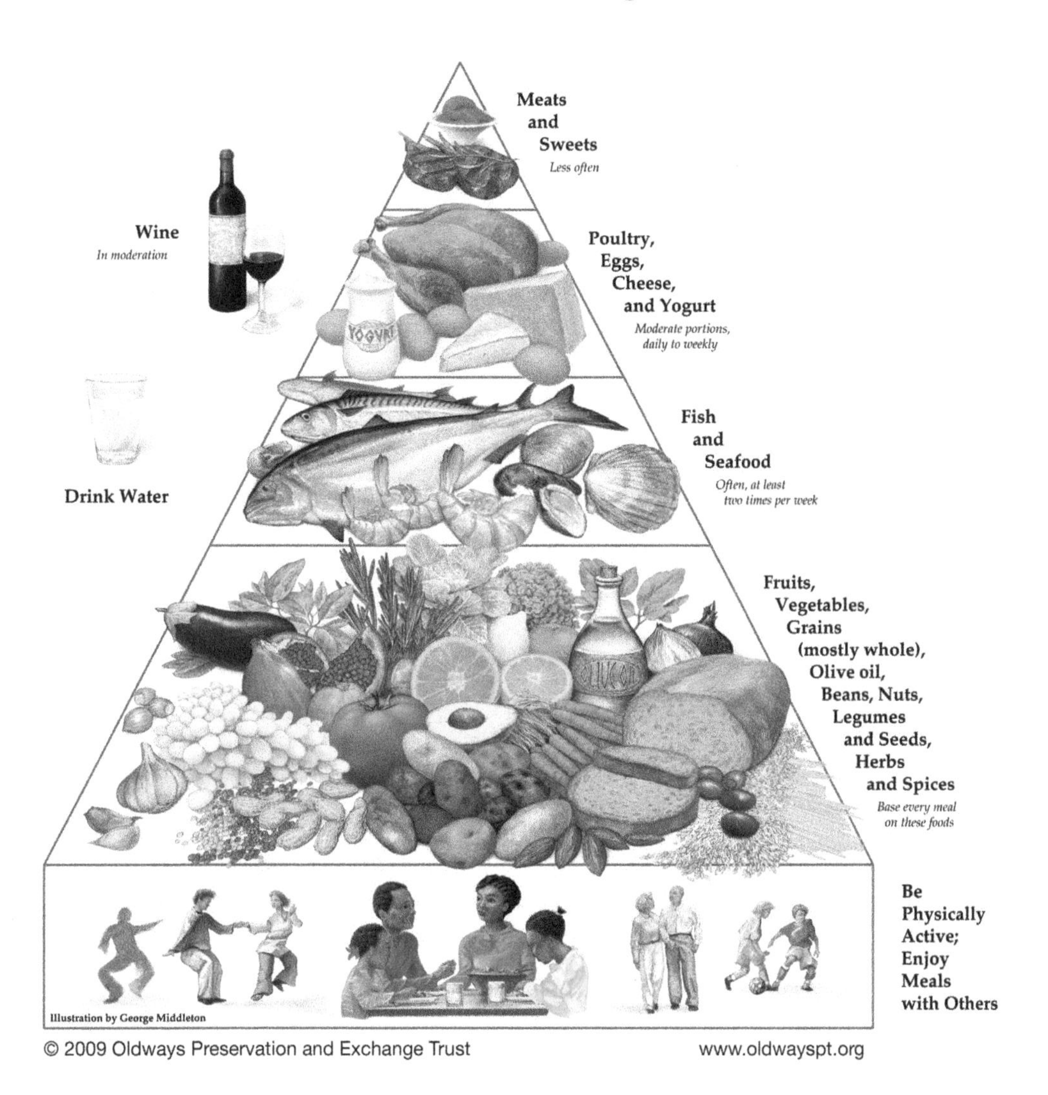

Figure 10.1 Mediterranean diet pyramid.

Behavioral Risk Factors and Common Health Problems Among Arab and Middle Eastern Americans

As a group, Arab and Middle Eastern Americans face the same health concerns as the majority of European Americans. Recent immigrants may be at greater risk for certain inborn genetic disorders as a result of interfamily marriages. Otherwise, their health risks mirror the majority of the population, with heart disease and cancer among the major morbidity factors. Smoking is highly ingrained in the Arab culture, and they have high smoking rates (Purnell, 2013). Due to modesty, screening rates are low. In a study conducted in California,

> Arab Americans had lower binge drinking (17.7 vs. 33.9%, $p < 0.001$) and alcohol consumption (40.1 vs. 51.2%, $p < 0.001$) prevalence in the past year than non-Hispanic Whites. Fewer Arab Americans received a flu vaccine (25.5 vs. 34.5%) and visited an emergency room (14.5 vs. 17.2%) in the past year than non-Hispanic Whites. Arab Americans had a higher prevalence of having two or more sexual partners in the past year (11.4 vs. 8.4%, $p = 0.022$) but lower prevalence of ever having contemplated suicide (3.7 vs. 6.3%, $p = 0.001$) than non-Hispanic Whites. (Abuelezam et al., 2019)

Considerations for Health Promotion and Program Planning for Arab and Middle Eastern Americans

Consider the following points when dealing with Arab and Middle Eastern Americans in health care:

- Arab and Middle Eastern Americans prefer treatment by a medical provider of the same gender, especially for women.
- Arab and Middle Eastern Americans consider nurses helpers, not health care professionals, and their suggestions and advice are not taken seriously.
- Arab and Middle Eastern Americans prefer treatment that involves prescribing pills or giving injections rather than simple medical counseling.
- Orthodox Muslims follow a halal (Muslim diet), which prohibits some types of meat, like pork, and medications and foods that contain alcohol. Meat needs to be prepared according to Islamic requirements. Also, provide for religious requirements for prayer as often as five times a day, starting before sunrise and ending at night, and provide fasting during the holy month of Ramadan between sunrise and sunset. Although those who are ill are exempted from this practice, devout Muslims may desire to fast anyway.
- Allow for receipt of food into the right hand for Muslim patients. The left hand is considered unclean because it is used for cleaning during toileting.
- Respect modesty and privacy.
- Allow for visits and input by the imam, a prayer leader.

Behavioral Risk Factors and Prevalent Health Problems

The top two leading causes of death in 2017 for Whites were cardiovascular diseases and cancer, which account for a combined 44.7% of all deaths among this population. The 10 leading causes of death are as follows:

1. Heart disease
2. Cancer

3. Chronic lower respiratory disease
4. Unintentional injuries
5. Stroke
6. Alzheimer's disease
7. Diabetes
8. Influenza and pneumonia
9. Suicide
10. Nephritis, nephrotic syndrome, and nephrosis (kidney diseases) (Elflein, 2021)

When compared to other race and ethnic groups, the White population has much higher death rates from suicide and drug and alcohol overdoses (Elflein, 2021).

Adult non-Hispanic Whites who smoke are 16.6% of the White population compared with the lowest rate being among Asians at 7% in 2015 (American Lung Association, 2020).

- Whites lead all other major populations with incidence of cancer (460.9/100,000; age-adjusted rate) compared to Blacks at 445.2/100,000 and Hispanics at 355.3/100,000 (National Cancer Institute, n.d.).
- The percent of men aged 20 and over with obesity is 41.7% and for women 39.7% (CDC, 2022).
- About half of the White population over 20 years of age has hypertension (52.7% of men and 45.4% of women) (CDC, 2021b).
- Non-Hispanic White teens have a pregnancy rate about half (13.2 per 1,000) that of non-Hispanic Black teens (27.5 per 1,000) and Hispanic teens (28.9 per 1,000) (CDC, 2019).
- The traditional Mediterranean diet incorporates the basics of healthy eating, plus some flavorful olive oil, and even a glass of red wine, and is characteristic of the traditional cooking style of countries bordering the Mediterranean Sea. This diet is associated with a reduced risk of death from heart disease and cancer, as well as a reduced incidence of Parkinson's and Alzheimer's diseases. The dietary guidelines for Americans recommends the Mediterranean diet (Mayo Clinic Staff, n.d.).

Tips for Working with European and Mediterranean American Populations

The European and Mediterranean American culture is diverse, so this section includes general tips for caring for peoples of all cultures. Every person is unique, so place yourself in your patients' shoes and consider their unique beliefs, needs, and concerns as you interact with them. Treat your patients as they would like to be treated.

Ask your patients if this is their first visit. If so, take a few moments to orient them. Patients who are new to the system may not know the roles of their health care team, how to report for an appointment, or other health care matters that patients who are already in the system may know.

If English is the patient's second language, or the patient is deaf or hard of hearing or has vision impairment, make sure to involve an interpreter in all your care discussions. Do not rely on family members to translate health information. Your patients may include many family members in their care decisions. Some may be related, and others may be friends your patients consider family and part of their support network.

Use the terms *partner* or *spouse* rather than *husband* or *wife* to avoid making assumptions about sexual orientation. Ask about preferences before acting. Pay attention to patient cues and follow their lead. If they do not establish eye contact or refuse to shake your hand, a cultural custom or spiritual belief may be guiding their behavior. Set the tone for your patient visits by asking questions.

Ask your patients how they would like to be addressed, and remember to continue calling them by their preferred names. Tell your patients why you think they are meeting with you after you ask them why they think they are there. Ask your patients what their goals are for their visit. Remind them they are active partners in their care plans.

Ask what cultural, religious, spiritual, or lifestyle beliefs may affect the kind of health care the patient wants to receive, and document these preferences so that other providers can honor them. Continuity of cultural appropriateness within the care team is essential. This is particularly important when you ask who else in their life needs to be involved in making medical decisions about care.

Ask patients to "teach back" the information you give them, and then document their understanding. Offer choices for treatment options. Use open-ended questions (instead of yes/no questions) to make sure you and your patients share a common meaning. Determine whether your explanation of the causes and likely course of the illness match your patients' perceptions and understanding of their illness. If there is a mismatch, some patients may rely on their own beliefs.

Acknowledge and respect your patients' interpretations of their illnesses. Listen carefully. When you talk with your patients, let them know you are listening by nodding your head that you understand, maintain eye contact if that is their norm, or avoid eye contact if that is their norm. Remain on the same physical level as much as possible with your patient.

Explain to your patients what you are writing as you take notes. After you are done taking their medical history, give your patients another opportunity to bring up something they may have omitted or did not feel comfortable talking about at first (especially if this is their first visit with you). They may feel more comfortable discussing something further into the visit. Tell your patients what you are doing and what they will feel if you are doing an exam, or procedure or performing other care that involves physically touching them (University of Washington Medical Center, 2011).

Summary

People who are characterized as European and Mediterranean Americans, or are generally associated with the group defined as White by the U.S. Census Bureau, are not composed of only those of northern European descent. They include people from very divergent backgrounds, such as the Amish, Roma, and those of Arab and Middle Eastern descent. It is important to remember that culture and ethnicity have a significant impact on people's health activities and on their perspectives on health, and merely characterizing a person as European, Mediterranean, or White does not describe those beliefs.

Review

1. Describe the health and illness beliefs of Amish and Roma Americans.
2. Prepare three recommendations to provide culturally competent care for a clinic that deals with Amish or Roma American clients.
3. Describe how Arab American clients might view American health practices differently from other patients.

Activity

Watch the video *Devil's Playground* (Cantor & Walker, 2002), a documentary film about the Amish. Write a three-page reaction paper to the video. What did you learn about the Amish? What surprised you? How would the knowledge about Rumspringa change how health care is provided to the Amish?

Case Study 1

Rebecca is a married Amish woman with six children. She is devout to her faith and her belief in shunning. Rebecca uses a horse and buddy to get to her medical appointments and does not use telephones, electricity, or television. Rebecca has strong family values and works hard. She does not have health insurance. She is not in agreement with getting vaccinations or using birth control.

Her daughter Susan, who is 11 years old, has cancer. Rebecca and her husband are refusing treatment. Susan got very ill, so as a last resort Rebecca took her to the hospital.

A social worker and physician spoke to Rebecca and her husband about future treatment and recommended chemotherapy. The providers informed them that their daughter has a highly curable form of cancer. Rebecca and her husband know that they will have to pay for the treatment and that financial assistance from their family and community would be needed. They also know that such treatment is costly.

1. What would be a way for the health care providers to share their concerns about Susan's condition and medical needs while still respecting Rebecca and her husband's religious and cultural beliefs?
2. How might your own religious and family background influence the way you react to this situation?

Adapted from Cox et al. (2020)

Case Study 2

A nurse found a Syrian patient on the floor when she entered her room. The nurse was concerned that the patient had fallen, and the patient became upset when the nurse tried to help her. Because the patient did not speak English, she could not explain to the nurse what she was doing. The nurse later learned that the patient was praying.

1. What information about the Muslim religion may have helped the nurse with understanding the situation?
2. Is there anything that the nurse could or should have done differently?

References

Abuelezam, N. N., El-Sayed, A. M., & Galea, S. (2019). Differences in health behaviors and health outcomes among non-Hispanic Whites and Arab Americans in a population-based survey in California. *BMC Public Health, 19*(892). https://doi.org/10.1186/s12889-019-7233-z

Altepeter, S. (2017). The effectiveness of Amish home remedies. *Nursing Capstones, 33*. https://commons.und.edu/nurs-capstones/33

American Association of Pediatrics. (2012). *Male circumcision*. https://publications.aap.org/pediatrics/article/130/3/e756/30225/Male-Circumcision. http://www.aap.org/en-us/about-the-aap/aap-press-room/Pages/Newborn-cMale-Circumcision.aspx#sthash.Rca4BHGr.dpuf

American Lung Association. (2020, October 14). *Tobacco use in racial and ethnic populations*. https://www.lung.org/quit-smoking/smoking-facts/impact-of-tobacco-use/tobacco-use-racial-and-ethnic

Cantor, S. (Producer), & Walker, L. (Director). (2002). *Devil's playground* [Documentary]. United States: Stick Figure Productions.

Centers for Disease Control and Prevention. (2014). Summary health statistics for U.S. Adults: National Health Interview Survey, 2012. *Vital and Health Statistics, 10*(260). http://www.cdc.gov/nchs/data/series/sr_10/sr10_260.pdf

Centers for Disease Control and Prevention. (2019, March 1). *About teen pregnancy*. https://www.cdc.gov/teenpregnancy/about/index.htm

Centers for Disease Control and Prevention. (2020, May 11). *Female genital mutilation/cutting (FGM/C)*. https://www.cdc.gov/reproductivehealth/womensrh/female-genital-mutilation.html

Centers for Disease Control and Prevention. (2021a, April 19). *Health equity considerations and racial and ethnic minority groups.* https://www.cdc.gov/coronavirus/2019-ncov/community/health-equity/race-ethnicity.html

Centers for Disease Control and Prevention. (2021b). *Health of White non-Hispanic population.* https://www.cdc.gov/nchs/fastats/white-health.htm

Centers for Disease Control and Prevention. (2022). *Health of White non-Hispanic population.* https://www.cdc.gov/nchs/fastats/white-health.htm

Cox, L. E., Tice, C. J., & Long, D. D. (2020). Case studies. In *Introduction to social work: An advocacy based profession.* https://edge.sagepub.com/cox2e/student-resources-0/chapter-1/case-studies

Elflein, J. (2021, August 13). *Distribution of the 10 leading causes of death among the U.S. White population in 2017.* Statista. https://www.statista.com/statistics/233304/distribution-of-the-10-leading-causes-of-death-among-whites-in-2016/

Feldman, J. M., & Bassett, M. T. (2020). The relationship between neighborhood poverty and COVID-19 mortality within racial/ethnic groups (Cook County Illinois). *medRxiv.* https://www.medrxiv.org/content/10.1101/2020.10.04.20206318v1

Frey, W. H. (2018, March 14). *The US will become "minority White" in 2045.* Brookings. https://www.brookings.edu/blog/the-avenue/2018/03/14/the-us-will-become-minority-white-in-2045-census-projects/

FXB Center for Health and Human Rights, Harvard University. (2020, November). *Romani realities in the United States: Breaking the silence, challenging the stereotypes.* https://cdn1.sph.harvard.edu/wp-content/uploads/sites/2464/2020/11/Romani-realities-report-final-11.30.2020.pdf

Henry, T. A. (2020, August 5). *Data from 10 cities show COVID-19 impact based on poverty, race.* AMA. https://www.ama-assn.org/delivering-care/health-equity/data-10-cities-show-covid-19-impact-based-poverty-race

Iraqi Refugees. (2002). http://www3.baylor.edu:80~Charles_Kemp/ Iraqi_refugees.htm

Julia, M. C. (1996). *Multicultural awareness in the health care professions.* Simon & Schuster.

Kitayama, S., Karasawa, M., Curhan, K. B., Ryff, C. D., & Markus, H. R. (2010). Independence and interdependence predict health and wellbeing: Divergent patterns in the United States and Japan. *Frontiers in Psycholology.* https://web.stanford.edu/~hazelm/publications/2010%20Kitayama%20et%20al%20Independence%20and%20interdependence%20predict%20health%20and%20wellbeing

Kluger, J. (2018, February 15). Amish people stay healthy in old age. Here's their secret. *Time.* https://time.com/5159857/amish-people-stay-healthy-in-old-age-heres-their-secret/

Lemon, B. C. (2006). Amish health and belief systems in obstetrical settings. *Journal of Multicultural Nursing & Health, 12*(3), 54–59.

Mather, M., & Feldman-Jacobs, C. (2016, February 5). *Women and girls at risk of female genital mutilation/cutting in the United States.* PRB. https://www.prb.org/us-fgmc/

Mayo Clinic Staff. (n.d.). *Mediterranean diet: A heart-healthy eating plan.* Mayo Clinic. http://www.mayoclinic.org/healthy-lifestyle/nutrition-and-healthy-eating/in-depth/mediterranean-diet/art-20047801

National Cancer Institute. (n.d.). *Cancer stat facts: Cancer disparities.* https://seer.cancer.gov/statfacts/html/disparities.html

Nolan, J. (1995). *Cultural diversity: Eating in America. Middle Eastern.* http://ohioline.osu.edu/hyg-Fact/5000/5256.html

NursingAnswers.net. (2018). *Health care in the Amish culture.* https://nursinganswers.net/essays/health-care-in-amish-culture-health-and-social-care-essay.php?vref=1

Ohio's Amish Country. (2021). *The health of the Amish.* https://www.ohiosamishcountry.com/articles/the-health-of-the-amish

Owings, M., Uddin, S., & Williams, S. (2013). *Trends in circumcision for male newborns in U.S. hospitals: 1979–2010.* CDC. http://www.cdc.gov/nchs/data/hestat/circumcision_2013/circumcision_2013.htm

Purnell, L. (2013). *Transcultural healthcare: A culturally competent approach* (4th ed.). F. A. Davis.

Roney, L. (2016, April 16). *10 US states are more than 90% White*. Newser. https://www.newser.com/story/223330/10-us-states-are-more-than-90-white.html

Ryczak, K., Zebreski, L., May, M., Traver, S., & Kemp, C. (n.d.). *Gypsy (Roma) culture health refugees immigrants*. Baylor University. http://bearspace.baylor.edu/Charles_Kemp/www/gypsy_health.htm

University of Washington Medical Center. (2011). *Culture Clue: Communication guide: All patients.*

U.S. Census Bureau. (n.d.). *Quick facts*. https://www.census.gov/quickfacts/fact/table/US/RHI825219#RHI825219

U.S. Census Bureau. (2011). *The White population, 2010*. http://www.census.gov/prod/cen2010/briefs/c2010br-05.pdf

CREDIT

CHAPTER 11

Nonethnic Cultures

We draw our strength from the very despair in which we have been forced to live. We shall endure.

—CESAR CHAVEZ

If God had wanted me otherwise, He would have created me otherwise.

—JOHANN WOLFGANG VON GOETHE

KEY CONCEPTS AND TERMS

Alien
Asylee
Baby boomers
Bisexual
Gay
Gender identity
Illegal alien
Immigrant
Lesbian
Millennials
Refugee
Sexual identity
Substance abuse
Transgender

LEARNING OBJECTIVES

After reading this chapter, you should be able to do the following:

1. Describe the differentiating characteristics of lesbian, gay, bisexual, transgender, queer or questioning, intersex, and asexual (LGBTQIA) people.
2. Discuss the health risks encountered by the LGBTQIA population.
3. Describe the problems often encountered by LGBTQIA people when accessing health care services.
4. Discuss health disparities of people with disabilities and ways to address their health needs.
5. Describe the challenges farmworkers encounter in obtaining health care.
6. Discuss ways to decrease farmworkers' health risks.
7. Discuss the unique situations of new immigrants and refugees and ways to address their health needs.
8. Discuss drug use in cultures and the culture of drugs.
9. Describe aspects of rural health that create health disparities from urban areas.
10. Describe differences in health concerns by different generations.

Introduction

Although culture can be easier to identify in ethnic and racial groups, it also exists in other human relationships. Culture is not restricted to race, ethnicity, or heritage; it includes customs, beliefs, values, and knowledge that influence our behavior and affect our health. Therefore, understanding the health of cultural groups not defined by race or ethnicity is just as important. A culture can develop within any group or community of people who share customs or beliefs. Athletes share a "sports culture," and illegal drug users may share a "drug culture."

This concept of culture becomes clear when we examine how the cultural relationships of LGBTQIA people, people with disabilities, farmworkers, new immigrants, refugees, drug users, rural residents and people from different generations affect their health. Cultures also can be based on common beliefs or lifestyles such as a culture of people suffering discrimination, a culture of consumers, and a culture of people living in poverty. Finally, cultures are affected by and affect other cultures.

People With Disabilities

People living with disabilities is a culture not defined by race or ethnicity. Steven Brown, the cofounder of the Institute on Disability Culture, states that those with disabilities have created a group identity. Brown (2002) describes the culture of disability as follows:

> We generate art, music, literature, and other expressions of our lives and our culture, infused from our experience of disability. Most importantly, we are proud of ourselves as people with disabilities. We claim our disabilities with pride as part of our identity. (p. 48)

Since the Americans With Disabilities Act was enacted in 1990, many social barriers have been removed or reduced for people with disabilities, and progress is continuing. Good health is important to be able to work, learn, and be engaged within a community.

DID YOU KNOW?

Deaf people typically do not view themselves as having lost their hearing or being handicapped, impaired, or disabled. The deaf celebrate and appreciate their culture, as it provides them with the unique privilege of sharing a common history and language.

The dominant cultural pattern in deaf culture is collectivism, and all deaf people are viewed as part of that culture. The group of deaf people is generally close-knit and connected. Deaf people find pleasure in being in the company of other deaf people and actively seek ways to accomplish this. When deaf people first meet, they typically begin the communication with identifying where the other person is from and whether they have deaf friends in common. A person's physical appearance is acknowledged and remembered, because it is the landscape for all signed communication. Sometimes a person's name is be revealed until the end of the conversation. Open communication is valued, and having secrets or withholding information is usually not done, as it does not support the interconnectedness that occurs in this collectivist culture (Siple et al., 2003).

Terminology

In section 504 of the Rehabilitation Act of 1973, a "person with a disability" includes any person who (a) has a physical or mental impairment, which substantially limits one or more of such a person's major life activities; (b) has a record of such impairment; or (c) is regarded as having such an impairment (Black Hawk College, 2014). Disabilities can affect people in different ways, even when one person has the same type of disability as another person. Some disabilities may be hidden and difficult to see. There are numerous types of disabilities, including these categories:

> *Physical disability* means a visual, hearing, mobility, or orthopedic impairment.
>
> *Communication disability* is an impairment in the processes of speech, language, or hearing.
>
> *Learning disability* is a persistent condition of presumed neurological dysfunction that may exist with other disability conditions. This dysfunction continues despite instruction in standard classroom situations.
>
> *Psychological disability* is a persistent psychological or psychiatric disorder or emotional or mental illness.

One in four adults in the United States is living with a disability for a total of approximately 61 million (see **Figure 11.1**) (CDC, 2018 a).

Adults with Disabilities: Ethnicity and Race
When it comes to the health of people with disabilities, it's important to know the health differences among racial and ethnic groups
Approximate number of adults with a disability by ethnicity and race
American Indian Alaska Native
3 in 10 have a disability
Black
1 in 4 have a disability
White
1 in 5 have a disability
Native Hawaiian Pacific Islander
1 in 6 have a disability
Hispanic
1 in 6 have a disability
Asian
1 in 10 have a disability
Percent of adults with a disability who are obese or smoke
60%
50%
40%
30%
20%
10%
0%
40.6%
41.2%
47.3%
28.1%
35.5%
28.7%
31.8%
28.2%
39.9%
20.6%
20.3%
12.8%
American Indian Alaska Native
Black
White
Native Hawaiian Pacific Islander
Hispanic
Asian

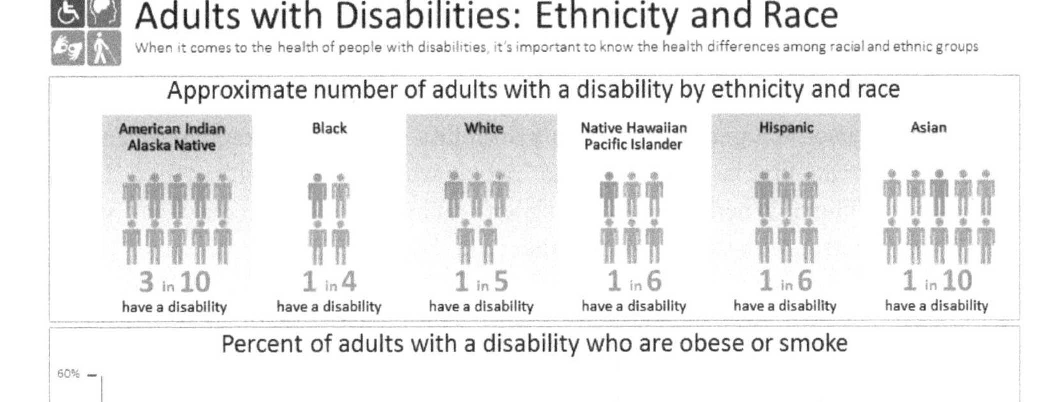

Figure 11.1 Adults with disabilities: Ethnicity and race.

Behavioral Risk Factors and Common Health Problems Among People with Disabilities

Disability is often equated with poor health, but people with disabilities can and should have the same opportunity for good health as people without disabilities. However, they report being in poorer health than those without disabilities.

Reports of fair or poor health among adults with a disability by race and ethnicity in 2018 were as follows:

- Hispanic: 48.6%
- Non-Hispanic Black or African American: 41.2%
- Non-Hispanic White: 39.1%
- Other/multiracial, non-Hispanic: 38.4% (CDC 2018a)

Smoking, lack of physical activity, lack of access to medical care due to cost, poor oral health, infrequent mammograms, and obesity all disproportionally affect people with disabilities. For example, in 2018 adults (age 18 and older) with disabilities were more likely to smoke (26.2%) than adults without disabilities (12.7%). This finding was observed in all states. In the same year, adults (age 18 and older) with disabilities were more likely to be obese (39.1%) than adults without disabilities (27.6%) (CDC, 2018b).

Considerations for Health Promotion and Program Planning for People with Disabilities

When working with people with disabilities, focus on their abilities, not on disabilities. Remember, a person is a person first, with a disability second. For example, whenever possible, use people-first language, such as "people who are blind" rather than "blind people" or "the blind." When communicating with an individual with a disability, speak directly to the person with the disability rather than the companion or interpreter. If you would like to offer assistance to a person with a disability, always ask first, wait until the offer is accepted, then listen patiently and follow instructions. If the offer of assistance is declined, respect the decision, and do not proceed to assist. If the person uses a service animal, do not pet or distract the animal. Consider the tips that follow for working with people who are deaf or hearing impaired, for people who are blind or have a visual impairment, and for people who have a mobile impairment.

Deaf or Hearing Impaired

Making eye contact

- Is essential for effective communication
- Is important because people who are deaf read the nuances of facial expressions and body language for additional information
- Is attention getting

- Hand waving is most common
- Tapping the shoulder or arm is acceptable
- Flickering lights on and off is also common
- Using a third person to relay attention in a crowded room can be effective

Blind or Visually Impaired

- DO identify yourself, especially when entering a room. Don't say, "Do you know who this is?"
- Speak directly to the individual. Do not speak through a companion. Unless they are hard of hearing, they can speak for themselves.
- Give specific directions like, "The desk is five feet to your right," as opposed to saying, "The desk is over there."
- Give a clear word picture when describing things to an individual with vision loss. Include details such as color, texture, shape and landmarks.
- Touch them on the arm or use their name when addressing them. This lets them know you are speaking to them, and not someone else in the room.
- Do not shout when you speak. They can't see but often have fine hearing.
- Do not be afraid to use words like "blind" or "see." Their eyes may not work, but it is still, "Nice to see you" (Wisconsin Department of Health Services, 2021).

Mobility Impairments

- Consider a person's wheelchair or walker as an extension of their body. Leaning on the wheelchair or walker, or placing your foot on a wheel, is not acceptable.
- Speak to a person who uses a wheelchair, walker, cane, or crutches in a normal voice in strength and tone.
- Talk to a person who uses a wheelchair at eye level whenever possible. Perhaps you can sit rather than stand.
- Feel free to use phrases such as "walk this way" with a person who cannot walk. Expressions such as this are commonly used by wheelchair users (University of Washington, 2015).

Farmworkers

Farmworkers in the United States are the backbone of the farming community and agriculture business. These workers and their families live a life driven by personal economic need, and a major commercial sector benefits from their lifestyle. Some farmworkers travel from one location to another due to changing locations of agricultural work opportunities. As farm labor shortages and wages have increased, fewer farmworkers are migrating and now work within driving distance from their homes. Nineteen percent of crop workers in 2015–2016 were migrant workers, compared to 27% in 2007–2009 and 42% in 2001–2002 (Farmworker Justice, 2019).

Farmworkers in the United States

It is difficult to track trends in this population as accurate statistics are problematic to find because 48% of all farmworkers in 2016 did not have authorization to work in the United States (U.S. Department of Agriculture [USDA], 2020). Because many workers and their families are unauthorized, they are reluctant to provide any demographic information about themselves or their community due to the risk of deportation.

Nevertheless, employment in agriculture has been on an upward trend since 2010, rising from 1.07 million in 2010 to 1.18 million in 2019, a gain of 11%. As fewer young immigrants are entering agriculture, the average age of foreign-born farmworkers has risen, thus increasing the average age for the farmworker workforce as a whole. The average age of immigrant farmworkers rose by 5 years between 2008 and 2018 to 41.5 years of age compared to U.S.-born workers with average age of 36.6. The average hourly wage for all agricultural occupations in 2019 was $14.91 (USDA, 2020).

The demand for farm labor increased dramatically between 2005 and 2019, with the number of H-2A foreign worker permit positions increasing. Between 2005 and 2019 H-2 certifications grew from just over 48,000 positions certified in fiscal year 2005 to nearly 258,000 in fiscal year 2019. The average duration of the permits in 2019 was 53 months, suggesting that the 258,000 positions certified represented approximately 114,000 full-year equivalents (USDA, 2020).

TABLE 11.1 Demographic Characteristics of All Hired Farmworkers

Demographic characteristics of hired farmworkers and all wage and salary workers, 2018					
Item	**Farm laborers, graders, and sorters**	**Farm managers, inspectors, and supervisors**	**All other occupations in agriculture**	**Agriculture: All occupations**	**All U.S. private wage and salary workers**
Percent female	25	13	32	26	45
Average age in years	39	43	42	40	40
Percent under age 25	22	13	15	19	18
Percent over age 44	38	46	47	41	41
Percent married	47	61	52	51	48

(continued)

TABLE 11.1 Demographic Characteristics of All Hired Farmworkers (*Continued*)

Demographic characteristics of hired farmworkers and all wage and salary workers, 2018					
Item	**Farm laborers, graders, and sorters**	**Farm managers, inspectors, and supervisors**	**All other occupations in agriculture**	**Agriculture: All occupations**	**All U.S. private wage and salary workers**
Race/Ethnicity/Ancestry					
Percent White, not Hispanic	32	64	59	43	60
Percent Black, not Hispanic	3	3	5	3	12
Percent other, not Hispanic	2	3	3	2	9
Percent Hispanic: Mexican origin	57	27	28	45	12
Percent Hispanic: Other	7	3	6	6	7
Percent born in United States (includes Puerto Rico)	45	76	75	57	80
Percent U.S. citizens	54	84	83	65	90
Education					
Percent lacking high school diploma	48	24	20	38	9
Percent with high school diploma (includes equivalency)	32	31	33	32	29
Percent with at least some college	20	45	47	30	62

Note: Counts all private sector wage and salary workers employed in the crop, livestock, and agricultural support industries.

Source: USDA (2020).

History of Hired Farmworkers in America

Mexican workers are the largest population of hired farmworkers in U.S. agriculture (U.S. Department of Labor, 2018). Farmworkers are also from other countries, including Guatemala, Honduras, Puerto Rico, the Dominican Republic, Southeast Asia, the Philippines, Jamaica, Haiti, and other Caribbean islands. Farm labor workers are predominantly Hispanic.

Mexican immigration began during the 1850s to geographic regions like California that were still considered part of Mexico. In the 1920s, the Mexican government addressed complaints of abuse with the United States by securing contracts with the United States to try to trace immigration and provide some type of labor protection to their citizens who traveled to the United States for work. The first was the de facto Bracero program, which allowed workers to bring their families. During World War II, the United States signed another Bracero treaty to legalize immigration for Mexican workers to fill the labor gaps left by soldiers who were participating in the war. Under this program, approximately 4 million Mexican farmworkers came to support the agriculture industry between 1942 and 1964. (National Center for Farmworker Health, 2020) Facts About Agricultural Workers http://www.ncfh.org/facts-about-agricultural-workers.html

More recently, the United States has entered trade agreements that directly affect farmworkers, including the General Agreement on Tariffs and Trade (GATT) and the North American Free Trade Agreement (NAFTA). The Immigration Reform and Control Act has also played a role in the legalization and fluctuation of farmworkers and their services. However, demand for labor continues to attract illegal workers who work without social or health services and live with some anxiety of deportation.

Behavioral Risk Factors and Common Health Problems Among Farmworkers

Many factors affect farmworkers' health. They tend to be geographically isolated, and some constantly move from place to place, which makes access to care difficult. In addition, a lack of health education contributes to poor knowledge of good health practices.

Most farmworkers cannot afford to take time off from work and also risk losing their jobs to attend doctor appointments. In 2015–2016 only 47% had health insurance (JBS International, 2018).

Farmworkers are exposed to many different types of diseases and injuries related to the sun, chemicals, and machinery they use, including musculoskeletal injuries, respiratory illness, tuberculosis, HIV, and others. Musculoskeletal injuries are very common in farmworkers. The labor done by farmworkers consists of heavy lifting and constant, quick movements of certain body parts, such as the wrists. Respiratory illnesses, including asthma, occur due to exposure to pesticides, dust, pollen, and molds. Exposure to these pollutants for long periods of time can have long-term effects on the workers.

Considerations for Health Promotion and Program Planning for Migrant Farmworkers

Guidelines for working with farmworkers include the following:

- Recognize the concern farmworkers have regarding immigration issues and the possibility of deportation.
- Ensure that appropriate translations services are available.
- Remember to include family members in decision-making.
- Determine a person's living situation before planning.
- Understand that fear and mistrust exist.

The motivation for economic improvement and participation in the United States economy continues today and among other groups of immigrants. We look at the lives of these new immigrants and refugees next.

Recent Immigrants and Refugees

Most Americans have descended from immigrants or refugees. Many noncitizen immigrants residing in the United States have lived here for decades and have adapted to life, either through acculturation or by maintaining their own cultures. However, recent immigrants and refugees confront the reality of living in another culture as new arrivals to the United States.

Terminology

A **refugee** is a person who has fled a home country because of fear of persecution. Under U.S. immigration law, a refugee is a person who has been or has a well-founded fear of being persecuted for reasons of race, religion, nationality, membership in a particular social group, or political opinion, and who is unable to receive the protection of that country. This definition focuses on persecution as the defining characteristic and excludes people who have been displaced because of civil war, ethnic strife, natural disaster, or economic reasons.

An **asylee** is a person who meet the definition for refugee—meaning having a well-founded fear of persecution based on one of the five enumerated grounds—and have been provided asylum. Asylum status and refugee status are closely related. Their major difference lies in where a person applies for asylum or refugee status. Applicants requesting refugee status do so outside the United States, whereas those seeking asylum status request it from within the United States. However, all people who are granted asylum must meet the definition of a refugee. Both refugees and asylees have the right to live and work indefinitely in the United States and to apply for lawful permanent residence after 1 year. In addition, both refugees and asylees are eligible for certain assistance from the

Department of Health and Human Services' Office of Refugee Resettlement. This assistance includes benefits such as cash and medical assistance, employment preparation and job placement, skills training, English language training, legal services, social adjustment, and aid for victims of torture.

The top 10 countries of refugee origin entering the United States between 2008 and 2016 were Mynmar, Iraq, Bhutan, Somalia, the Democratic Republic of the Congo, Cuba, Iran, Syria, Eritrea, and Sudan (Haynie, 2017). The overall number of refugees allowed into the United States each year had been drastically reduced from 85,000 per year in 2016 to 15,000 in 2020 (Migration Policy Institute, 2020). However, in 2021 the quota was increased to 62,500 (Shear & Kanno-Youngs, 2021).

An **immigrant** is a person who migrates to another country, usually for permanent residence. Under this definition, an immigrant is an alien admitted to the United States as a lawful permanent resident. The emphasis in this definition is on the presumptions that (a) the immigrant followed U.S. laws and procedures in establishing residence in the country; (b) the immigrant wishes to reside here permanently; and (c) the immigrant swears allegiance to the country or at least solemnly affirms to observe and respect the laws and the constitution. The overall annual number of immigrants between 2018 and 2019 totaled 204,000 (Migration Policy Institute, 2021).

By contrast, an **alien** is generally understood to be a foreigner—a person who comes from a foreign country—who does not owe allegiance to our country. An **illegal alien** is a foreigner who (a) does not owe allegiance to the country and (b) who has violated laws and customs in establishing residence in the country. The illegal alien is therefore a criminal under applicable U.S. laws. The term *undocumented immigrant* is an oxymoron (the parts conflict). An immigrant is synonymous with a *permanent legal resident.* Proper terms for the undocumented are *illegal alien* or *undocumented alien, unauthorized worker.* There were approximately 11 million undocumented aliens in the United States in 2018, and Homeland Security reported 531,300 removals and returns of undocumented aliens during fiscal year 2019 (Migration Policy Institute, 2021).

Behavioral Risk Factors and Common Health Problems Among People Who Are Immigrants or Refugees

Many health conditions may affect the health of refugees; therefore, the CDC provides guidelines for health care providers who may see refugees at any point during the resettlement process. These guidelines aim to do the following:

- Promote and improve the health of the refugee
- Prevent disease
- Familiarize refugees with the U.S. health care system

Because of the vast diversity of immigrants and refugees and the varied ways in which they enter the United States, a national snapshot of their health status is not available.

DID YOU KNOW?

The CDC (2021) maintains an online set of refugee health profiles for various refugee groups, including the Bhutanese, Burmese, Central Americans, Congolese, Iraqi, Somali, and Syrian.

Each profile addresses the following:

- Priority health conditions
- Background
- Population movements
- Health care and conditions before arrival
- Medical screening of U.S.-bound refugees
- Post-arrival medical screening
- Health information

Current information may be found at the following link: https://www.cdc.gov/immigrantrefugeehealth/profiles/index.html.

Considerations for Health Promotion and Program Planning for People Who Are Immigrants or Refugees

Considerations for health promotion for newly arrived immigrants and refugees follows the same pattern as for people from different cultures. A foundation of cultural awareness must be developed to understand the means of communication, values, attitudes, and cultural practices. Cultural awareness and competence are not only useful for delivering health care services but likely will also be appreciated and facilitate the delivery of care or acceptance of prevention measures.

The diversity of nationalities, ethnic groups, religions, and other dimensions is apparent in many refugee settings. Urban refugee populations often consist of people from numerous national, ethnic, and religious backgrounds. In these situations, target audience segmentation is challenging. One approach is to develop simple messages in languages that are most common in that setting. Visual communication materials, such as pamphlets and brochures, featuring neutral images that are not specific to any particular group, are preferred. In some settings, neutral cartoon characters have been well received. It is important to ensure representation of all groups in formative assessment, the pretesting of materials, and interpersonal communication channels. During pretesting, the target group's responses to draft communication materials should be sought and materials revised to ensure comprehension and acceptability and to promote effectiveness.

Differences between displaced and host communities also significantly affect access to effective communication. Similarly, refugees and internally displaced people often come from areas of long-standing conflict with interruptions in schooling, resulting in low levels of basic education and literacy.

One unfortunate aspect of the discussion about immigration in the United States is the repeated arguments that immigrants, and particularly undocumented aliens, are a source, if not the primary source of drugs in the United States. Yet, this is simply wrong. In 2016, approximately 70% all drug trafficking offenders were U.S. citizens (71.5%), with the rate varying on the type of drug (U.S. Sentencing Commission, 2016). Drugs are indeed a problem for the United States, and we will discuss the associated drug culture in the next section.

Users of Drugs

The drug culture includes (a) how cultures use drugs and (b) the culture among users of legal and illicit drugs. Some see the medical system as a drug culture, stating that medical providers and pharmaceutical companies push and encourage drug use.

Drugs have been part of various cultures for thousands of years. The Catholic Church has used wine in religious ritual for 2,000 years, the Caribbean Indians were using tobacco as medicine when Columbus arrived in America, American Indians used peyote, and the Aztec used alcohol rituals. Drugs were not usually used to excess, nor was use of them seen as separate from the main culture. The Aztecs, for instance, used ritual alcohol, but use by commoners was a capital offense, with commoners executed in front of young men and the elite executed in private.

The Aztec emperor said upon his election:

> that drink which is called octli (alcohol), is the root and the origin of all evil and of all perdition; for octli and drunkenness are the cause of all the discords and of all the dissension, of all revolt and of all troubles in cities and in realms. It is like the whirlwind that destroys and tears down everything. It is like a malignant storm that brings all evil with it. Before adultery, rape, debauching of girls, incest, theft, crime, cursing and bearing false witness, murmuring, calumny, riots, and brawling, there is always drunkenness. All those things are caused by octli and by drunkenness. (Fresno County Hispanic Commission on Alcohol and Drug Abuse Services, Inc., 2016)

While culture impacts drug use, drug users and those in recovery have their own culture. Identification with a drug culture enables its members to view substance use disorders as normal. Drug use may become a source of rebellious pride and sense of independence, and people may celebrate their drug-related identity with other members of that culture. The disapproval that general society attaches to substance abuse can unconsciously increase a user's engagement with drug culture, decreasing the chances they will seek treatment. Drug use behaviors have a reinforcing effect that can distract users from other life issues they may need to address, such as other mental health issues like depression, posttraumatic stress disorder, or personality disorder. People may use drugs and/or alcohol as a way to self-medicate. Self-medicating refers to the misuse of drugs or alcohol in an attempt to manage the distressing symptoms of a mental health disorder or other health condition. Feelings of alienation from society and a firm rejection of authority can cause youth to look outside the traditional cultural institutions, allowing youth to seek acceptance in a drug culture where they can learn skills to avoid being caught and thereby continue their use. The more an individual's needs are met within drug culture, the harder it will be to leave that culture behind and find recovery (Scoles, 2020).

Is easy to dismiss the members of the drug culture as merely a deviant subculture. But the scale of this culture affects society across the board. The U.S. government budget for drug control in 2020 was $35 billion; 14.8 million have an alcohol use disorder, 58.8 million people use tobacco, and 31.9 million use illegal drugs (National Center for Drug Abuse Statistics, n.d.). Tobacco use has itself taken a great deal of talent from society. While purporting to be cool, sexy, and macho many figures, known by their cigarette use, died of lung cancer brought on by smoking:

> Humphry Bogart, Walt Disney, "The Marlboro Man," Rod Serling, Peter Jennings, Paul Newman, George Harrison, Dean Martin, Vincent Price, Robert Mitchum, Donna Summer, George Peppard, Nat King Cole, Steve McQueen, Gary Cooper, Chuck Conners, Don Knotts, Chad Everett, Ann Miller, Buster Keaton, Joe DiMaggio, John Updike, Duke Ellington, Alan King, Joe Paterno, Audrey Meadows, Yul Brynner, Bette Grable, Jean Simmons, Ray Milland, Foster Tucker, Robert Taylor, Anthony Burgess, Roddy McDowell, Dezi Arnaz, James Whitmore, Jason Robards, Robert Ryan, Lou Rawls, Freddy Fender, Frank Gorshin, Suzanne Pleschette, Tex Avery, Scatman Crothers, Zeppo Marx, Roger Miller, Patricia Neal, Alan J. Lerner, Rosemary Clooney, Pat Nixon, Doug McClure Gypse Rose Lee, Sarah Vaughn, E. G. Marshall, Jesse Owens, LLoyd Nowlan, Chet Huntley, and Edward R. Murrow. (Ranker.com, 2021)

BOX 11.1 Facts About Drug Use

- There were 700,000 drug overdose deaths in the United States between 2000 and 2019.
- The federal budget for drug control in 2019 was $35 billion.
- Almost 20% of people have used illicit drugs at least once.
- Among Americans aged 12 years and older, 31.9 million are current (2019) illegal drug users (used within the last 30 days).
- With alcohol and tobacco included, in 2019 165 million (60.2%) Americans aged 12 years or older used drugs (i.e., used within the last 30 days).
    - 139.8 million Americans 12 and over drank alcohol.

(continued)

BOX 11.1 Facts About Drug Use (*Continued*)

- 14.8 million (10.6%) Americans 12 and older who drank alcohol had an alcohol use disorder.
- 58.8 million people used tobacco.
- 31.9 million used illegal drugs.
- 8.1 million (25.4%) illegal drug users had a drug disorder.

- Two million illegal drug users (24.7%) have an opioid disorder; this includes prescription pain relievers, or pain killers, and heroin.
- Persons previously abusing drugs and recently released from prison were at the highest risk for overdose as their tolerance to the drug dropped while incarcerated.
- "Club drugs" such as ecstasy, meth, cocaine, ketamine, LSD, and GHB are primarily used in higher income settings by young people.
- Among lower income users, the most commonly used drugs are inhalants such as paint thinner, gasoline, paint, correction fluid, and glue.
- In 2019, $193 billion was incurred in overall costs for illegal drugs in addition to $78.5 billion for prescription opioids.
- In 2019, $11 billion was incurred in health care costs related to the use of illegal drugs and $26 billion for prescription opioids.
- There were 326,000 hospitalizations for nonfatal drug poisonings or overdoses in 2016, including unintentional, undetermined intent, and intentional self-harm.
- There were 577,794 emergency room visits for nonfatal drug poisonings or overdoses in 2016, with most patients experiencing opioid poisoning.
- In 2020, the National Drug Control Budget requested $34.6 billion across five areas of drug control functions: operations, prevention, treatment, interdiction, and law enforcement.

Source: National Center for Drug Abuse Statistics (n.d.).

The drug recovery process is another subculture. For example, Alcoholic Anonymous has its own culture that includes norms such as an addiction topic for each meeting and the 12 steps to recovery.

Some will say that the drug culture is not all bad, as drug use is sometimes attributed to performance enhancement and exceptional creativity. It is not particularly clear how much value to society can be attributed to the drug culture. Some attribute contributions, such as enhancing creativity, reducing pain, increasing energy and productivity, and improving social interaction, to drug use. For example, caffeine can increase alertness and enhance sports performance. A common myth is that Walt Disney must have been on drugs when he created Fantasia, despite the fact it took hundreds of sober, hard-working animators, musicians, and other talented people to create the work. Overall, the drug culture finds benefit within itself, including the drug dealers and commercial sellers, rather than contributing positively to general society.

Behavioral Risk Factors and Common Health Problems

In addition to the well-known health hazards of drug behaviors such as overdosing, inadvertent suicide, cirrhosis of the liver, lung cancer, and diminishment of brain function, there is a greater chance of contracting viral infections such as hepatitis or HIV:

- Drug abuse affects symptoms and adversely changes the outcomes of infectious diseases.
- Abusers who inject their drugs account for one in 10 HIV diagnoses.
- In 2016, 20% of HIV cases (150,000) among men were attributed to injection drug use.
- In 2016, 21% of HIV cases (50,000) among women were attributed to injection drug use.
- Nearly 2,000 children were diagnosed with perinatal HIV in 2016.
- Over 10,000 adults were living with perinatal HIV in 2016 (National Center for Drug Abuse Statistics, n.d.).

Considerations for Health Promotion and Program Planning

Consider a person's cultural background when assessing for substance abuse or dependence. Five major items may be considered: cultural identity, cultural explanation of the illness, cultural factors related to psychosocial environment and levels of functioning, cultural elements of the relationship between the individual and the clinician, and overall cultural assessment for diagnosis and care (Abbott & Chase, 2008).

The considerations related to a patient's cultural identity are cultural reference groups, involvement with culture of origin, language, and cultural factors of development. For example, for American Indians it is important to note the tribe the individual is part of and what tribe or ethnic group the person identifies with. Another factor that should be considered is what the person's native language is and what first language was spoken. Often, individuals can feel alienated from their host culture if they do not speak their native language fluently or at all. This can be a barrier to those wishing to seek care from traditional healers. It is also important to note what involvement a person has had with an original host culture and to what degree the perons's family is involved with their culture (Abbott & Chase, 2008).

One aspect of recovery treatment is cultural recovery, in which the person needs to reidentify with original cultural norms outside the drug culture in order to engage with supportive aspects that do not allow reentry into drug behavior. For instance, family interaction is important when working with Hispanic and American Indian communities.

The drug culture affects all cultures and is not the only pan-culture that has members from all other cultures. One that is also visible but not anywhere near as disruptive to society in general is the LGBTQIA community. We address the health aspects of this culture in the next section.

LGBTQIA

There are more than 8 million adults in the United States who are lesbian, gay, or bisexual, comprising 5.6% of the adult population, and approximately 18 million Americans identify as LGBTQIA when transgender persons are included. For those 18 to 23 years, 1 in 6 (15.9%) identify as LGBTQ. In each older generation, LGBTQ identification is lower, including 2% or less for people born before 1965. Among LGBTQ adults, a majority, or 54.6%, identified as bisexual. About a quarter, or 24.5%, identify as gay; 11.7% as lesbian; 11.3% as transgender; and 72% as bisexual (Miller, 2021).

Terminology

Gay people, referred to as individuals who are LGBTQIA, exist in all cultures, communities, and subgroups of American society. Therefore, biologically and ethnically LGBTQIA persons tend to be as different as the varied cultures from which they arise. However, LGBTQIA culture has its own values, beliefs, traditions, and behaviors.

It is often difficult to identify members of this culture without their self-identification. Historically, the secrecy of the culture has been an effort at self-preservation. Today, the LGBTQIA culture is emerging and being given a place in society.

Key to understanding this population is to understand some terms. **Sexual identity** is usually defined as a person's physical, romantic, emotional, and spiritual attraction to another person. **Gender identity** references a person's internal, personal sense of being male or female, boy or girl, man or woman. Gender identity and sexual identity are not the same. For **transgender** people, their physical, birth-assigned gender does not match their internal sense of their gender. Transgender is usually defined as individuals who live full- or part-time in the gender role opposite to the one in which they were physically born. **Bisexual** refers to those whose sexual identity is to both men and women. **Gay** individuals' gender identity is consistent with their physical sexual characteristics, but their sexual identity is to persons of the same sex, and it usually refers to gay males specifically. **Lesbian** refers to gay women specifically.

Behavioral Risk Factors and Common Health Problems Among LGBTQIA Americans

While there are a great number of variations among LGBTQIA individuals, there are some aspects that may be helpful to understand when working with this cultural group.

Gender Correction Surgery

Optional therapies and surgeries are sometimes sought to "confirm" or convert physical attributes to personal identities. The integration of LGBTQIA persons in the military has led to some political resistance due to perceived cost of such treatments to the military health system. While debate continues, current policy is to accept LGTBQIA persons into the Armed Services and to allow treatment when approved. The participation of transgender and transsexual people in competitive sports is also a controversial issue.

At another level, debate also continues around the "confirmation" treatment of minors. Certain practices, such as conversion therapy, have been banned in some places, and medical treatment of minors has been banned by statute by 2020 in 20 states (Society for the Psychology for Sexual Orientation and Gender Identity, 2020).

Health disparities are linked to societal stigma and discrimination. Much of the negative response by other people results from reaction to the group member's own risky health behaviors that have become highly associated with the HIV/AIDS epidemic and the fear, dread, and expense associated with the disabling health condition it represents. Yet, discrimination against LGBTQIA persons has been associated with high rates of psychiatric disorders, substance abuse, and suicide. Violence and victimization are relatively common for LGBTQIA individuals and have a long-lasting impact on the individual and the community. Family, and social acceptance of sexual orientation and gender identity affects the mental health and personal safety of LGBTQIA individuals (Office of Disease Prevention and Health Promotion, n.d.).

LGBTQIA health requires specific attention from health care and public health professionals to address a number of disparities, including the following:

- LGBTQIA youth are two to three times more likely to attempt suicide.
- LGBTQIA youth are more likely to be homeless.
- Lesbians are less likely to get preventive services for cancer.
- Gay men are at higher risk of HIV and other sexually transmitted diseases (STDs), especially among communities of color.
- Lesbians and bisexual females are more likely to be overweight or obese.
- Elderly LGBTQIA individuals face additional barriers to health because of isolation and a lack of social services and culturally competent providers (Office of Disease Prevention and Health Promotion, n.d.).

Transgender individuals have a high prevalence of HIV/STDs, victimization, mental health issues, and suicide and are less likely to have health insurance than heterosexual or LGBTQIA individuals (Office of Disease Prevention and Health Promotion, n.d.).

LGBTQIA populations have the highest rates of tobacco, alcohol, and other drug use. Youth who identify as other than heterosexual (sexual minority youths) report more violence victimization, substance use, and suicide risk than do other youths. This can be due to minority stress resulting from stigma (Johns et al., 2018).

The onset of acquired immunodeficiency syndrome (AIDS) in the 1980s brought devastation to the lives of gay men. Although discrimination and a belief that these men deserved their fate was the initial response to the epidemic, with time a better understanding of the disease and its risk factors have enlightened the discussion. The importance of distinguishing between sexual identity and sexual behavior has been emphasized in dealing with this disease.

Changing behavior remains the primary way of reducing the spread of the human immunodeficiency virus (HIV). Education about safer sex practices has been strongly supported within the gay community, and research has shown that most gay men report having protected sex most of the time.

Cancer

Gay men and lesbians are at higher risk for certain cancers: Kaposi's sarcoma (KS), non-Hodgkin's lymphoma (NHL), cervical cancer, Hodgkin's lymphoma, anal cancer, lung cancer, and liver cancer. Gay men are at higher risk for Kaposi's sarcoma, which is associated with HIV infection, and AIDS-related non-Hodgkin's lymphoma (Smart, 2015). More effective treatments for HIV/AIDS are improving the survival rate by treating the infections associated with HIV/AIDS and Kaposi sarcoma (Cancer.net, 2021).

Lesbians have been found to be at higher risk for breast cancer than heterosexual women due to increased risk factors, including alcohol consumption, obesity, and not having children. Lesbians receive less frequent gynecologic care and breast cancer screening.

Substance Use

When compared with the general population, LGBTQIA individuals

- are more likely to use alcohol and drugs,
- have higher rates of substance abuse,
- are less likely to abstain from alcohol and drug use, and
- are more likely to continue heavy drinking into later life (CDC, 2016).

Alcohol and drug use among some men who have sex with men may be a reaction to homophobia, discrimination, or violence they experienced due to their sexual orientation and can contribute to other mental health problems. Substance abuse is associated with a wide range of mental health and physical problems. It can disrupt relationships and employment and threaten financial stability.

Mental Health

As previously noted, being gay was declassified as a mental illness in 1973. However, the LGBTQIA population is at increased risk for certain mental health issues as a result of stressors related to antigay societal attitudes and internalization of negative social attitudes. Significant among the problems encountered by this group are mental disorders and distress, substance use, and suicide. As with other health issues faced by this population, few scientifically significant studies are available in this area.

Considerations for Health Promotion and Program Planning for LGBTQIA Americans

To investigate U.S. hospitals' policies and procedures related to LGBTQIA concerns, the Human Rights Campaign Foundation and the Gay and Lesbian Medical Association (Henderson, 2007) devised the Healthcare Equality Index to evaluate how the health care community responds to the needs of the LGBTQIA community. The focus of the inquiry was on five criteria: patient nondiscrimination, hospital visitation, decision-making, cultural competence training, and employment policies.

The project began in 2007, and all participants were given anonymity for their responses. Requests for participation were sent to 1,000 hospitals. Responses from 78 hospitals in 20 states were obtained. The results showed that 50 hospitals had policies providing the same access to same-sex partners as is provided to married spouses, 56 allowed the designation of a domestic partner or someone else as medical surrogate, only 45 had a policy allowing same-sex parents the same access to medical decision-making for their minor children as married spouses, and 57 provided staff training on specific issues affecting LGBTQIA patients and their families (Henderson, 2007).

Efforts to improve LGBTQIA health include the following:

- Implementing antibullying policies in schools
- Providing supportive social services to reduce suicide and homelessness risk among youth
- Appropriately inquiring about and being supportive of a patient's sexual orientation to enhance the patient-provider interaction and regular use of care
- Providing medical students with access to LGBTQIA patients to increase provision of culturally competent care
- Expansion of domestic partner health insurance coverage
- Establishment of LGBTQIA health centers
- Dissemination of effective HIV and STD interventions (CDC, n.d.)

The LGBTQIA community experiences barriers to accessing care. The lack of health insurance for individuals and their partners, cultural barriers, and a poor understanding of their health care needs all affect the health of this group. For health promotion to occur, efforts need to be made to address these problems. Cultural competence must be addressed within the provider community as well. **Table 11.2** provides objectives for creating LGBTQIA cultural competence.

TABLE 11.2 Recommended Community Standards for Gay, Lesbian, and Transgender Persons

Create and promote open communication and a safe and nondiscriminatory workplace.
Create comprehensive policies to ensure that services are provided to LGBTQIA clients and their families in a nondiscriminatory manner.
Have procedures available for clients to resolve complaints concerning violation of policies.
Prepare and implement assessment tools to meet the needs of LGBTQIA clients and their families.
Maintain a basic understanding of LGBTQIA issues within the organization.
All personnel who provide direct care to LGBTQIA clients shall be competent to identify and address the health issues encountered by LGBTQIA clients and their families and be able to provide appropriate treatment or referrals.
The organization shall ensure the confidentiality of client information.
Community outreach shall include the LGBTQIA community.
The board of directors of the organization should have an LGBTQIA representative.
The organization shall provide appropriate and safe care and treatment to all LGBTQIA clients and their families.

Source: Adapted from Gay and Lesbian Medical Association (2001).

Rural and Urban Residents

There are significant differences in health care delivery between rural and urban areas. Obviously distance and sparse population can limit access to health care in rural areas. But due to demand for health workers, many providers choose the rich economic, social, and cultural opportunities of urban areas. Due to economics, major health care resources and specialty providers are located in urban areas. The availability of those resources in turn draws people from rural areas as well as the urban area to have access to better health care.

Rural–Urban Health Disparities

Rural Americans are a population group that experiences significant health disparities when compared to the overall population. There is a higher incidence of disease and/or disability, increased mortality rates, lower life expectancies, and higher rates of pain and suffering. Factors leading to these health disparities include geographic isolation, lower socioeconomic status, higher rates of health risk behaviors, limited access to health care specialists, and more limited job opportunities and thus a decreased likelihood of having employer-provided health insurance coverage. The rural poor are often not covered by Medicaid (Rural Health Information Hub, 2019). In addition, there is generally a shortage of people interested in working in health care in rural areas because there are many opportunities in urban areas. Fewer than 8% of all physicians and surgeons choose to practice in rural settings (National Center for Health Workforce Analysis, 2014). Transportation systems are also not as well developed in rural areas and can limit access to distant health resources.

Causes of Rural–Urban Health Disparities

To begin to understand some of the magnitude of differences between urban and rural, the map in **Figure 11.2** depicts an area of rural America that encompasses the same-sized population as New York City. The physical distance between people is a contributing factor to cultural differences. For instance, although there are small concentrations of rural people in towns and small cities, many live on remote land. This necessitates greater self-reliance, advanced planning for stocking supplies of food and medicine, and challenges to reach a medical provider and in many cases no access at all to medical specialists without extensive travel. On the other hand, urban residents may become overly confident in the availability of medical resources. For instance, some may forego medical insurance and rely on the local emergency room for care.

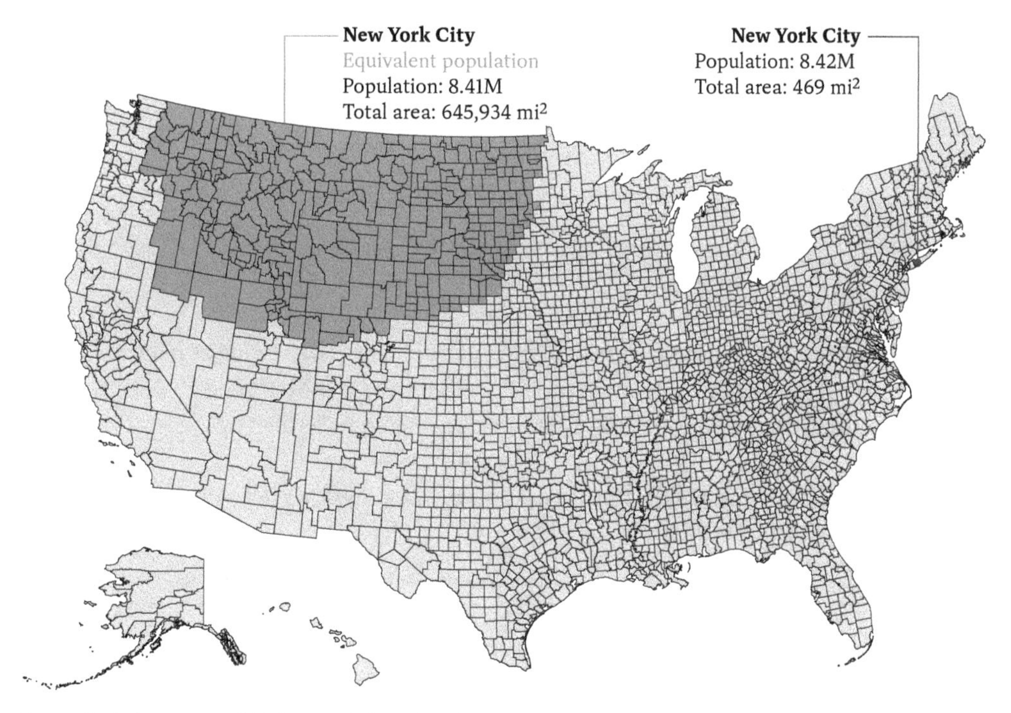

Figure 11.2 Extremes of U.S. population density.

Health Behaviors

Adoption of constructive health behaviors can impact rural-urban health disparities. In its 2017 report "Health-Related Behaviors by Urban-Rural County Classification—United

States, 2013," published in 2017, the CDC reviewed five key health-related behaviors and compared urban and rural areas. Urban residents were more likely to report four or five of the positive health behaviors (see **Table 11.3**).

TABLE 11.3 Positive Adult Health Behaviors and Geography by Percent, 2013

Behavior	Large metro center	Large fringe metro	Medium metro	Small metro	Micropolitan	Non-core
Current nonsmoking	83.9%	82.3%	80.5%	77.5%	76.5%	74.9%
No or moderate drinking	61.1%	59.9%	63.3%	64.3%	67.3%	68.6%
Maintaining normal body weight	36.5%	35.3%	33.3%	32.9%	30.6%	28.9%
Meeting aerobic activity recommendations	51.4%	51.4%	51.1%	50.7%	49.2%	46.7%
Sufficient sleep	62.4%	61.7%	62.4%	62.1%	61.1%	61.5%
Reported four or five of these health-related behaviors	31.7%	30.2%	30.5%	29.5%	28.8%	27.0%

Source: Kevin A. Matthews, et al., "Health-Related Behaviors by Urban-Rural County Classification—United States, 2013," *MMWR Surveillance Summaries*, vol. 66, no. 5, p. 5. 2017.

One study showed that teenagers in rural areas are more than twice as likely to smoke (13%) as their peers in large central metropolitan counties (5%) (Meitt et al., 2014). Overall, health disparities are evident in CDC statistics, as shown in **Table 11.4**.

TABLE 11.4 Age-Adjusted Death Rates for the Five Leading Causes of Death per 100,000 Population: United States, 2014

Cause of Death	Nonmetro Areas	Metro Areas
Heart Disease	193.5	161.7
Cancer	176.2	158.3
Unintentional injury	54.3	38.2
Chronic lower respiratory disease	54.3	38.0
Stroke	41.5	35.4

Source: Adapted from Ernest Moy, et al., "Leading Causes of Death in Nonmetropolitan and Metropolitan Areas — United States, 1999–2014" *MMWR Surveillance Summaries*, vol. 66, no. 1, p. 4. 2017.

Efforts to address rural-urban disparities include plans to enhance broadband capabilities, approve telemedicine practices, enhance physical infrastructure, and provide tuition incentives to college students who promise to work for at least a limited time in rural areas.

The need for cultural competence among young college graduates providing service to rural areas is magnified by the fact that rural areas are predominantly the more mature generations in society. Therefore, it may be important to understand the differences between "generations" in both rural and urban areas.

Generations

It is easy to think that people of all ages belonging to one culture share common values and beliefs within that culture. That is true, but as we have seen, people can belong to more than one culture at a time. An individual may be disabled, Hispanic, and LGBTQIA and be part of an urban culture all at once. As the country has begun to strive to bring together and respect the many cultures making up the American mixing bowl (rather than melting pot), certain protections have been given to bias or discrimination based on sex, race, age, disability, and other individual characteristics. Legally these characteristics should not matter. For age, since the late 1940s unique characteristics of "generations" have been identified and analyzed. The first group, the baby boomers, are distinguished by being born between the end of World War II and 1964, resulting from soldiers coming home from war. Prior to this generations had generally been defined in 20-year increments, but the designation of a generation as the "13th" generation seems unlucky, so the term Generation X was created for the 1965 to 1980 group. The Millennial generation includes those coming of age at the turn of the 21st century, and Generation Z membership begins in 1997. By population they line up as follows:

- Baby boomers: Born between 1946 and 1964 (71.6 million in the United States)
- Gen X: Born between 1965 and 1979/80 (65.2 million people in the United States)
- Millennials: Born between 1981 and 1994/1996 (72.1 million in the United States)
- Gen Z: Born between 1997 and 2012/2015 (nearly 68 million in the United States) (Kasasa, 2021)

Generations have some distinguishing characteristics: Baby boomers have learned to us new technologies as productivity tools rather than for the social connectivity that developed as Millennials emerged. Baby boomers generally attempt to follow the rules, to achieve the American Dream.

Generation X (1965 to 1980) focuses more on work-life balance than climbing career ladders. Gen Xers, also labeled "latch-key kids," were the first "daycare" generation, with two working parents or a single or divorced parent. They have focused on self-development rather than marriage and children.

Millennials developed after GenXers and are often seen as technology experts who generate innovations, create startups, and work out of coffee shops. They were born between 1980 and 2000. Because they want it all, they seem confident and entitled. Millennials negotiate their own the rules rather than emulate their parents. The generation is successful and ambitious. However, dependance on social networking technology has had a negative effect on interpersonal skills and, as a result, depression is not unusual. As opposed to baby boomers, Millennials are interested in flexibility rather than simply additional pay as an incentive. They seek more vacation time, casual dress, and flexibility to work from home.

Finally, Generation Z members developed between 1995 and 2012. While still evolving, this under-20 group has always known computers and mobile technology (Ryback, 2016).

The relationship between generations and their related health has only recently been the subject of studies. A common view was health behaviors and status resulted from "Like father, like son" or a "chip off the old block." It has been generally accepted that lifestyle behavior is, and is often expected, to pass from parents to children in the same way as ethnic culture. In the health field, there is often an effort to break the generational connection of perceived behaviors that lead to ill health, such as eating fatty foods or smoking. This is sometimes tied to efforts to address poverty in which lack of resources and lack of education result in limited food and health care choices and limited knowledge of unhealthy outcomes. Multigenerational strategies have been proposed to break up the cycle where generation after generation are living in the same unhealthy lifestyle (Cheng et al., 2016).

Nevertheless, understanding the differences among generations has been the subject of several studies. One study conducted by OnePoll on behalf of Know Diabetes by Heart, a joint undertaking of the American Heart Association and the American Diabetes Association, in part surveyed the role health plays in experiencing different life moments across generations. The results were as follows:

Top "life moments": Generation Z (ages 18–23)

1. Travel somewhere new: 23.8% (tied 1, 2, and 3)
2. Buy a house: 23.8% (tied 1, 2, and 3)
3. Earn a diploma, degree, or certification: 23.8% (tied 1, 2, and 3)
4. Spend more time with friends: 23%
5. Reach a health goal: 22.2% (tied 5 and 6)
6. Have a child/children: 22.2% (tied 5 and 6)

Top "life moments": Millennials (ages 24–39)

1. Have a child/children: 36%
2. Buy a house: 31.6%

3. Travel somewhere new: 30%
4. Reach a health goal: 29.8%
5. Get married: 26.8%

Top "life moments": Generation X (ages 40–55)

1. Have a child/children: 42.6%
2. Get married: 37.2%
3. Buy a house: 34.2%
4. Travel somewhere new: 33.6%
5. Watch my child(ren) graduate: 32.8%

Top "life moments": Baby boomers (ages 56+)

1. Have a child/children: 40.6%
2. Get married: 39.2%
3. Watch my grandchildren grow up: 38%
4. Watch my child(ren) graduate: 35.4%
5. Retire: 35.2%

Source: Haaland (2020).

Considerations for Health Promotion and Program Planning

Generational differences result in differing perspectives on health care and approaches to well-being.

Baby Boomers

Boomers are becoming aged, are not necessarily in the best of health, are affected by being too sedentary, have too much stress, and eat with diets rich in sugary food. Boomers generally want health care that is relational rather than transactional. They also expect to communicate with medical professionals face-to-face, and they expect technological solutions to many of their health care needs. More than other generations, boomers want personal relationships with providers and expect solutions that help them stay active and feel young. They grew into using the internet from a life without it, but now routinely will research health issues on their own. As they are becoming aged, many are becoming caregivers to their parents or others. One study found that in a group of over 100,000 baby boomers, 24.2% were caretakers involved with care at least 20 hours per week and represented 38.5% of all caregivers (Miyawaki et al., 2020). With a greater life expectancy than previous generations, baby boomers have higher rates of chronic disease, more disability, and lower self-rated health. But they are less likely to smoke cigarettes and have lower rates of emphysema and myocardial infarction (King et al., 2013).

Generation X

Gen X is relatively demanding, and members of this generation, as the market model U.S. health system dictates, readily shop for health care as if they were shopping for retail goods and services. They expect to be allies in their care and will pursue second opinions as a matter of course. They are also sensitive to time and want to know exactly how long a visit or a treatment will take. Gen Xers are the key decision-makers for everybody, from their silent and boomer parents to their Gen Z kids—yet they are an often-ignored generation.

Millennials

Millennials typically avoid visits to a medical professional, and they try to eschew activities like checkups. More often they will use the internet to find out the reason for a health issue. They are particularly interested in convenience and low cost. Millennials have an easier relationship with authority than Gen Xers and may be more compliant with medical authority once engaged. Millennials lived entirely within the internet age and are highly technical and interactive and thus are open to technical solutions such as telemedicine.

Gen Z

Members of Gen Z still have much of their health care decisions made by their parents. The slightly older ones tend not to trust Big Pharma and health care systems. Gen Zs are enthusiastic about wearables and customization (Sandle, 2017).

Summary

In this chapter we discussed the barriers to care and the challenges encountered by cultures not defined by race or ethnicity in achieving good health and their interactions with health care services. Some cultures, such as LGBTQIA, are less likely to seek care because of fear of discrimination, and they tend to have higher incidences of diseases as a result. Farmworkers account for approximately 3 to 5 million people in the United States. They are mostly Hispanic people who work in almost every state. Poverty, unsettlement, legal issues, low education level, and harsh working conditions are their main challenges. They are at major risk for skin diseases and exposure to the sun and pesticides. AIDS is common among farmworkers due to lack of education, an increase in sexually transmitted diseases, and prostitution.

People face a wide variety of disabilities. People with disabilities have health challenges related to access to medical care and preventive services, oral health, high rates of smoking, and obesity.

Immigrants and refugees may have low literacy skills and have an array of physical and mental health issues. Refugees, in particular, are displaced peoples, and they may be unfamiliar with U.S. culture and face fear, depression, and other mental health issues, as well as physical problems such as poor nutrition.

The drug culture draws people from their racial and ethnic cultures into a group who believe their behavior is smart, fashionable, gratifying, or creative when in fact the culture fosters great harm to its members' health, whether it be smoking, legal or illegal pharmaceuticals, or alcohol. It places a large burden on the health system.

While members of all race and ethnic cultures are engaged in the drug culture, they are also part of a generational set of the population that has its own perspective and view of lifestyle and health care. The attributes of generational culture can affect how health care providers interact with their patients.

Review

1. Describe three roadblocks to accessing health care that are encountered by the LGBTQIA community and farmworkers.
2. Prepare three cultural competence recommendations for a clinic that provides services to farmworkers.
3. Outline what areas should be covered in a staff training session to address the needs of LGBTQIA clients.
4. Describe how discrimination toward farmworkers and LGBTQIA people affects their health and health care.
5. Describe some types of disabilities and cultural considerations to be considered when providing health services.
6. Define immigrant, asylee, alien, and refugee.
7. Explain how the drug culture affects the health care system.
8. Generally, in what years were following generations born: baby boomers, Generation X, Millennials, and Generation Z?

Activities

1. Select a nonethnic subculture, such as athletes, veterans, or prison inmates, and write a paper about the group. Discuss topics such as their demographics, culture, health issues, practices, and beliefs.
2. Watch the video "ASL and Deaf Culture" (https://www.youtube.com/watch?v=witq6X-zLWQk) and write a brief paper about the differences between hearing and nonhearing cultures and ways that the hearing culture can communicate with those who have impaired hearing.

3. Watch the video "The Hidden Crisis in Rural America" (https://www.youtube.com/watch?v=EIkqx-sAHpw) and write a brief summary about mental health services in rural America and some ideas on how to resolve the mental health crisis.

Case Study 1

Carlos is a 22 year old Salvadoran female to male transgender person. His parents died shortly after his birth and he was given into adoption to a well -known family in San Salvador City. Carlos was sexually abused throughout his childhood by his step-father. At 9 years old he began feeling distressed about his assigned female sex at birth and the gender roles that his family expected him to follow. Then at 13 years old he started cross-dressing. Since his arrival in the US, about 4 years ago he has been working as a bartender in a nightclub. He has been with the same sexual partner for the past six months. Today he is visiting the clinic for a transgender health assessment.

1. What methods can the provider use to establish a relationship with Carlos as a patient in a culturally sensitive manner?
2. How do you gather the general health history for a Female to Male transgender patient and how do you perform the physical exam?
3. Identify ways the provider can gain insight into Carlos's lifestyle and his knowledge about HIV.
4. Should the provider encourage Carlos to have an HIV test?
5. What Primary Health Prevention and Screening tests should you recommend to Carlos?
6. Should you do a screening for depression at this visit?
7. Carlos is considering hormone therapy, what issues about fertility and sexual function should you discuss?

Source: AETC-NMC, "Case Study 17: Addressing HIV Care and Latino Model," https://www.aetcnmc.org/documents/case-study-17.pdf.

Case Study 2

Mary, a 33-year-old Native American male to female transgender person, wants to look into services you provide. She has not legally changed her name, so her documents display her given male name, Mark. She is new in transition and dresses in high heels and tight skirts. She produces facial hair (which is exposed). She looks to be very nervous and shy and does not look anyone in the eyes. Mary has been diagnosed HIV positive for 3 years and has just begun a relationship with Robert, who is HIV negative.

1. How can the provider establish a sense of trust with the patient?
2. What can the provider do to gain a sense of Mary's knowledge about HIV, how it is contracted, and how it is treated?
3. What social support, if any, should Mary be offered?
4. How can the provider fulfill their ethical responsibility to Mary and her partner(s)?
5. Discuss other cultural competence issues that may impact retention into care and treatment.

Source: AETC-NMC, "Case Study 37: Addressing HIV Care and Transgender Communities," https://www.aetcnmc.org/documents/case-study-37.pdf. Copyright © by AIDS Education and Training Center-National Multicultural Center (AETC-NMC) at Howard University. Reprinted with permission.

References

Abbott, P., & Chase D. (2008). Culture and substance abuse: Impact of culture affects approach to treatment. *Psychiatric Times, 25*(1). https://www.psychiatrictimes.com/view/culture-and-substance-abuse-impact-culture-affects-approach-treatment

AIDS Education and Training Center, National Multicultural Center, Howard University. (n.d.b.). *Case study adapted from addressing HIV care and transgender communities #37.* https://www.aetcnmc.org/documents/case-study-37.pdf

Black Hawk College. (2014). *Types of disabilities.* https://www.bhc.edu/student-resources/disability-services/types-and-definitions

Brown, S. E. (2002). What is disability culture? *Disability Studies Quarterly, 22*(2), 34–50.

Cancer.net. (2021). *Sarcoma - Kaposi: Statistics.* https://www.cancer.net/cancer-types/sarcoma-kaposi/statistics

Centers for Disease Control and Prevention. (2016). *Substance abuse.* https://www.cdc.gov/msmhealth/substance-abuse.htm

Centers for Disease Control and Prevention. (2018a). *Disability and health data system.* https://dhds.cdc.gov/LP?CategoryId=GENHLTH&IndicatorId=HEALTH&ShowFootnotes=true&View=Table&yearId=YR3&stratCatId1=DISSTAT&stratId1=DISABL&stratCatId2=RACE&stratId2=&responseId=YESNO01&dataValueTypeId=AGEADJPREV&MapClassifierId=quantile&MapClassifierCount=5

Centers for Disease Control and Prevention. (2018b). *Disability and health data system fact sheet.* https://www.cdc.gov/ncbddd/disabilityandhealth/documents/DHDS_FactSheet-508.pdf

Centers for Disease Control and Prevention. (September 16, 2020a). https://www.cdc.gov/ncbddd/disabilityandhealth/materials/infographic-disabilities-ethnicity-race.html

Centers for Disease Control and Prevention. (2020b). *Adults with disabilities: Ethnicity and race.* https://www.cdc.gov/ncbddd/disabilityandhealth/materials/infographic-disabilities-ethnicity-race.html

Centers for Disease Control and Prevention. (2021). *Refugee health profiles.* https://www.cdc.gov/immigrantrefugeehealth/profiles/index.html

Cheng, T., Johnson, S. B., & Goodman, E. (2016). Breaking the intergenerational cycle of disadvantage: The three generation approach. *Pediatrics, 137*(6), e20152467. https://pediatrics.aappublications.org/content/137/6/e20152467

Farmworker Justice. (2019). *Selected statistics on farmworkers (2015–16 data).* http://www.farmworkerjustice.org/wp-content/uploads/2019/05/NAWS-Data-FactSheet-05-13-2019-final.pdf

Festa, A. (2020, September 5). *7 most common health conditions among baby boomers.* Healthgrades. https://www.healthgrades.com/right-care/aging-well/7-most-common-health-conditions-among-baby-boomers

Fresno County Hispanic Commission on Alcohol and Drug Abuse Services, Inc. (2016). *The Aztecs and alcohol.* http://hispaniccommission.org/index.php/en/the-aztecs-and-alcohol

Gay and Lesbian Medical Association. (2001). *Healthy People 2010 companion document for lesbian, gay, bisexual and transgender (LGBT) health.* https://lgbtqi2stoolkit.net/pdf/GLMA_LGBT-Healthy-People_2010.pdf

Haaland, M. (2020, July 7). Study shows Gen Z is more concerned about their health than boomers. *NY Post.* https://nypost.com/2020/07/07/gen-z-more-concerned-about-their-health-than-boomers-according-to-study

Haynie, D. (2017, February 9). 10 Countries with the most refugees in the U.S. *U.S. News and World Report.* https://www.usnews.com/news/best-countries/slideshows/10-countries-with-the-most-refugees-in-the-us

Henderson, W. (2007, October 7). *HRC, GLMA release inaugural Healthcare Equality Index.* The Advocate. http://www.advocate.com/health/health-news/2007/10/02/hrc-glma-release-inaugural-healthcare-equality-index

Howard University College of Medicine. (n.d.). Addressing HIV care and health literacy. https://www.aetcnmc.org/documents/case-study-38.pdf

JBS International. (2018). *Findings from the National Agricultural Workers Survey (NAWS) 2015–2016.* https://www.dol.gov/sites/dolgov/files/ETA/naws/pdfs/NAWS_Research_Report_13.pdf

Johns, M. M., Lowry, R., Rasberry, C. N., Dunville, R., Robin, L., Pampati, S., Stone, D. M., & Mercer Kollar, L. M. (2018). Violence victimization, substance use, and suicide risk among sexual minority high school students—United States, 2015–2017. *Morbidity and Mortality Monthly Report, 67*(43), 1211–1215. https://www.cdc.gov/mmwr/volumes/67/wr/mm6743a4.htm?s_cid=mm6743a4_e

Kasasa. (2021). *Boomers, Gen X, Gen Y, and Gen Z explained.* https://www.kasasa.com/articles/generations/gen-x-gen-y-gen-z

King, D., Matheson, E., Chirina, S., Shankar, A., & Broman-Fulks, J. (2013). The status of baby boomers' health in the United States: The healthiest generation? *JAMA Internal Medicine, 173*(5), 385–386. https://jamanetwork.com/journals/jamainternalmedicine/fullarticle/1568518

Matthews, K. A., Croft, J. B., Lui, Y., Lu, H., Kanny, D., Wheaton, A. G., Cunningham, T. J., Kahn, L. K., Caraballo, R. S., Holt, J. B., Eke, P. I., & Giles, W. H. (2017). Health-related behaviors by urban-rural county classification—United States, 2013. *Morbidity and Mortality Weekly Report, 66*(5), 1–8. https://www.cdc.gov/mmwr/volumes/66/ss/ss6605a1.htm

Meitt, M., Knudson, A., Gilbert, T., Yu, A. C.-.T., Tanenbaum, E., Ormson, E., TenBroeck, S., Bayne, A., Popat, S., & NORC Walsh Center for Rural Health Analysis. (2014). *2014 update of the rural-urban chartbook.* https://ruralhealth.und.edu/projects/health-reform-policy-research-center/pdf/2014-rural-urban-chartbook-update.pdf

Migration Policy Institute. (2020). *U.S. annual refugee resettlement ceilings and number of refugees admitted, 1980–present.* https://www.migrationpolicy.org/programs/data-hub/charts/us-annual-refugee-resettlement-ceilings-and-number-refugees-admitted-united

Migration Policy Institute. (2021, February 11). *Frequently requested statistics on immigrants and immigration in the United States.* https://www.migrationpolicy.org/article/frequently-requested-statistics-immigrants-and-immigration-united-states-2020

Miller, S. (2021, February 24). Society is changing: A record 5.6% of US adults identify as LGBTQ, poll shows. And young people are driving the numbers. *USA Today*. https://www.usatoday.com/story/news/nation/2021/02/24/lgbtq-gallup-poll-more-us-adults-identify-lgbtq/4532664001/

Miyawaki, C. E., Bouldin, E. D., Taylor, C. A., & McGuire, L. C. (2020). Baby boomers as caregivers: Results from the Behavioral Risk Factor Surveillance System in 44 states, the District of Columbia, and Puerto Rico, 2015–2017. *Preventing Chronic Disease, 17*. https://www.cdc.gov/pcd/issues/2020/20_0010.htm

Moy, E, M.D., Garcia, M., Bastian, B., Rossen, L., Ingram, D., Faul, M., Massetti G., Thomas, C., Hong, Y., Yoon, P., & Iademarco, M. (2017). Leading causes of death in nonmetropolitan and metropolitan areas—United States, 1999–2014. *Morbidity and Mortality Weekly Report, 66*(1), 1–8.

National Center for Drug Abuse Statistics. (n.d.). *Home page*. https://drugabusestatistics.org/

National Center for Farmworker Health. (2020). Facts About Agricultural Workers, http://www.ncfh.org/facts-about-agricultural-workers.html

National Center for Health Workforce Analysis. (2014). *Distribution of U.S. health care providers residing in rural and urban areas*. U.S. Department of Health and Human Services. https://www.ruralhealthinfo.org/assets/1275-5131/rural-urban-workforce-distribution-nchwa-2014.pdf

Office of Disease Prevention and Health Promotion. (n.d.). *Lesbian, gay, bisexual, and transgender health*. https://www.healthypeople.gov/2020/topics-objectives/topic/lesbian-gay-bisexual-and-transgender-health

Ranker.com. (2021). *Famous people who died of lung cancer*. https://www.ranker.com/list/famous-people-who-died-of-lung-cancer/reference

Routley, N. (2021). *These powerful maps show the extremes of U.S. population density*. Visual Capitalist. https://www.visualcapitalist.com/maps-extremes-us-population-density/

Rural Health Information Hub. (2019). *Rural health disparities*. https://www.ruralhealthinfo.org/topics/rural-health-disparities

Ryback, R. (2016, February 26). From baby boomers to Generation Z, a detailed look at the characteristics of each generation. *Psychology Today*. https://www.psychologytoday.com/us/blog/the-truisms-wellness/201602/baby-boomers-generation-z

Sandle, T. (2017, July. 6). *Boomers, Gen Xers, millennials, Gen Z: Healthcare expectations*. Digital Journal. https://www.digitaljournal.com/life/boomers-gen-xers-millennials-gen-z-healthcare-expectations/article/497028

Scoles, P. (2020, July 1). *Drug culture and the culture of recovery*. The Sober World. https://issuu.com/soberworld/docs/july20_issue, p. 11.

Shear, M., & Kanno-Youngs, Z., (2021, May. 3). In another reversal, Biden raises limit on number of refugees allowed into the U.S. *The New York Times*. https://www.nytimes.com/2021/05/03/us/politics/biden-refugee-limit.html

Siple, L., Greer, L., & Holcolm, B. R. (2003). Deaf culture. *PEPNet 2*. http://www.pepnet.org/sites/default/files/71PEPNet%20Tipsheet%20Deaf%20Culture.pdf

Smart, T. (2015). *Study finds high risk of cancer among older people living with HIV*. http://www.aidsmap.com/Study-finds-high-rates-of-cancer-among-older-people-living-with-HIV/page/2950216/

Society for the Psychology for Sexual Orientation and Gender Identity. (2020, April). *A growing number of states ban sexual orientation change efforts*. https://www.apadivisions.org/division-44/publications/newsletters/division/2020/04/ban-conversion-therapy

Time. (2013). Millennials: The me-me-me-generation. https://time.com/247/millennials-the-me-me-me-generation/

University of Washington. (2015). *Strategies for working with people who have disabilities*. http://www.washington.edu/doit/strategies-working-people-who-have-disabilities

U.S. Department of Agriculture. (2020a). *Farm labor*. https://www.ers.usda.gov/topics/farm-economy/farm-labor

U.S. Department of Labor. (2018). *Who works America's farms?* https://sites.tufts.edu/deborahschildkraut/files/2020/05/Who-Works-Americas-Farms.pdf

U.S. Sentencing Commission. (2016). *Quick facts: Drug trafficking offenses.* https://www.ussc.gov/sites/default/files/pdf/research-and-publications/quick-facts/Quick_Facts_Drug_Trafficking_2016.pdf

Wisconsin Department of Health Services. (2021) *Do's and Don'ts When Interacting with a Person who is Blind.* (https://www.dhs.wisconsin.gov/obvi/adjustment/dos-donts.htm)

CREDITS

Fig. 11.1: Source: https://www.cdc.gov/ncbddd/disabilityandhealth/materials/infographic-disabilities-ethnicity-race.html.

Fig. 11.2: Source: Adapted from https://www.visualcapitalist.com/maps-extremes-us-population-density/.

CHAPTER 12

The Macro Cultures Related to Health and the Health Care System

America's health care system is neither healthy, caring, nor a system.
— WALTER CRONKITE

I've been asked a lot for my view on American health care. Well, "it would be a good idea," to quote Gandhi.
— PAUL FARMER

KEY CONCEPTS AND TERMS

Capitalism
Class
Commerce
Lower class
Middle class
Targeted marketing
Upper class
Value pricing

LEARNING OBJECTIVES

After reading this chapter, you should be able to do the following:

1. Explain how commerce can affect health.
2. Identify how capitalism can reduce access to health care.
3. Explain how health consumer values affect health.
4. Describe why government is involved in health care research.

Introduction

The overarching culture in the United States has its own ideology of what is healthy. For example, some view a tan as healthy in the United States while other cultures see paler skin as healthy. Smaller body sizes are viewed as healthy, yet that is not the case in all cultures. In addition, there are many symbols related to health, such as a pink ribbon signifying breast cancer awareness.

The health care system has its own culture as well. It has its own language and symbols as well as structures and hierarchies. It follows the biomedical disease model, has different levels of care, and has a complex system; providers and patients have roles and responsibilities; and it emphasizes technology. The health insurance companies, pharmaceutical companies, governments and other macroeconomic participants wield a strong influence on the system that, in turn, impacts how we view, access, prioritize, and pursue health.

In this chapter we look at the interrelated economic associated beliefs and perspectives of commerce, social classes, and capitalism. After a short introduction, terminology is described before a brief description of each "subculture" of commerce, social class, and capitalism is provided. The differences between them are explained and the nature of their relationship to all patients in the country are discussed. Behavior risk factors and common health problems are addressed, followed by suggestions for health promotion and program planning.

The United States is built on an economic philosophy brought to America by Europeans. That is our economic culture, and it affects how health care is paid for and delivered. The Europeans brought the modern, free enterprise, marketplace economic model, and everyone interacts with this fundamental cultural framework of the country. In fact, the U.S. Constitution was drawn up after 10 years of experience with the Articles of Confederation, in part to facilitate the free flow of goods and services across state lines.

Some free enterprise activities that emerged from **commerce** (the exchange of goods and services for money or other items of value) have improved the health of all peoples. For instance, drug manufacturing, physical fitness gymnasiums, vitamin companies, hospitals, and health insurance companies have all flourished under the free enterprise system and contributed to improved health in one way or another. In addition, the development and sale of nonhealth-related commodities such as cell phones and computers have enabled improved communication with health providers through email and texting, while telemedicine has greatly improved the delivery of health care for many people. Commerce has led to negative health consequences as well. In this section, we look at commerce's impact on three nonethnic populations affected by the culture of commerce: consumers; members of the upper, middle, and lower classes; and everyone, as a group, living under the culture of capitalism.

Terminology

Health care is a business. Health products and services are everywhere in our lives, and people spend a tremendous amount of money on health. To understand some of the complex interactions of business on all people in America, regardless of ethnicity or race, it is important to clarify the meaning of certain terms. As stated previously, commerce is the exchange of goods and services for money or other items of value. Commerce has existed throughout history and across all civilizations to one extent or another. Every country in the world has some approach to providing health care yet approaches health care differently. Most developed countries in the world do not have as "free" a market as the United States, as their government often has a significant role in setting standards, conducting unprofitable basic research, and paying for direct medical services. These differences in approaches are related to culture. Culture drives commerce as cultural values help determine what is purchased, how it is purchased, and who pays for it.

Social **class** is another attribute that affects health in most cultures but differs substantially by country. Class results in essentially three categories, each with different general characteristics. There is an **upper class** with the most wealth and a concentration of power, a **middle class** that generally has a comfortable or acceptable financial means for life with some access to power, and the **lower class** that is generally trading their labor for wages that provide minimal lifestyle options if even subsistence.

In the United States, the economic philosophy of **capitalism** has a particular presence in health care. Capitalism is based on the general concept that capital (resources) is best used to engage in activities that can produce goods and services that potential buyers find of value and can be exchanged for what the goods and products cost to produce and include an additional premium return called profit. Not all efforts or investments of capital ultimately returns profit, but the potential to do so drives many efforts to attain success despite the general experience that only one in five business that start survive more than 5 years. It is the anticipation of profit that drives the activities in this economy. Sometimes the effort to invest capital, produce a product, market it, sell it, and obtain a profitable result is not possible (e.g., research on the effects of herbs on health). In the health care field this has led to the government funding some "basic research" through such entities as the National Institutes of Health. For example, research into deoxyribonucleic acid (DNA), ribonucleic acid (RNA), and antibodies, paid for by the government, was used by major pharmaceutical manufactures to undertake risky capital investments to develop COVID-19 vaccines. But most of the time, free enterprise capitalism allows a wide range of choice for people to invest capital in everything, from expensive innovations such as magnetic resonance imaging to street corner health clinics, or to even cell phone applications to measure heart rates.

To entice buyers to purchase something, including health care goods and services, producers use marketing and advertising in one form or another to present the value of their items to potential buyers, also known as consumers. Often marketing becomes focused on certain types of people with certain types of health issues or to particular types of people by age or culture through **targeted marketing**. Everyone reading this book fits into this overall economic and social structure by obtaining health care goods and services through exchanging something of value as a buyer/consumer. This is why by being a member of an ethnic or racial culture you are also a member of a social class, living in a capitalist economy with ever-present commercial activity.

Usually, consumers make choices based on concepts of quality and price such that the value to us is worth the amount exchanged for it. The uniqueness of a product or service may simply be determined by the seller who judges the highest price consumers will tolerate and still generate enough volume to support business goals. This is often the case with items that are protected by patents (e.g., for medications or unique or very specialized services). To reach particular consumers a recent practice has been to justify price based on the "value" to the person of avoiding the dire medical consequences of not using the product regardless of production costs. This "value pricing" is discussed more later in this chapter.

Health care services often do not follow this typical economic pattern of decision-making based on price and quality. Because in the U.S. culture health insurance is offered by most employers, price shopping does not typically occur, and providers do not openly list prices. For example, if someone has a $25 copay for a medication, that copay is usually the same the regardless of the cost of the medication. Therefore, consumers do not price shop as their out-of-pocket cost is the same regardless of the cost of the medication. Some items are difficult to place a value on. How do we compare the value of an X-ray at one facility over the value of the X-ray at another facility? And finding the price to be charged of an X-ray is not easy.

Consumers and Their Health

People from every culture in the United States confront the influence of commerce. They are consumers who are enticed to make purchases related to their health. Consumers are subjected to enticements to buy both helpful healthy products (e.g., pedometers) and services, as well as those that are unhealthy, such as cigarettes or supersized portions of fast food. This process occurs because of our capitalistic culture.

Americans spend a great deal of money on health care. In 2019, Americans' per capita health care expenses were about $11,100, the highest spending among two dozen or so of the most affluent countries (Peter G. Peterson Foundation, 2020).

In theory a full and free open commercial marketplace can optimize the availability of goods and services and minimize cost. While the United States does not have a fully open marketplace due to factors affecting availability and price, such as patents and tariffs, it has created a vast opportunity for consumers at all levels. However, marketing and peer pressure in a consumer-oriented society can compel people to remain engaged in an unceasing stressful struggle to make money and spend it. Yet there is little correlation between increased income and increased happiness across society. Evidence suggests that greater consumption beyond that necessary for basic subsistence does not create significant satisfaction and happiness. Research has shown that, across many nations, there is no correlation between increased income and increased happiness (Etzioni, 2017).

Some negative health consequences of consumers responding positively to commercial enticements continued and even increased engagement in unhealthy activities and products. Examples include negative impacts from tobacco use and lung cancer, automobile smog and asthma, and supersized fast food and obesity. The fast-food industry has capitalized on the fast-paced culture, and rates of obesity, diabetes, and other health problems are on the rise. The fast-food industry spends a large amount of money on advertising, leading to an annual exposure to consumers of thousands of commercials for junk food and fast food. In addition, television (TV) time can mean decreased physical activity. There is evidence that food and beverage marketing on TV may be responsible for the TV-obesity correlation (Harvard T.H. Chan School of Public Health, 2021). Medical research confirms that the more television children watch, the more likely they are to be overweight (IS Global, 2019). The potential conflict with their children over which purchases to make may contribute to parents' overall long-term stress levels (University of Arizona, 2020).

Internet advertising is larger than TV advertising in amount spent and is growing. For 2018, online advertising cost about $107.5 billion, $36 billion higher than the cost of television advertising ($71.0 billion) (Top Media, 2019). Food companies spent $11 billion on TV ads in 2017, and 80% of that, about $8.8 billion, was spent on their unhealthy products, including sugary soda, fast food, candy, and unhealthy snacks (Weber, 2019). It was estimated that medical marketing reached $30 billion in 2016, an increase of $12 billion from 1997. Prescription drug advertisements appeared 5 million times in just 1 year (Tanner, 2019).

Although cigarette ads are no longer permitted on TV, ads directed at potential consumers for prescription drugs have increased dramatically. The United States and New Zealand are the only two developed countries that allow direct-to-consumer ads on TV, radio, and billboards, and in magazines and newspapers. Expansion into broadcast direct-to-consumer ads climbed due to a change in federal regulations in the late 1990s. The new regulations require broadcast ads to include only "major statements" of the risks and benefits of the drug, along with directions to alternate information sources for full disclosure.

With all the exposure to ads related to health, it is important that accurate information is presented. The government takes steps to assure consumers have enough accurate information to make informed decisions as opposed to being led into purchasing based solely on enticing ads. For instance, the Food and Drug Administration inspects and grades certain foods and medicines, there are some truth-in-advertising measures in place, food packaging must include calorie and nutrition information, and warnings are required to be on certain drugs as well as alcohol and tobacco products. Even fast-food chains are required to provide calorie counts on their menus to help inform the public.

The ads can entice the purchasing of good and services. The increase in purchases of items, such as medications and services, contribute to rising health care costs. These increases can be passed on to consumers through methods such as higher copays, deductibles, and cost sharing for insurance coverage. This has an impact on health. For example, high drug prices contribute to medication nonadherence among patients, with a quarter of patients not filling a prescription for themselves or a family member due to cost (Ellis, 2019).

Since World War II, per-capita income has tripled, but levels of life satisfaction remain about the same. Studies also indicate that many consumers within capitalist cultures feel unsatisfied, because other people make and spend even more, creating a sense of relative deprivation (Etzioni, 2017).

Americans' Reports of Postponing Medical Care Due to Costs, 2001-2019

Within the last twelve months, have you or a member of your family put off any sort of medical treatment because of the cost you would have to pay? (If yes) When you put off this medical treatment, was it for a condition or illness that was very serious, somewhat serious, not very serious, or not at all serious?

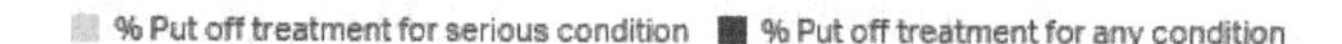

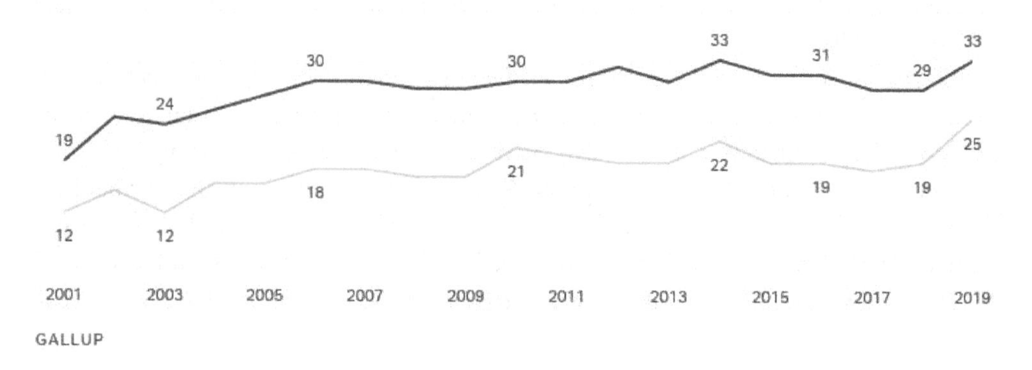

Figure 12.1 Postponing medication care due to costs, 2001–2019.

In one study, 32% of survey respondents indicated that they could not afford to live a healthy lifestyle (Stewart, 2018). In 2014, an American Psychological Association survey on stress in the United States found 54% of Americans thought they had just enough or not enough money each month to meet their expenses and that money was the nation's greatest source of stress. Seventy-two percent of adults reported feeling stressed about money at least some of the time, with nearly 25% judging their stress "extreme" (Bethune, 2015).

Since 2001, there has been about a 50% increase in the percentage of Americans saying that they chose not to seek medical care because of costs to them. These choices can lead to more severe care needs later and have a significant impact on health care services. One indicator of the stress that delayed care can put on health care is the use of hospital emergency departments. According to the American Hospital Association, patient visits to emergency departments in community hospitals increased 19% between 2001 and 2016 and has likely continue climbing. While this may be due in part to the aging of the population and proximity to hospitals, it may also be indicative of a greater need for emergency care due to lack of routine care (Saad, 2019).

These rising costs are changing consumer behavior. Instead of routinely looking to health care professionals for answers, American consumers are now looking for more cost-effective options, including self-care and self-treatment. However, consumers want choices such as nondrug treatments, and producers are responding to provide drugs, dietary supplements, and even devices to meet consumer interests. Partly in response to the COVID-19 pandemic, consumers are relying more on internet-based information of all kinds, including health. Expanded online research and searches for health care products have been augmented by new government expansion of access to telehealth. As consumer behavior reduces profit for traditional health care, some companies, such as Merck, Boehringer Ingelheim, and Pfizer, are moving from traditional consumer health to concentrate on more highly profitable prescription drugs. This has created opportunities for more traditional consumer-packaged goods and food companies to move to the consumer health space to meet changing consumer expectations (McKinsey, 2021).

An ongoing issue is how American consumers want to obtain their health care when they need it. According to a 2015 survey by The Commonwealth Foundation, *The New York Times*, and Harvard University, the majority of U.S. consumers believe Americans should have a right to health care. They also believe that not all Americans are receiving the same care, and most believe all people should receive the same quality and access to care as White Americans. They do not think it should go so far as to be the same as available to the upper class. A strong majority of Americans highly approve of Medicare and Medicaid but are cautious of federal government operations. A majority of Americans (60%) would like to either improve the existing Affordable Care Act or move to a Medicare-for-all program (Harvard T.H. Chan School of Public Health, 2019).

They also support health care delivered by nonprofit hospitals. But values are different for other aspects of health care. A definite minority, who are generally affluent, employed, covered by private health care plans and opposed to new taxes, believe a state-run health care system would be the best option (Harvard T.H. Chan School of Public Health, 2010).

The impact of the changing consumer expectations related to health has not been uniform across U.S. cultural groups, but it has affected everyone from all cultures. In the next section, we describe how the culture of multiple classes impacts individual health and access to health care.

Social Classes and Health

Despite some profound differences between cultures, all share a stratification of social classes. Understanding social class as culture is a relatively recent idea, with research demonstrating the influence class position can have on individual behavior and identity (Bittman, 2016).

A 2020 survey from Gallup found 72% of Americans said they belonged to the middle or working classes. In determining their social class, people often do not just think about income, but include other factors, including education, location, and family history (Snider & Kerr, 2020).

The size of someone's paycheck or income is only one factor contributing to overall sense of wealth. Many times, net worth is considered as well. Net worth is everything owned minus all liabilities. For instance, net worth is calculated by taking the value of a home, cars, retirement funds, financial accounts, and other assets and subtracting any debts or payments owed.

The Upper Class

The upper class, from an economic point of view, have better access to higher quality health care. They have resources to travel to care provider locations and even partake, if so inclined, in medical tourism and seek care worldwide if necessary. Health insurance may not be needed as individuals in this class may rely on their own resources. Lifestyle habits affecting health are usually well within their control. They have the best access to healthy food, opportunities for exercise, and choices for constructive social interaction; can engage with the best available health care, even if at remote locations; purchase health gadgets to protect and monitor health; and live in healthy neighborhoods. This is not to say that the rich all see health care the same way or live a healthy lifestyle.

Within the upper class culture, two distinct factions have conflicted and have had important consequences for all health care consumers. Historically, the New England elite have amassed significant wealth but had a cultural philosophy different from the culture derived from the Southern elite. The New England elite generally the idea that once a fortune is made, the concept of *nobleese oblige* requires that some effort be made to take care of the greater good and the less fortunate, including their health. Members of the community had a strong moral duty to care for the sick, support education and provide for the poor to maximize each person's liberty to live in dignity and achieve their potential. This view of "ordered liberty" is still an active element of American class culture. This is reflected in philanthropies funded by the Carnegie, Ford, Rockefeller, Gates, and Kennedy families that fund health programs and research. However, the Southern elite did not share the *noblesse oblige* philosophy (Robinson, 2013).

Nobody had the authority to tell a Southern aristocrat what to do with resources under the aristocrat's direct control. When a Southern conservatives fear losing liberty (the power or scope to act as one pleases) it is the loss of control over the people and property under their control that is concerning. Anything given to lower status people reduces the freedom of the upper classes to use those people as they please. Thus, expansion of rights and services is not acceptable, resulting in, for one, traditional Southern opposition to universal health care. This general conflict is fundamental to the resistance to national health care. This difference significantly limits changes sought by most health care consumers, such as eliminating denial of services to people with preexisting health conditions.

The Middle Class

The middle class has more restrictions on its access to health care than the upper class. Most are employees or small business owners who usually do need health insurance to fully engage with health care resources and do not have as much ability to access specialists. The middle class generally will have resources to purchase healthy food and to keep healthy if they chose. However, middle-class economic progress has not kept up with that of the upper or the lower class. There is growth in middle-class income that is due to the rise in women's labor force participation rates, as increased effort is made to keep up, which impacts parenting, relationships, and health (Maciolek & Van Drie, 2021).

Despite middle-class families working more with only modest financial gains, health actually became worse. For example, between 2000 and 2018 the percentage of middle-class persons with diabetes increased from 7.1 to 10.5 (Maciolek & Van Drie, 2021).

The Lower Class

The lower class usually are employees who make minimal salaries or could be among the unemployed. They are fortunate if they have access to health care insurance. It is not that the poor chose not to have health insurance, but without access to employer-paid health insurance reliance is placed on government-provided Medicaid; support from family, friends, and neighbors; or even full reliance on emergency room services. They tend to purchase unhealthy fast food due to cost and availability. They generally are unable to afford items to help them stay healthy such as gym memberships.

Obesity, diabetes, heart disease, kidney disease, and liver disease are all two to three times more common in families whose income is less than $35,000 when compared to those who have a family income greater than $100,000 (Stewart, 2018).

Among low-educated, middle-aged Whites, the death rate in the United States increased between 1999 and 2018 and is unique among advanced economies. Supporting the trend was the rapid increase in what has been called "deaths of despair" by the CDC, which includes suicides and alcohol- and drug-related deaths (Colpe, 2020).

DID YOU KNOW?

In 2018, 72% of smokers lived in low-income areas. There are about 375,000 tobacco retailers in the United States, which is almost 27 times more than McDonald's and 28 times more than Starbucks, and they are disproportionately situated in low-income communities. Low-income neighborhoods are also more likely to have tobacco retailers near schools than other neighborhoods (The Truth Initiative, 2018).

Capitalism and Health

Crossing all aspects of health care, including all cultures, is the fundamental principles of capitalism. Capitalism is an economic system characterized by private or corporate ownership of capital, by investments that are determined by private decision, and by prices, production, and the distribution of goods that are determined mainly by competition in a free market (Merriam-Webster, n.d.). While commerce involving exchanging goods and services for compensation has occurred throughout history and across all cultures, capitalism has developed since the decline of feudalism in the Middle Ages. The concept of has been especially championed in the United States, where the culture of individual autonomy, freedom, strong work ethic, and self-reliance have contributed to the United States having the most robust economic system in the world. In America, these cultural attributes have led to affluent private sector health company interests blocking public funding for health except for very basic services. In many other countries the interplay between capital and labor has resulted in mixed public/private health care system (Goodman, 2013).

As stated previously, health care costs in the United States continue to rise. A relatively recent trend in marketing health care products and services is the move from "cost plus fee" pricing for patient services to "**value pricing**" aimed specifically at patient emotions and fears. The move to value-based pricing posed the possibility that health care costs could dramatically increase. Particularly in the pharmaceutical area value is increasingly determined by the seller, with a shift from cost-based sales to a more emotional-based decision regarding "what it's worth to the patient." For instance, the allergic reaction preventative product EpiPen price increased more than 600% between 2007 and 2015 with little or no improvement in the product itself, because the EpiPen is a potentially life-saving device so there is a high value to the product. U.S. patients disproportionately use more drugs for legal medical care than other countries, and prices can be 80–150% more than elsewhere for identical drugs with the same health results (Ellis, 2019).

Another feature of our capitalistic and commercial culture is the U.S. workers' willingness to commute long distances to make an income. These choices can be harmful to health, mental health, and well-being. Lengthy commutes can cause obesity, neck pain, stress, insomnia, loneliness, and divorce. A study found that a commute of 45 minutes or longer by one spouse increased the chance of divorce by 40% (Stewart, 2018).

Another consideration is the availability of care providers. The United States has been in last place five times among health care systems in high-income countries (see **Figure 12.2**), yet doctors are paid almost twice as much as in other countries. This

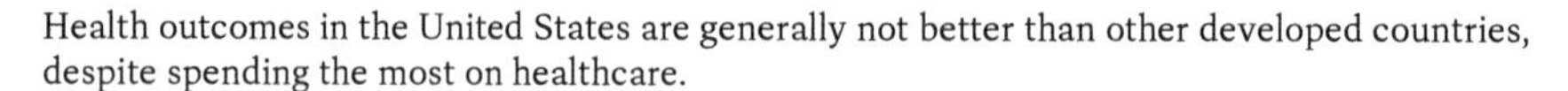

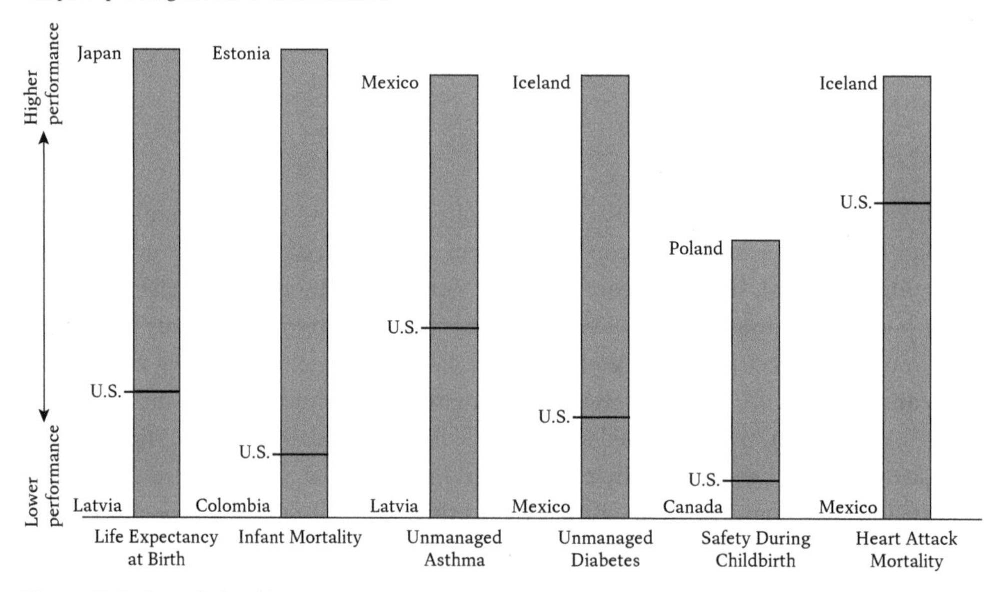

Figure 12.2 Country health outcomes.

may, in part, be due to cartel-like nature of U.S. medical professions, their influence on the number of training positions at medical schools, the availability of residencies, the licensing of foreign-trained doctors, and the role of nurse practitioners. Physician organizations and other professional organizations can limit the competition to their own members (Stewart, 2018).

But the competitive free enterprise culture, in cooperation with government, can work impressively. In response to the COVID-19 pandemic in 2020, major drug companies responded to expedite the development of effective vaccines as large financial incentives existed. Building on science discoveries identified in prior government research, and with the government waiving a number of regulations, several vaccines were developed within 1 year when often a vaccine for a new illness can take 5 years. And capitalism worked best to develop effective solutions.

Behavioral Risk Factors and Common Health Problems

In response to commercial marketing, Americans of all walks of life have responded for the profit-oriented companies, and Americans' health continues to decline as a result. Smoking, drinking alcohol, drinking sugary drinks, and fatty fast-food enticements such as triple-layer burgers with bacon and double cheese have driven increases in many health conditions. Research by the World Health Organization found increased fast-food sales related directly to an increase in body mass index, and it makes up about 11% of the average American diet (De Vogli et al., 2014). Another study demonstrated that added sugars from items like soda and energy drinks make up at least 10% of the calories the average American eats in a day, and about one in 10 people obtain one quarter or more of their calories from added sugar (Corliss, 2014). So it is not just how much we eat, but what we eat.

Lung cancer, alcoholism, diabetes, and heart disease are endemic to the overall American culture of commerce. In response, there are hundreds of ads directed at consumers who are asked to talk to their doctor, urge the prescribing of pharmaceuticals to address food- and drug-induced illnesses with the assurance that if a person cannot pay the full price, the company will take what it can get and offer some kind of discount. Additionally, it has created business opportunities for treatment centers, rehabilitation programs, diet programs, and gymnasiums to counter the problems developed through individual choices driven by commercial efforts to sell unhealthy food and drugs.

The overall leading causes of death in the United States do not track our topic of commerce, class, and capitalism specifically, but because all people in the United States are subject to this culture, the causes of death for all Americans are presented here. There are surprising causes on this list, except of course COVID-19, which cut unevenly across all segments of society. In 2020, The United States had the most incidents and deaths in the world due to COVID-19. One aspect of national experience was the cross messaging on how to address the pandemic. The national government

BOX 12.1 The 10 Leading Causes of Death Among all Americans in 2020

Heart disease

Cancer

COVID-19

Unintentional injury

Stroke

Chronic respiratory disease

Alzheimer's disease

Diabetes

Influenza and pneumonia

Kidney disease

Source: Ahmad et al. (2021).

gradually established a simple message, based on "following the science" to wear a face mask, keep a social distance of 6 feet or more between people in public, and wash hands regularly. There was widespread resistance to government recommendations that generally aligned with the geographical distribution of "conservative attitudes" based on the historic Southern upper class culture opposing government, demanding individual rights and autonomy, and opposing restrictions on freedoms. It has yet to be determined how much impact this cultural conflict had on the overall outcomes. Certain "science-based" facts are indisputable; the old, people with preexisting conditions, and care providers were substantially at risk and were among the most impacted. We have seen how the capitalistic free enterprise system effectively developed science-based preventive vaccines, but the cultural conflict over messaging and personal responsibility has yet to be fully assessed.

WHAT DO YOU THINK?

Health care marketing impacts you, one way or another, every day. Often the ads suggest potential consumers should ask their doctor about the product being advertised. Do you think it is useful to you to "educate" your doctor about medicines you are not allowed to buy yourself? Are you improving your health while sharing commercial messages to your providers? Are you relieving your provider from the responsibility to keep up with treatments for any conditions you may have?

QUICK FACTS

1. Nearly three in four judge their own diet to be healthier than that of the average American.
2. Nearly one in five Americans are using a mobile health monitoring device or app, and two thirds of those say it has led them to make healthy changes in their life.
3. Half of Americans say that whether a food is processed impacts their purchasing decision, a factor that has gained traction over the past decade.
4. Sixty-three percent of consumers with an income greater than $35,000 describe their health as excellent/very good, but 39% of those with incomes below $35,000 do not hold that belief.
5. The factors that drive food purchasing decisions have remained quite stable over the past decade, but when you ask consumers themselves how their decision-making compares, more than half say healthfulness matters more to them now (International Food Information Council, 2020).
6. The federal government is expected to spend about $49.1 billion on health-related research and development in its 2020–2021 budget (Chantrill, 2021).
7. In 2019 about two thirds (65%) had a positive view of "capitalism," and a third viewed it negatively (Pew Research Center, 2019).
8. Research found consumption and sale of processed and high-fat/-sugar foods increased by 30% during the 2020 COVID-19 pandemic (Deloitte, 2020). Our cultural differentiation makes a difference when viewing health in other advanced economies. In the United States, African Americans are generally less affluent and are targets of specific advertising for unhealthful products. In Rhode Island, where Black life expectancy was highest, it ranked lower than the averages in 20 advanced economies. Life expectancy for non-Hispanic Blacks in 2007 was lower than 31 of 34 advanced countries. Whites in the United States compared somewhat better. But Hispanic Americans' life expectancy was higher than that of any other advanced country, even Japan, the healthiest population of the advanced economies. America's Asian population is even healthier, as Asian Americans live about 5 years longer than Japanese citizens. If the United States were only Hispanic and Asian Pacific minorities, it would be the healthiest country on earth, even though the country would also have higher poverty rates and greater economic inequality than it does today (Eberstadt, 2015).

It cannot be said that the United States is an unhealthy place to live, but based on a competitive economy, cultural differences, and evolving lifestyles it can be said that the United States does not lead other advanced societies as far as health.

Consideration for Health Promotion and Program Planning

Studies have determined that inequalities in health status between those of lower and higher socioeconomic status should be recognized in assessing patients, and clinicians should view their clients from a perspective that includes socioeconomic factors in diagnostic and management decisions (Fein, 1995).

There is no end to advice on how to live a healthy lifestyle, but there is strong competition in messaging from advertising. Everyone living within this economy should be reminded that their health depends on their own individual decisions and that while the culture of America encourages autonomy and self-reliance, they must "own" responsibility for their personal health despite the endless commercial and social enticements to take up offers to engage in unhealthy behaviors.

Providers should also recognize that, unless volunteering, their service is a commercial transaction. The provider may not be directly involved in the monetary aspects of patient and health plan payments, but the patients will still be having a "customer" experience. Providers may, at the same time, by having a "seller's experience, being aware of implied warranties for service and goods, which may subject them to malpractice claims. Caution may call for more time with the patient, but the business model calling for profitable delivery of service may call for minimizing time with patients so that others may be also seen. Being culturally competent and aware of perspectives on both sides of the patient-provider relationship will help achieve a successful balance.

Providers may also encourage patients to take opportunities to maximize their "consumer power." While not always possible, patient/consumers can have some choice in their health insurance plan, particularly during open-enrollment periods. Within different plans, individuals may usually be able to have some choice of providers and select among several choices within a plan based on checking credentials and experience. Quality control and assessment of services can be enhanced now that personal health records can be available. Patients may perform some quality control and assessment by checking the accuracy of their own records and consider if changes in their records and providers should occur. Patients may seek to confirm the accuracy of their information held by the Medical Information Bureau, which provides information to insurance companies on individuals to assure accuracy and mitigate against risk. In addition, as an autonomous consumer, patients should also be informed of potential complementary and alternative (CAM) options in the nonallopathic health market.

WHAT DO YOU THINK?

In some geographic regions, a higher sales tax is imposed on certain unhealthy products, such as tobacco, soda, and alcohol. Do you think that is ethical? What products, if any, should have a higher sales tax and why? Does a higher sales tax infringe on people's personal choices? Should some items, such as alcohol, be made illegal? What role does the culture of commerce have on these laws and policies?

Changing Views of Health Care: Establishing a Culture of Health

Health insurance essentially started by capitalistic employers to help their employees be effective workers and to retain them in the workforce. This practice was supported by the government granting tax-free status to insurance provided to employees. While very popular among individuals there were problems when people moved from one employer to another. In 1996 this issue was addressed by the national Health Insurance Portability and Accountability Act (HIPAA) legislation to help provide continuity of care for people moving between employers and different health care systems. However, by articulating this need for improved access to health records enormous change followed. To achieve the ability to move file information around, major changes in technology were needed. But as technology allowed confidential transfer of health records, it became apparent that patients themselves wanted access to the records. It was then possible and difficult to deny a patient access when the health care system had already moved away from the position that patient records belonged to the doctor or health care provider. This was a reflection of the culture shift from following the doctor's orders to being involved with health decisions and participating in managing one's own care.

Electronic personal health records were invented, and later computer access was expanded to smartphone web-based applications. This further increased the involvement of Americans engaged in the smartphone culture and deepened patient knowledge of their personal care and involvement in treatment.

As part of the change in expectations for consumer/patient culture, Americans have increasingly looked to the nongovernmental sector to help reduce the human cost of correctable factors contributing to health disparities among various populations. As a result there has been a move by health care professionals to create a "culture of health" among health care institutions that would address the root causes of disease and promote healthy living among all Americans. Since 1999, a number of conferences were convened among leading health care leaders. Rather than traditional business metrics, a concept of an "Organizational Therapeutic Index" could measure therapeutic value to patients and would be based on core values and also be central to an American culture of health. Initially, the core values selected were justice, truth, hope, mercy, and autonomy for individual patients and providers. Later patient access to records and involvement in care were added to the concept of an appropriate "caring enterprise." The basic idea is that there should be some metric that can allow patients and providers to assess how they are performing in the context of basic human values (Bulger, 2015).

It is now generally agreed among providers and patients that the social contract for the health care sector includes values supporting competence (including safety), compassion, hope for successful treatment (including merciful assistance in a dignified death if cure or remission is not possible), justice and equity, and full respect and dignity for all patients, while including them and their close family in the decision-making. More organizations are making commitments to collaborating with other health professionals on the therapeutic teams essential to patient care and reliance (Bulger, 2015).

Summary

Commerce is necessary in any society, and all cultures in America are subsumed within the class-based capitalistic commercial culture that dominates America. Americans tolerate massive amounts of advertising, which includes a great deal of health and health care–related solicitations. Some ads are targeted more specifically to certain subcultures and populations than others. Many health behaviors are influenced by advertising, and the choices made by consumers can lead to both positive and negative health outcomes.

Americans rely on capital investments to advance medicine and develop health facilities and services but have also authorized the government to explore unprofitable research that is impractical for free enterprise business to pursue. Capital resources are concentrated within the American upper class. Governmental health policy and private health care delivery reflects the cultural perspective of the upper class, which brings great medical advances and services. Yet the process does not deliver health outcomes as well as other developed economies in the world. This is in part due the competing commercial activities that entice consumers to engage in very recognized poor health behaviors and product purchases that create endemic health issues throughout American society. This then creates mass market demand for health remedies that encourage additional commercial responses to patient cultural practices.

Review

1. Discuss how the culture of capitalism impacts health behaviors and costs.
2. Discuss how consumers impacts health care.
3. Discuss why upper class attitudes and perspectives impact health care in the American capitalistic society.
4. Discuss why basic research conducted by government is crucial to advancing medicine in the American context of a capitalism.
5. Discuss why profit motive is important to your health as a resident of the United States.

Activities

1. Watch the video titled Opioids, Inc. (https://www.pbs.org/video/opioids-inc-x1xeg9/) and write a summary of your thoughts on how culture affects drug use.

2. Watch the YouTube video "What the Health" (https://youtu.be/6opXP4bGBY0) and write a brief essay on your understanding of the impact of commerce on health.

Case Study 1

An example of the culture of commerce is television advertising for prescription drugs targeted at the general population. Viewers cannot buy any of these products without a prescription from the consumer's doctor. The United States is only one of two countries that allows direct-to-consumer ads (Levine, 2016). In 2016 alone, there were 771,368 drug ads televised (Kaufman, 2017).

1. Do you think advertisers generally create ads primarily to improve consumers' health or to promote product sales?
2. Why do you think ads are directed at patients who cannot directly buy the products rather than to doctors who authorize purchases?

Case Study 2

Sally was unemployed and recently turned 65 years old. She knew she needed to select her Medicare program options. She understood that Medicare was highly regarded by most Americans and had thought in her older years she would enjoy having almost free single-payor insurance as she had heard in political debates. She was surprised to find that there were monthly fees, copays, gaps in coverage, time limits for enrollment to avoid increased costs for life, and, depending on choices, some geographic restrictions. She was a little surprised to find that the government did not actually operate any services directly but had patients receive services from private providers. She could use her own consumer skills to figure out the numerous options, or she could engage a free private Medicare consultant to help her understand the various choices and requirements. Her choices included a large number of items and considerations: Part A (hospital coverage) had no monthly cost but had copays and deductibles; Part B (medical services) could be delayed if she had been working but there were time limits for selecting whether to use "traditional Medicare" or Part C (Medicare advantage HMO, including drug coverage) with enhanced services but geographic and provider limitations and/or chose Part D (drug coverage). Parts a through g include six tiers of drug coverage and Sally needed to consider purchasing a private "supplement" insurance plan to cover some of the 20% copay required for traditional Medicare. And she learned there was a "donut hole" where after her drug plan spent a certain amount of money for covered drugs, she would have to pay all costs out of pocket for future drugs, up to a yearly limit, at which point coverage was reinstated.

Sally had been bombarded by numerous ads on TV and mailings for several months. She decided to engage one of many free private advice services off the internet to help her understand her choices and select her options in time to not have penalties imposed. She was glad that Medicare plan costs could be deducted from her monthly Social Security payments once she became eligible and was pleased she met the enrollment deadlines so that she did not have to pay additional costs for the rest of her life.

1. As a consumer, do you think it is helpful to a number of choices in selecting Medicare services?
2. Can you think of reasons the government does not provide services directly but relies on private providers?
3. The federal government controls Medicare reimbursement rates to private providers, and providers often indicate the rates are low and costs need to be shifted to non-Medicare patients. If this is so, why is there so much competition to attract Medicare customers?

References

Ahmad, F. B., Cisewski, J. A., Miniño, A., & Anderson, R. N. (2021). Provisional number of leading underlying causes of death. *Morbidity and Mortality Weekly Report, 70*(14), 519–522. https://www.cdc.gov/mmwr/volumes/70/wr/mm7014e1.htm

Bethune, S. (2015). Money stress weighs on Americans' health. *Stress in America*, 46(4), https://www.apa.org/monitor/2015/04/money-stress

Bittman, A. (2016, August 12). *Understanding social class as culture.* Behavioral Scientist. https://behavioralscientist.org/understanding-social-class-as-culture/

Bulger, R. (2015). Establishing a national culture of health and its values. *Journal of Thoracic Disease,* 7(1), 111–114. https://www.ncbi.nlm.nih.gov/pmc/articles/PMC4311072/

Chantrill, C. (2021). *Government spending details 2021.* https://www.usgovernmentspending.com/year2021_0.html

Colpe, L. (2020). *Deaths of despair: How connecting opioid data extends the possibilities for suicide research.* CDC. https://www.cdc.gov/surveillance/blogs-stories/deaths-of-dispair.html

Corliss, J. (2014, February 6). *Eating too much added sugar increases the risk of dying with heart disease.* Harvard Health Publishing. https://www.health.harvard.edu/blog/eating-too-much-added-sugar-increases-the-risk-of-dying-with-heart-disease-201402067021

De Vogli, R., Kouvenen, A., & Gimeno, D. (2014). *The influence of market deregulation on fast food consumption and body mass index: A cross-national time series analysis.* http://dx.doi.org/10.2471/BLT.13.120287

Deloitte. (2020). *Are consumers already living the future of health?* https://www2.deloitte.com/content/dam/insights/us/articles/6851_Consumer-survey-and-FOH/DI_Consumer-survey-and-FOH.pdf

Eberstadt, N. (2015, December 10). *Race, class, and health in the 21st century.* National Review. https://www.nationalreview.com/2015/12/race-class-health-21st-century/

Ellis, L. D. (2019, March 14). *The need to treat the ailing U.S. pharmaceutical pricing system.* Harvard T. H. Chan School of Public Health. https://www.hsph.harvard.edu/ecpe/united-states-pharmaceutical-pricing/

Etzioni, A. (2017, December 6). The crisis of American consumerism. *Huffington Post.* https://www.huffpost.com/entry/the-crisis-of-american-co_b_1855390

Fein, O. (1995). The influence of social class on health status: American and British research on health inequalities. *Journal of General Internal Medicine, 10*(10), 577–586. https://pubmed.ncbi.nlm.nih.gov/8576775/

Goodman, B. (2013). *Marxism and healthcare.* https://www.academia.edu/3250126/Marxism_and_Health_Care

Harvard T. Chan School of Public Health. (2019). Americans' values and belief about national health insurance reform. https://cdn1.sph.harvard.edu/wp-content/uploads/sites/94/2019/10/CMWF-NYT-Harvard_Final-Report_Oct2019.pdf

Harvard T. H. Chan School of Public Health. (2021). *Television watching and "sit time."* https://www.hsph.harvard.edu/obesity-prevention-source/obesity-causes/television-and-sedentary-behavior-and-obesity/

International Food Information Council. (2020). *Food and health survey.* https://foodinsight.org/wp-content/uploads/2020/06/IFIC-Food-and-Health-Survey-2020.pdf

IS Global. (2019, December 10). Barcelona Institute for Global Health. https://www.isglobal.org/documents/10179/7035461/Press+Release+Children+obesity+%26+TV/c5ce6b4c-88ef-462b-b1f5-

Kaufman, J. (2017, December 24). Think you see more drug ads on TV? *The New York Times.* https://www.nytimes.com/2017/12/24/business/media/prescription-drugs-advertising-tv.html

Levine, B. (2016, March 14). *Why we ignore the litany of potentially deadly side effects in TV ads for drugs.* Salon. https://www.salon.com/2016/03/14/drug_ads_2_partner/

Maciolek, A., & Van Drie, H. (2021, February 11). *The future of the middle class: How the middle class is really doing.* Brookings. https://www.brookings.edu/blog/up-front/2021/02/11/monitoring-the-middle-class-how-the-american-middle-class-is-really-doing/

McKinsey & Company. (2021). *Looking ahead in US consumer health: An interview with Scott Melville.* https://www.mckinsey.com/industries/consumer-packaged-goods/our-insights/looking-ahead-in-us-consumer-health-an-interview-with-scott-melville#

Merriam-Webster. (n.d.). *Capitalism.* https://www.merriam-webster.com/dictionary/capitalism

Peter G. Peterson Foundation. (2020, July 14). *How does the U.S. healthcare system compare to other countries?* https://www.pgpf.org/blog/2020/07/how-does-the-us-healthcare-system-compare-to-other-countries

Pew Research Center. (2019, October 7). *In their own words: Behind Americans' views of "socialism" and "capitalism."* Pew Research Center. https://www.pewresearch.org/politics/2019/10/07/in-their-own-words-behind-americans-views-of-socialism-and-capitalism/

Robinson, S. (2013). *Southern Aristocracy, How a brutal strain of American aristocrats have come to rule America.* ThePeopleAreComing.org. https://thepeoplearecoming.wordpress.com/tag/southern-aristocracy/

Saad, L. (2019). *More Americans delaying medical treatment due to cost.* Gallup. https://news.gallup.com/poll/269138/americans-delaying-medical-treatment-due-cost.aspx

Snider, S., & Kerr, E. (2020, December 8). Where do I fall in the American economic class system? *U.S. News & World Report.* https://money.usnews.com/money/personal-finance/family-finance/articles/where-do-i-fall-in-the-american-economic-class-system

Stewart, M. (2018, June). The 9.9 percent is the New American aristocracy. *The. Atlantic.* https://www.theatlantic.com/magazine/archive/2018/06/the-birth-of-a-new-american-aristocracy/559130/

Tanner, L. (2019, January 8). *US medical marketing reaches $30 billion, drug ads top surge.* AP News. https://apnews.com/article/health-us-news-business-nh-state-wire-ap-top-news-f44a7baa710d458ca50edd66affc1b91

Top Media (n.d.). *Social media vs traditional media statistics.* https://topmediadvertising.co.uk/social-media-vs-traditional-media-statistics/

Top Media. (2019, June 24). *US on-line and traditional media advertising outlook 2019–2023.* https://www.marketingcharts.com/advertising-trends-108995

The Truth Initiative. (2018, January 24). *Why are 72% of smokers from lower-income communities?* https://truthinitiative.org/research-resources/targeted-communities/why-are-72-smokers-lower-income-communities

University of Arizona. (2020, November 10). *When kids watch a lot of TV, parents may end up more stressed.* Medical Xpress. https://medicalxpress.com/news/2020-11-kids-lot-tv-parents-stressed.html

Weber, L. (2019, January 15). Junk food companies spend billions of dollars on ads targeting Black children. *Huffington Post.* https://www.huffpost.com/entry/junk-food-ads-black-children_n_5c3d063be4b0922a21d7c3c5

CREDITS

Fig. 12.1: Source: https://news.gallup.com/poll/269138/americans-delaying-medical-treatment-due-cost.aspx.

Fig. 12.2: Source: Adapted from https://www.pgpf.org/blog/2020/07/how-does-the-us-healthcare-system-compare-to-other-countries.

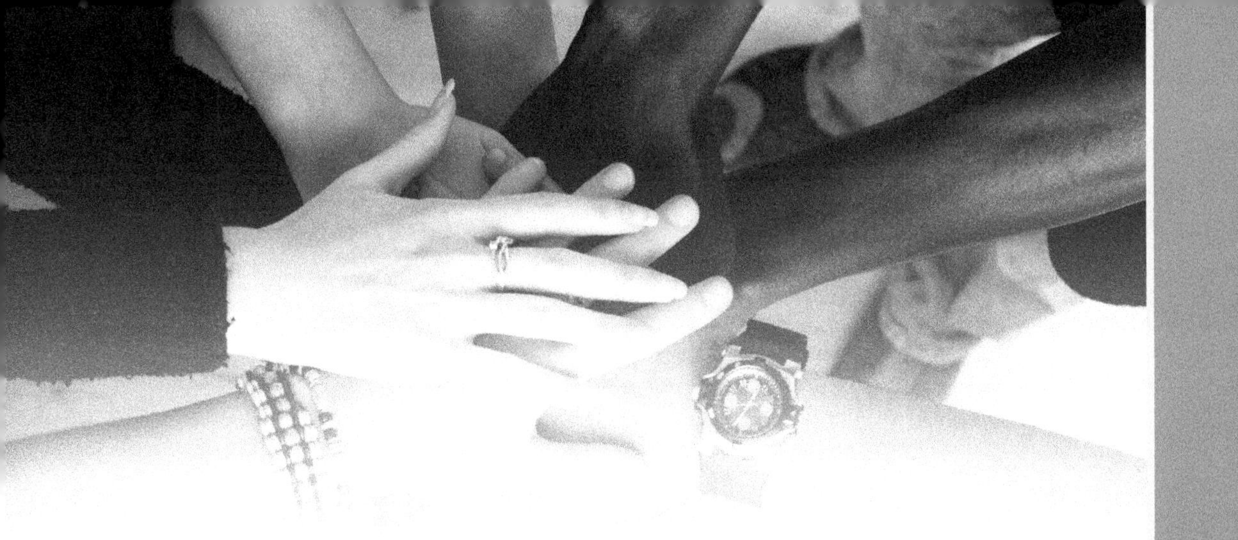

UNIT III

Looking Ahead

CHAPTER 13

Closing the Gap: Strategies for Eliminating Health Disparities

It is time to refocus, reinforce, and repeat the message that health disparities exist and that health equity benefits everyone.

—KATHLEEN G. SEBELIUS, SECRETARY, HEALTH & HUMAN SERVICES (U.S. DEPT OF HEALTH AND HUMAN SERVICES, N.D.A.)

The future health of the nation will be determined to a large extent by how effectively we work with communities to reduce and eliminate health disparities between non-minority and minority populations experiencing disproportionate burdens of disease, disability, and premature death.

—GUIDING PRINCIPLE FOR IMPROVING MINORITY HEALTH (OFFICE OF MINORITY HEALTH & HEALTH DISPARITIES, 2007)

KEY CONCEPTS AND TERMS

Best practices | Cultural competence | Telehealth

LEARNING OBJECTIVES

After reading this chapter, you should be able to do the following:

1. Describe at least six strategies for reducing or eliminating health disparities.
2. Explain the role of the Affordable Care Act is reducing inequalities.

Health disparities in the United States are extensive, as has been demonstrated by the differences in the incidence and consequences of diseases and mortality rates for various populations. The causes of health disparities are complex, systemic, personal, integrated, and multifactorial, and there are no easy and immediate solutions to reduce or eliminate them. The complexity of the problem should not deter our efforts to work on reducing, and eventually eliminating, these differences in health because these disparities have a negative impact on the people of our nation. The changing demographics anticipated over the next decade will amplify these problems, hence the importance of addressing disparities in health today. Groups currently experiencing poorer health status are expected to grow as a proportion of the U.S. population, and the future health of the United States as a whole will be influenced substantially by our success in improving the health of these groups. A national focus on health disparities exists as discrimination and impacts of COVID-19 have been highlighted. There may be years of research and subsequent planning resulting from the COVID-19 pandemic, which became the third highest cause of death nationwide in 2020. Disparities were markedly evident for certain populations such as the elderly, but also for certain minority populations including especially American Indians and African Americans. Part of this may have been due to underlying comorbidities, such as obesity, but there are many questions that remain to be answered and addressed in the future.

The government has recognized the need to reduce health disparities, and this focus is reflected in the Healthy People 2030 objectives. Healthy People 2030 is designed to achieve five overarching goals:

1. Attain healthy, thriving lives and well-being free of preventable disease, disability, injury, and premature death.
2. Eliminate health disparities, achieve health equity, and attain health literacy to improve the health and well-being of all.
3. Create social, physical, and economic environments that promote attaining the full potential for health and well-being for all.
4. Promote healthy development, healthy behaviors, and well-being across all life stages.
5. Engage leadership, key constituents, and the public across multiple sectors to take action and design policies that improve the health and well-being of all (HHS, n.d.c.).

Healthy People 2030 objectives are organized into topics. The topic areas of Healthy People 2030 are listed in **Box 13.1**.

In April 2011, the HHS announced a nationwide plan to reduce health disparities. The plan has not been updated and is described in the "National Stakeholder Strategy for Achieving Health Equity," which is a common set of goals and objectives for public and private sector initiatives and partnerships to help racial and ethnic minorities and other underserved groups reach their full health potential. The strategy incorporates ideas, suggestions, and comments from thousands of individuals and organizations across the country. The five goals outlined in the document are as follows:

Goal 1: Awareness: Increasing awareness of the significance of health disparities, their impact on the nation, and the actions necessary to improve health outcomes for racial, ethnic, and underserved populations.

BOX 13.1 Healthy People 2030 Topic Areas

Health Conditions

- Addiction
- Arthritis
- Blood disorders
- Cancer
- Chronic kidney disease
- Chronic Pain
- Dementia
- Diabetes
- Foodborne illness
- Health care-associated infections
- Heart disease and stroke
- Infectious disease
- Mental health and mental disorders
- Oral Conditions
- Osteoporosis
- Obesity
- Pregnancy and childbirth
- Respiratory disease
- Sensory or communication disorders
- Sexually transmitted infections

Health Behaviors

- Child and adolescent development
- Drug and alcohol use
- Emergency preparedness
- Family planning
- Health communication
- Injury prevention
- Nutrition and healthy eating
- Physical activity
- Preventive care
- Safe food handling
- Sleep
- Tobacco use
- Vaccination
- Violence prevention

Populations

- Adolescents
- Children
- Infants
- LGBTQIA
- Men
- Older adults
- Parents or caregivers
- People with disabilities
- Women
- Workforce

Settings and Systems

- Community
- Environmental health
- Global health
- Health care
- Health insurance
- Health IT
- Health policy
- Hospital and emergency services
- Housing and homes
- Public health infrastructure

(continued)

BOX 13.1 Healthy People 2030 Topic Areas (*Continued*)

- Schools
- Transportation
- Workplace

Social Determinants of Health

- Economic stability
- Education access and quality
- Health care access and quality
- Neighborhood and built environment
- Social and community context (HHS, n.d.b.)

Source: U.S. Department of Health and Human Services, "Healthy People 2030."

Goal 2: Leadership: Strengthen and broaden leadership for addressing health disparities at all levels.

Goal 3: Health system and life experience: Improve health and healthcare outcomes for racial, ethnic, and underserved populations.

Goal 4: Cultural and linguistic competency: Improve cultural and linguistic competency and the diversity of the health-related workforce.

Goal 5: Data, research, and evaluation: Improve data availability, coordination, utilization, and diffusion of research and evaluation outcomes. (National Partnership for Action to End Health Disparities, 2011, p. 108)

In November 2010 the HHS (n.d.a.) was charged with developing a department-wide action plan for reducing racial and ethnic health disparities. The outcome was the document titled "HHS Action Plan to Reduce Racial and Ethnic Health Disparities." The action plan included transforming health care and expanding access, building on the provisions of the Affordable Care Act related to expanded insurance coverage and increased access to care. The plan also called for more opportunities to increase the number of students from populations underrepresented in the health professions, train more people in medical interpretation to help serve patients with a limited command of English, and train community workers to help people navigate the system.

Within the framework of the HHS action plan, the five overall goals for reducing disparities and associated action steps included the following:

1. Transform health care: Action steps include expanding insurance coverage, increasing access to care through the development of new service delivery sites, and introducing quality initiatives such as increased utilization of medical homes.
2. Strengthen the nation's health and human services workforce: Action steps include a new pipeline program for recruiting undergraduates from underserved communities for public health and biomedical sciences careers, expanding and improving health care interpreting and translation, and supporting more training of community health workers, such as *promotoras*.

3. Advance the health, safety, and well-being of the American people: Action steps include implementing the CDC's new community transformation grants and additional targeted efforts to achieve improvements in cardiovascular disease, childhood obesity, tobacco-related diseases, maternal and child health, flu, and asthma.
4. Advance scientific knowledge and innovation: Action steps include implementing a new health data collection and analysis strategy authorized by the Affordable Care Act and increasing patient-centered outcomes research.
5. Increase the efficiency, transparency, and accountability of HHS programs: Actions steps include ensuring that assessments of policies and programs on health disparities become part of all HHS decision-making. Evaluations will measure progress toward reducing health disparities.

The "National Stakeholder Strategy" and the HHS action plan call for federal agencies and their partners to work together on social, economic, and environmental factors that contribute to health disparities. Many other federal agencies and states have developed strategic plans to eliminate health disparities. For example, the Centers for Medicare and Medicaid Service's (2021) equity plan for Medicare is built around a framework that consists of three core elements:

1. Increasing understanding and awareness of disparities
2. Developing and disseminating solutions to achieve health equity
3. Implementing sustainable actions to achieve health equity

These plans can be useful to organizations when they are developing their own objectives and interventions.

Eliminating health disparities will require enhanced efforts and changes in research, improving the environments of people who are affected by health disparities, increasing access to health care, improving the quality of care, and making policy and legal changes. These plans are the spokes of the overarching goal of this chapter, which is to provide information about strategies for reducing health disparities.

WHAT DO YOU THINK?

What is your opinion of these national priorities to reduce health disparities? Are there any you would add or remove? Do you think any of the goals are a higher priority than the others? What steps would you take to achieve these national goals?

Strategies for Reducing or Eliminating Health Disparities

A variety of approaches are needed to reduce health disparities. This task requires a systematic, coordinated, and collaborative effort to effectively implement the strategies.

The methods necessitate implementation at different ecological levels with community, local, state, and national organizations and politicians at the helm.

Cultural Competence

Implementing change does not mean imposing a uniform solution. Cultural differences and a variety of approaches to achieving good health should be utilized and encouraged to ensure optimal results. This approach involves a course to culturally competent understanding. In health care, there is no universally accepted definition of cultural competence. In general, **cultural competence** is "a set of congruent behaviors, attitudes, and policies that come together in a system, agency, or among professionals that enables effective work in cross-cultural situations" (Prevention Information Network, 2021). Cultural competence requires skills in individuals and systems that allow for an increased understanding and appreciation of cultural differences and the demonstrated skills necessary to work with and serve diverse individuals and groups.

Indicators of a culturally competent organization include the following:

- Recognizing the power and influence of culture, and that most organizations were constructed according to white supremacist culture
- Understanding how each of our backgrounds affects our responses to others
- Not assuming that all members of cultural groups share the same beliefs and practices
- Acknowledging how past experiences affect present interactions
- Building on the strengths and resources of each culture in an organization
- Allocating resources for leadership and staff development in the area of cultural awareness, sensitivity, and understanding
- Actively eliminating prejudice in policies and practices
- Willing to share power among leaders of different cultural backgrounds
- Evaluating the organization's cultural competence on a regular basis (Community Tool Box, n.d.).

DID YOU KNOW?

The National Center for Cultural Competence at Georgetown University (http://nccc.georgetown.edu/) has a wealth of resources on cultural competence. Its site includes information about projects and initiatives and data vignettes. There is a large variety of self-assessment tools as well as resources. In addition, there is information about distance learning opportunities and promising practices.

Cultural competence entails the willingness and ability of individuals and a system to valuc the importance of culture in the delivery of services to all segments of the population at all levels of an organization. It includes activities such as policy development and implementation, governance, education, promoting workforce diversity, and the reduction of language barriers.

Becoming culturally competent is an ongoing process. It requires a dedication to growing with a changing society that is becoming more diverse and to serving the individuals and communities with the most culturally appropriate, and hence highest quality, care possible.

Improving cultural competence levels should begin with an assessment to determine where an individual or organization can improve. It can assist with directing training and education for the workforce, policy development, and other systematic changes. We included an individual and an organizational cultural competence assessment tool in Chapter 2.

Research

Eliminating health disparities requires new knowledge about the determinants of disease, causes of health disparities, effective interventions for prevention and treatment, and innovative ways of working in partnership with health care systems. From a culturally informed perspective, the advances in knowledge about topics such as genetics and best practices need to be put into action and applied to the health care industry and not just lie in the pages of professional journals.

Best practices of disparity-reduction initiatives and programs are being identified and shared. This needs to continue and be magnified. Government organizations and researchers need to continue to work to document and publicize those programs and policy changes that have been proven to be effective, but it is just as important to identify programs that do not work. Most of what is published in journals and on websites illustrates the successes, but the unsuccessful programs and policies add to the knowledge as well. Knowing what does not work helps prevent health care professionals from channeling valuable resources to interventions that have already been shown not to produce positive effects.

Data on specific populations also is needed. A majority of the data report on broad categories of race and ethnicities, such as Asians and American Indians. In addition, much of the research combines groups, such as Asians with Pacific Islanders and American Indians with Alaska Natives. There is great diversity within these groups, so more specific data is needed to help identify the health problems within the subpopulations and successful strategies for reducing them. This problem also can obscure successful health strategies among subpopulations. Researchers and government agencies are encouraged to collect and report data for racial and ethnic subgroups instead of the current commonly used broad categories.

In the United States, socioeconomic status has traditionally been measured by education and income. Surveys also should capture information about a range of contextual variables that have been found to be explanatory in health differences, such as social support, social networks, family supports, levels of acculturation, social cohesion, community involvement, perceived financial burdens, discrimination, and differences in the health status of foreign-born versus U.S.-born individuals, which at times also are linked to socioeconomic status.

Improving the Environments of People Affected by Health Disparities

Health disparities have complex origins. Not all are due to traditional concepts of social culture. For instance, the cultures of poverty, discrimination, and commerce have significant cross-cultural importance. There is little doubt that neighborhood characteristics are important elements associated with health. Residents of socially and economically deprived communities experience worse health outcomes on average than those living in more prosperous neighborhoods. Neighborhoods may influence health through relatively short-term influences on behaviors, attitudes, and health care utilization, thereby affecting health conditions that are more immediate. Neighborhoods also can influence health on a long-term basis through "weathering," whereby the accumulated stress, lower environmental quality, and limited resources of poorer communities experienced over many years negatively affect the health of residents.

Members of minority cultures are more likely to live in poor neighborhoods. These neighborhoods often have poor performing schools, high crime rates, substandard housing, few health care providers and pharmacies, more alcohol and tobacco advertising, and limited access to grocery stores with healthy food choices. These social determinants of health can accumulate over the course of a life and can be detrimental to physical and emotional health.

Increasing Access to Health Care

Lack of access to the modern health care system is generally based on economic barriers. In March 2010, President Obama signed comprehensive health reform into law, the Patient Protection and Affordable Care Act (ACA). The law was intended to make preventive care—including family planning and related services—more accessible and affordable for many Americans. Tax credits, mandates (which have been overturned), and covering those with preexisting conditions are some ways the original law was intended to improve access to care and make it more affordable. Research indicates that the ACA narrowed racial and ethnic disparities in insurance coverage (Chaudry et al., 2019). Blacks and Hispanics had the highest uninsured rates prior to the law's passage and have made the largest gains. The uninsured rate for Black adults dropped from 24.4% in 2013 to 14.4% in 2018, while the rate for Hispanic adults decreased from 40.2% to 24.9% (The Common Wealth Fund, 2020). This progress reduced the difference between the two groups and White adults.

Access to care is also related to having health care providers within every geographic region. There are imbalances in how the health care workforce is distributed, and this leads to lower access to care in some geographic regions of the United States. Poor neighborhoods tend to have a lower person-to-health care provider ratio than more affluent regions. **Telehealth** is the use of technology to remotely deliver health care, health information, or health education at a distance. Examples include telepsychiatry, in which mental health services are provided using video conferencing, and teleradiology, in which films are electronically forwarded to providers in remote locations. Telehealth can be used to provide medical services to medically underserved geographic regions.

Government incentives programs also help improve access to care. These programs offer incentives and competitive salaries to providers who work in low-income and medically underserved regions.

Improving Quality of Care

Improving quality of care is related to the training of health care providers, providing equal care, reducing language barriers, and increasing diversity in the workforce. Each of these four areas is discussed in the following paragraphs.

With regard to training health care providers, fostering a culturally competent health care system that reflects and serves the diversity of America must be a priority for health care reform. States and academic centers that train health care professionals can develop, and some already have, requirements for training in this area. This can assist with providing equal treatment.

The groundbreaking report "Unequal Treatment: Confronting Racial and Ethnic Disparities in Healthcare" (Smedley et al., 2003) showed that racial and ethnic minorities receive lower quality health care than Caucasians, even when insurance status, income, age, and severity of conditions are comparable. More recently, the 2019 National Healthcare Quality and Disparities Report showed that overall, some disparities were getting smaller from 2000 through 2016–2018, but disparities persist, and some even worsened, especially for poor and uninsured populations in all priority areas.

Racial and ethnic disparities vary by group:

- For about 40% of quality measures, Blacks (82 of 202) and American Indians and Alaska Natives (47 of 116) received worse care than Whites. For more than one third of quality measures, Hispanics (61 of 177) received worse care than Whites.
- For nearly 30% of quality measures, Asians (52 of 185) received worse care than Whites, but Asians received better care than Whites for nearly one third (56 of 185) of quality measures.
- For one third of quality measures, Native Hawaiians/Pacific Islanders (24 of 72) received worse care than Whites.

- For a little less than 20% of quality measures, medium and small metropolitan residents received worse care than residents of large fringe metropolitan areas (Agency for Healthcare Research and Quality; December 2020).

Language barriers can lead to numerous problems, such as damage to the patient-provider relationship, miscommunication with regard to the health problem and treatment approach, medication and correct dosage mistakes, and legal problems. Health care has a language of its own and can make communication with people with limited English proficiency skills even more difficult. Barriers can be reduced by multilingual signage, providing interpretive services, noting a patient's native language and communication needs, and having documents (e.g., consent forms and educational materials) available in languages that reflect the demographics of the region served.

Diversity in the workforce is another goal. The health care workforce is underrepresented by people who are non-White, yet people of color are more likely to practice in federally designated underserved areas, to see patients of color, and to accept Medicaid patients.

Policy Changes and Laws

The ACA, as stated previously, intends to provide more affordable coverage and put an end to preexisting condition limitations as well as to limits on care and coverage cancellations (The White House, n.d.). In addition to the ACA, policies and laws that mandate cultural competence training for medical professionals have been implemented. For example, in 2005, New Jersey became the first state to address the issue of equity in health care and cultural competence training of physicians (Senate Bill [SB] 144). The law requires medical professionals to receive cultural competence training to receive a diploma from medical schools located in the state or to be licensed or relicensed to practice in the state. Each medical school in New Jersey is required to provide this training. California has taken several steps to ensure cultural competence across the state's health care infrastructure. In 2005, Assembly Bill 1195 required mandatory continuing medical education courses to include cultural and linguistic courses. The state of Washington enacted SB 6194 in 2006, which requires all medical education curricula in the state to include multicultural health training and awareness courses. All these laws strive to establish cultural competence among health care professionals.

There are many more current laws designed to reduce health disparities. For example, the Health Equity and Accountability Act of 2018 (HEAA) is comprehensive, broadly supported legislation to eliminate racial and ethnic health disparities. HEAA is the only legislation that holistically addresses health inequalities, their intersections with immigration status, age, disability, sex, gender, sexual orientation, gender identity and expression, language, and socioeconomic status, along with obstacles associated with historical and contemporary injustices (Asian & Pacific Islander American Health Forum, 2018). Another example is the Henrietta Lacks Enhancing Cancer Research Act of 2019, signed by the president on January 5, 2021. The bill requires the Government Accountability Office to complete a study reviewing how federal agencies address barriers to participation in federally funded cancer clinical trials by individuals from underrepresented populations and provide recommendations for addressing such barriers.

Summary

To achieve quality and affordable health care for all, health care reform must include concrete steps to reduce health disparities. Ensuring access to coverage is only part of the answer. Other strategies include reducing barriers to quality health care for people of differing cultures by requiring cultural competence training of medical professionals, recruiting a diverse workforce, eliminating language barriers, coordinating public and private programs that target disparities, providing more funding to community health centers, and improving chronic disease management programs by making them more responsive to minorities. Health disparities reflect and perpetuate the inequity and injustice that permeates American society. Eliminating health disparities will help create equal opportunity for all Americans in all sectors of our society.

In this chapter, a variety of methods for reducing health disparities are presented. These include strategies such as diversifying the health care workforce, changing policies, training health care professionals in the area of cultural competence, and conducting additional research. These changes can help reduce the gap in health among Americans, and this needs to continue to be a priority for our nation, particularly in light of the changing demographics of the United States.

Cultural competence is a process, and there is still much to learn. No one can learn all there is to know about the numerous cultural groups in the United States, but it is important that you are aware of the major differences, challenge your assumptions, respect and embrace values and beliefs that are different from your own, and provide the same high standards of care to all people, regardless of race, ethnicity, gender, sexual preference, or other attribute. Our hope is that you will go beyond this by advocating for equality and striving to improve health care systems to help close the gaps in the levels of health that exist among certain groups. We leave you with this final thought:

> *Cultural differences should not separate us from each other, but rather cultural diversity brings a collective strength that can benefit all of humanity.*
>
> —ROBERT ALAN

Review

1. Describe what cultural competence is and why it is important.
2. List at least four national goals for eliminating health disparities.
3. Describe strategies to reduce or eliminate health disparities.

Activity

Write a letter to the president of the United States. Provide suggestions about how to reduce the health disparities in the United States. What changes need to be made in terms of policy, training, or other areas?

Case Study 1

Cambridge Health Alliance set out to increase mammography rates among women 50 to 69 years of age. Screening rates for all women were below 60% when the initiative began. The initiative focused on three areas: developing patient tracking systems and other information systems (e.g., improving communication within and between facilities), improving access by enhancing the capacity of the radiology department to reduce appointment wait times, and conducting outreach to difficult-to-reach and unscreened patients.

The outreach process included staff and patient education. Outreach staff work individually with the 15 clinics, reviewing their breast health screening rates and lists of patients due for mammograms and identifying factors that contribute to unscreened patients. This review assisted the clinic staff with understanding the clinic population. The clinic and outreach staff worked together and sent unscreened patients a personalized letter from their primary care provider. The content of the letter encouraged the patient to go to the clinic for a screening.

After the letter was sent, a follow-up personal phone call was made to the patient. The patient was called up to three times. During the call, the staff offered to schedule, and occasionally transport, women to the clinic for their screening. Letters and phone calls were provided to patients in their own languages.

Special Saturday events took place to assist working women with having the screening. The patients were often able to attend a session with friends. The Saturday sessions provided group education and individual screenings.

At the end of the initiative, screening rates were at 86%, and rates for all language groups were above 80%; the screening rate for Spanish speakers was 92%, and the screening rate for Portuguese speakers was 94% (American Hospital Association, n.d.).

1. Why do you think these initiatives were successful?
2. Do you think these program changes would be helpful with other groups? Why or why not?
3. What health outreach program changes have you seen other programs make (e.g., on billboards, on television) to improve the health among specific groups?

Case Study 2

COVID-19 vaccine distribution raised concerns about inequities. Preventing racial disparities in the uptake of COVID-19 vaccines was important to help mitigate the disproportionate impacts of the virus for people of color and prevent widening racial health disparities going forward.

1. Why do think that the vaccination rates were lower among minorities when they had higher case rates than Whites?

2. How would you organize the vaccination distribution to avoid or mitigate the disparities in vaccination rates?

References

Agency for Healthcare Research and Quality. (2020, December). *2019 National healthcare quality & disparities report.* https://www.ahrq.gov/sites/default/files/wysiwyg/research/findings/nhqrdr/2019qdr-final-es.pdf

American Hospital Association. (n.d.). *Eliminating disparities in care.*

Asian & Pacific Islander American Health Forum. (2018, April). *The Health Equity and Accountability Act of 2018.* https://www.apiahf.org/resource/the-health-equity-and-accountability-act-of-2018/

Centers for Medicare and Medicaid. (2015–2021). *Paving the way to equity: A progress report.* https://www.cms.gov/files/document/paving-way-equity-cms-omh-progress-report.pdf

Chaudry, A., Jackson, A., & Glied, S. A. (2019, August 21). *Did the Affordable Care Act reduce racial and ethnic disparities in health insurance coverage?* The Commonwealth Fund. https://www.commonwealthfund.org/publications/issue-briefs/2019/aug/did-ACA-reduce-racial-ethnic-disparities-coverage

Community Tool Box. (n.d.). *Chapter 27.* https://ctb.ku.edu/en/table-of-contents/culture/cultural-competence/culturally-competent-organizations/main#:~:text=%20Building%20Culturally%20Competent%20Organizations%20%201%20Valuing,of%20difference%0AMany%20factors%20can%20affect%20cross-cultural...%20More%20

National Partnership for Action to End Health Disparities. (2011, April). *National stakeholder strategy for achieving health equity.* U.S. Department of Health and Human Services, Office of Minority Health.

National Prevention Information Network. (2021, September 10). *Cultural competence in health and human services.* https://npin.cdc.gov/pages/cultural-competence

Office of Minority Health & Health Disparities. (2007). *Eliminating racial & ethnic health disparities.*

Smedley, B. D., Stith, A. Y., & Nelson, A. R. (Eds.). (2003). *Unequal treatment: Confronting racial and ethnic disparities in health care.* National Academies Press.

The Common Wealth Fund. (2020, January 16). *How the Affordable Care Act has narrowed racial and ethnic disparities in access to health care.* https://www.commonwealthfund.org/publications/2020/jan/how-ACA-narrowed-racial-ethnic-disparities-access

The White House. (n.d.). *Health care that works for Americans.*

U.S. Department of Health and Human Services. (n.d.a). *HHS action plan to reduce racial and ethnic health disparities.* http://minorityhealth.hhs.gov/assets/pdf/hhs/HHS_Plan_complete.pdf

U.S. Department of Health and Human Services. (n.d.b.). *Healthy People 2030 framework.* https://health.gov/healthypeople/about/healthy-people-2030-framework

U.S. Department of Health and Human Services. (n.d.c.). *Healthy People 2030.* https://health.gov/healthypeople/objectives-and-data/browse-objectives

Glossary

***aAma* and *aDuonga*:** Vietnamese belief of balance in all things, similar to yin and yang in traditional Chinese medicine.

acculturation: The process of adapting to another culture by acquiring elements of the majority group's culture.

acupuncture: Traditional Chinese medicine treatment that involves stimulating specific points along the meridians to achieve a therapeutic purpose. The usual practice involves inserting a needle into one of the acupoints along a meridian that is associated with an organ or function.

advance directive: Pertains to treatment preferences and the designation of a surrogate decision-maker in the event that a person should become unable to make medical decisions on their own behalf.

ahimsa: A Buddhist and Hindu doctrine that expresses belief in the sacredness of all living creatures and urges the avoidance of harm and violence.

alien: A person who is generally understood to be a foreigner (i.e., comes from a foreign country) and does not owe allegiance to the United States.

alternative medicine: A variety of therapeutic or preventive health care practices, such as homeopathy, naturopathy, chiropractic, and herbal medicine, that do not follow generally accepted medical methods and may not have a scientific explanation for their effectiveness; used instead of Western medicine.

assimilation: The process of becoming absorbed into another culture, adopting its characteristics, and developing a new cultural identity.

asylee: A person granted legal status in the United States based on applying, upon arrival in the United States, for refugee status due to a well-founded fear of persecution (must meet the criteria for a refugee).

autonomy: The ethical principle that embodies the right of self-determination.

Ayurvedic system: India's ancient and traditional natural system of medicine that provides an integrated approach to preventing and treating illness through lifestyle interventions and natural therapies.

beneficence: The state or quality of being kind and charitable; a principle that requires doing good or removing harm.

best practices: The assertion that there is a strategy that is more effective at delivering a particular outcome than any other technique, method, or process.

biomedical (allopathic) medicine: The system of medicine that uses pharmacologically active agents or physical interventions to treat or suppress symptoms or pathophysiologic processes of diseases or disorders.

bisexual: Individuals whose sexual preference is to both men and women.

brauche: Amish practice whereby healers lay their hands over a patient's head or stomach while quietly reciting verses to "pull out" the ailment.

Candomblé: A religion developed in Brazil by enslaved Africans that involves rituals such as animal sacrifice, drumming, and dancing.

collectivism: The view that the group should be the priority rather than the individual.

commerce: The exchange of goods and services for money or other items of value.

complementary medicine: Treatments that are utilized in conjunction with conventional Western medical therapies prescribed by a physician.

cultural adaptation: The degree to which a person or community has adapted to the dominant culture or retained its traditional practices.

cultural competence: The ability to interact effectively with people of different cultures; a set of congruent behaviors, attitudes, structures, and policies that come together to work effectively in intercultural situations.

cultural relativism: The principle that one's beliefs and activities should be interpreted in terms of one's own culture and that no culture is superior to another.

culture: The set of learned behaviors, beliefs, attitudes, values, and ideals that are characteristic of a particular society or population.

curandero **(male) or** ***curandera*** **(female):** A traditional folk healer or shaman who is dedicated to curing physical and spiritual illnesses.

discrimination: The practice of treating people differently on a basis other than merit.

dominant culture: The total, generally organized way of life, including values, norms, institutions, and symbols that reflect the largest culture.

doshas: In Ayurvedic medicine, the three vital energies that regulate everything in nature.

drabarni: Roma women who have knowledge of medicines.

durable power of attorney: A legal document that gives someone that you select the ability to make decisions for you when you are not able to do so for yourself.

Ellis–van Creveld syndrome: Genetic disorder found among the Amish in which there is a defective recessive gene from each parent.

empacho: In the Hispanic culture, a description of stomach pains and cramps.

espiritismo: A Latin American and Caribbean belief that good and evil spirits can affect human life, such as one's health and luck.

ethnicity: Large groups of people who are classified according to common racial, national, tribal, religious, or linguistic traits or cultural origin or background.

ethnocentricity: When a person believes that their culture is superior to that of another.

euthanasia: Act or practice of ending the life of an individual who is suffering from a terminal illness or an incurable condition.

evil eye: Also referred to as **mal de ojo**. In the Hispanic culture, an illness thought to be caused by jealousy; the Spanish translation is "bad eye." This belief is held by many migrant farmworkers.

***familismo*:** A strong loyalty and identification with one's nuclear and extended family.

fate versus free will: The belief that events are predetermined and cannot be changed (fate or destiny) versus humans being able to determine the direction of their life (free will).

fidelity: Ethical principle that entails keeping one's promises or commitments.

five elements: The traditional Chinese medicine theory based on the perception of the relationships among all things. These patterns are grouped and named for the five elements: wood, fire, earth, metal, and water.

***fotonovela*:** An illustrated novel.

***gadje*:** All things non-Roma; considered not clean.

gay: Term that refers to those who are sexually and emotionally attracted to people of the same gender and is usually used to refer to males specifically.

gender identity: A person's internal, personal sense of being male or female, boy or girl, man or woman.

germ theory: The theory that microorganisms in the body cause specific diseases.

health disparities: Also referred to as health inequalities. Gaps in the quality of health and health care across racial, ethnic, sexual orientation, and socioeconomic groups.

Healthy People 2030: A program that provides a prevention framework for the United States. It is a statement of national health objectives designed to identify the most significant preventable threats to health and to establish national goals to reduce these threats.

heritage consistency: The degree to which people identify with their culture of origin.

Hill–Burton Act: Also referred to as the Hospital Survey and Construction Act of 1946. It provided federal assistance to state governments for the construction and modernization of hospitals and other health care facilities. The original statute required recipient hospitals to make services available "to all persons residing in the territorial area of the application, without discrimination on account of race, creed, or color."

Hispanic paradox: The apparent contradiction reflected in the fact that Hispanics generally have better health and live longer than more affluent non-Hispanic Whites and other cultural groups within the United States.

Hmong: Mountain-dwelling people from Cambodia and Vietnam.

holistic medicine: An approach to well-being that integrates the whole person (body, mind, and spirit).

hydrotherapy: A treatment used by naturopathic practitioners based on the therapeutic effects of water. Thought to assist in ridding the body of waste and toxins, it utilizes hot and cold baths, compresses, wraps, and showers as treatment modalities.

illegal alien: A foreigner who (a) does not owe allegiance to the United States and (b) who has violated U.S. laws and customs in establishing residence in the United States.

immigrant: A person who migrates to another country legally and who usually seeks permanent residency.

individualism: The outlook that places high importance on the individual and individual self-reliance.

justice: The ethical principle stating that people should be treated equally and fairly.

karma: The total effect of a person's conduct during the successive phases of existence, which is expected to determine the person's destiny.

***Ki* or chi force:** Korean belief in a life force similar to chi in traditional Chinese medicine; it is important in maintaining health, and efforts are made to balance this force and not to engage in activities that could diminish it.

lesbian: Term that refers to women who are attracted to women specifically.

living will: A set of instructions that documents a person's wishes about medical care.

lower class: Generally trading their labor for wages that provide minimal lifestyle options if even subsistence.

***mal de ojo*:** Also referred to as evil eye. In the Hispanic culture, an illness thought to be caused by jealousy; the Spanish translation is "bad eye."

***marime*:** Roma concept of impurity, which is foundational to their health beliefs.

medicine bundle: A wrapped package containing objects such as tobacco, a flute, eagle feather, or other items thought to contain spiritual significance; used by American Indians for religious and healing purposes.

medicine wheel: A symbol that represents harmony and peaceful interaction.

meditation: A group of mental techniques intended to provide relaxation and mental harmony as well as to quiet one's mind and increase awareness.

meridians: The traditional Chinese medicine concept of channels through which qi, blood, and information flow to all parts of the body.

middle class: Generally has a comfortable or acceptable financial means for life with some access to power.

mind–body integration: Seeing the mind and body as a consolidated unit.

mindfulness meditation: The concept of increasing awareness and acceptance of the present.

minority: A group that is smaller in number than another group; a part of a population that differs in characteristics, often resulting in differential treatment.

multicultural evaluation: Integrates cultural considerations into an evaluation's theory, measures, analysis, and practice.

multicultural health: The provision of health services in a sensitive, knowledgeable, and nonjudgmental manner with respect for people's health beliefs and practices when they are different from your own.

naturalistic theories of disease: The belief that illness is caused by a person's imbalance with the natural environment.

naturopathy: Healing practice based on ancient beliefs in the healing power of nature and that natural organisms have the ability to heal themselves and maintain health. The body strives to maintain a state of equilibrium, known as homeostasis, and unhealthy environments, diets, physical or emotional stress, and lack of sleep or fresh air can disrupt that balance. Natural remedies, such as herbs and foods, are used instead of surgery or drugs.

nonmaleficence: The principle that one should practice competently.

organizational health literacy: The degree to which organizations equitably enable individuals to find, understand, and use information and services to inform health-related decisions and actions for themselves and others.

orishas: A spirit that reflects one of the manifestations of God in Yoruba religion and is expressed in practices such as Santeria.

personal health literacy: The degree to which individuals have the ability to find, understand, and use information and services to inform health-related decisions and actions for themselves and others.

personalistic belief system: The belief that illness is caused by the intervention of a supernatural being or a human being with special powers and is related to one's behavior.

peyote: A spineless, dome-shaped cactus (*Lophophora williamsii*) native to Mexico and the southwest United States. The plant has buttonlike tubercles that are chewed fresh or dry as a narcotic, hallucinogenic drug by certain Native American peoples.

prakriti: The combination of the doshas at the time of conception that are unique to each individual.

***promotores* (male) or *promotoras* (female):** Community members who promote health in their own communities.

proxemics: The scientific study of the amount of space that people feel is necessary to have between themselves and others.

qi: In traditional Chinese medicine, the vital life force that animates all things.

qigong: Translates to "energy work." A part of traditional Chinese medicine that involves movement, breathing, and meditation that is intended to improve the flow of qi through the body.

race: The concept of dividing people into populations or groups on the basis of visible traits and beliefs about common ancestry.

racism: The belief that some races are superior to others by nature.

reciprocity: The exchange of like or similar things of value for mutual benefit.

refugee: A person who has fled another country due to fear of persecution because of their race, religion, nationality, social group, or political opinion and requests legal status before entering the United States.

Reiki: A form of alternative medicine in which the healer uses their hands to channel healing energy.

religion: An organized collection of beliefs, cultural systems, and worldviews that explain the meaning of life and the universe.

respect: A sense of admiration, honor, value that invokes a belief that a person or object should be treated seriously and with courtesy.

***respeto*:** A Spanish word meaning respect.

Romany: A language derived from Sanskrit that is spoken by the Roma people.

Rumspringa: An Amish practice that allows adolescents to be free to explore the world outside of the Amish culture.

sand painting: The art of creating paintings using sand for the purpose of healing.

Santeria: An African-based religion that combines the worship of traditional Yoruban deities with the worship of Roman Catholic saints.

sexual identity: A person's physical, romantic, emotional, and spiritual attraction to another person.

Shintoism: The formal state religion of Japan, which is based on a belief in the importance of developing harmony and balance in life and with other people with the help of the spiritual beings, including some that are within nature and objects such as trees and stones.

stereotype: The mistaken assumption that everyone in a given culture is alike.

susto: In the Hispanic culture, an illness thought to be caused by soul loss or fright.

sweat lodge: A kind of sauna, usually a domed or oblong hut, that is used in a spiritual ritual by some American Indians.

tai chi: A traditional Chinese medicine exercise designed to improve the flow of qi through the body and encourage balance and harmony.

targeted marketing: When marketing becomes focused on certain types of people with certain types of health issues or to particular types of people by age or culture.

telehealth: The use of technology to remotely deliver health care, health information, or health education at a distance.

temporal relationship: A relationship involving time.

***timbang*:** Filipino belief in a range of "hot" and "cold" humoral balances in the body and food and dietary balances.

transcendental meditation: A technique that allows a practitioner to experience ever-finer levels of thought until the source of thought is experienced.

transgender: Individuals who live full- or part-time in the gender role opposite to the one in which they were physically born. They may be heterosexual or gay or lesbian.

upper class: The people with the most wealth and a concentration of power.

veracity: An ethical principle that involves being truthful.

vitalistic system: The theory or doctrine that life cannot be explained entirely as physical and chemical phenomena and that life is partially self-determining through one's energy or soul.

voodoo: A religion that originated in Africa and was influenced by Roman Catholics in which a supreme God rules deities, deified ancestors, and saints who communicate with believers in dreams, trances, and ritual possessions.

worldview: The overall perspective from which one sees and interprets the world.

wuzho: A Roma belief of what is pure, which is a foundation of their health traditions.

yin and yang: The traditional Chinese medicine theory that everything is made up of two polar energies.

yoga: An ancient system of exercises and breathing techniques designed to encourage physical and spiritual well-being.

Index

D

G

H

Q

R

S

Y

About the Authors

Lois A. Ritter earned a doctorate in education and master's degrees in health science, health care administration, and cultural and social anthropology. She has taught at the university level for more than 25 years and has led national and regional research studies on a broad range of public health topics.

Donald H. Graham is an attorney and holds a master's degree in urban affairs. He has developed and managed client-centered and culturally appropriate health and human service programs for more than 30 years.

CPSIA information can be obtained
at www.ICGtesting.com
Printed in the USA
LVHW052332211122
733733LV00002B/5